The Anti-Inflammatory D

The Anti-Inflammatory Diet cookbook

The best beginner's guide, over 1000 Easy Recipes to Heal the Immune System and Restore Overall Health

Gary Volgel

Sommario

Introduction 1

BreakFast 2

1. **Quinoa Bread** 2
3. **Blueberry Muffins** 2
4. **Savory Bread** 3
5. **Crepes with Coconut Cream & Strawberry Sauce One** 3
6. **Honey Pancakes Satisfying** 3
7. **Zucchini Pancakes** 4
8. **Blueberry & Cashew Waffles** 4
9. **Arugula & mushroom Frittata** 4
10. **Baked Eggs with Spinach** 5
11. **Spiced Apple Omelet** 5
12. **Baked Oatmeal** 5
13. **Banana Porridge** 5
14. **Ham & Bell Pepper Muffins** 6
15. **Eggs In Avocado Cup** 6
16. **Veggie Poached Eggs** 6
17. **Apple Omelet** 6
18. **No-Bake Veggie Fritatta** 7
19. **Almond Mascarpone Dumplings** 7
20. **Almond Scones** 7
21. **Apple Bread** 8
22. **Apple Oatmeal** 8
23. **Bake Apple Turnover** 8
24. **Banana Cashew Toast** 9
25. **Grams Banana-Oatmeal Vegan Pancakes** 9
26. **Beef Breakfast Casserole** 9
27. **Blueberry-Bran Breakfast Sundae** 9
28. **Breakfast Pitas** 10
29. **Carrot Bread** 10
30. **Cauliflower and Chorizo** 10
31. **Cheesy Flax and Hemp Seeds Muffins** 11
32. **Grams Chicken Muffins** 11
33. **Cilantro Pancakes** 11

34.	Cinnamon-Apple Granola with Greek Yogurt	12
35.	Coco-Tapioca Bowl	12
36.	Cranberry and Raisins Granola	12
37.	Crepes with Coconut Cream & Strawberry Sauce	13
38.	Egg Muffins with Feta and Quinoa	13
39.	Fennel Seeds Cookies	13
40.	Fruity Muffins	14
41.	Grapefruit-Pomegranate Salad	14
42.	Ham and Veggie Frittata Muffins	14
43.	Honey Pancakes	15
44.	Kale Turmeric Scramble	15
45.	Grams Mango Granola	15
46.	Maple Toast and Eggs	15
47.	Mini Breakfast Pizza	16
48.	Nutty Oats Pudding	16
49.	Oatmeal-Applesauce Muffins	16
50.	Banana Breakfast	16
51.	Peaches with Honey Almond Ricotta	17
52.	Poached Salmon Egg Toast	17
53.	Pumpkin Pancakes	17
54.	Quinoa & Veggie Croquettes	17
55.	Quinoa Breakfast Bowl	18
56.	Salmon Burgers	18
57.	Savory Bread	18
58.	Shirataki Pasta with Avocado and Cream	18
59.	Spicy Marble Eggs	19
60.	Spinach Mushroom Omelet	19
61.	Strawberry Yogurt treat	19
62.	Sun-Dried Tomato Garlic Bruschetta	19
63.	Sweetened Brown Rice	20
64.	Tomato and Avocado Omelet	20
65.	Tuna & Sweet Potato Croquettes	20
66.	Vegan-Friendly Banana Bread	20
67.	Weekend Breakfast Salad	21

68.	Whole Grain Blueberry Scones	21
69.	Yummy Steak Muffins	21
70.	Zucchini Pancakes	21
71.	Cherry & Apple Bowl	22
72.	Healthy Bread	22
73.	Fruity Muffins	22
74.	Gingered Carrot & Coconut	22
75.	Savory Veggie Muffins	23
76.	Spicy Ginger Crepes	23
77.	Cilantro Pancakes	23
78.	Pumpkin & Banana Waffles	23
79.	Zucchini Quiche	24
80.	Kale & Bell Pepper Frittata	24
81.	Tomato Omelet	24
82.	Kale Scramble	24
83.	Oats & Seeds Granola	25
84.	Millet Porridge	25
85.	Baked Simple Eggs	25
86.	Eggs In Mushrooms Caps	25
87.	Baked Veggie Omelet Definitely	26
88.	Smoked Salmon Scramble	26
89.	Almond Pancakes with Coconut Flakes	26
90.	Breakfast Frittata	27
91.	Apple Bruschetta with Almonds and Blackberries	27
92.	Apple, Ginger, and Rhubarb Muffins	27
93.	Baked French Toast Casserole	28
94.	Banana Pancakes	28
95.	Barley Breakfast Bowl with Lemon Yogurt Sauce	28
96.	Blueberry & Cashew Waffles	29
97.	Breakfast ArrozHot	29
98.	Breakfast Sausage and Mushroom Casserole	29
99.	Carrot Cake Overnight Oats	30
100.	Cheddar and Chive Souffles	30
101.	Cherry Chia Oats	30

102.	Choco-Banana Oats	30
103.	Cinnamon Pancakes with Coconut	31
104.	Coconut & Banana Cookies	31
105.	Cornmeal Grits	31
106.	Cream Cheese Salmon	31
107.	Edamame Omelet	32
108.	Fantastic Spaghetti Squash with Cheese and Basil Pesto	32
109.	Flaxseed Porridge with Cinnamon	32
110.	Gingerbread Oatmeal Breakfast	32
111.	Greek Yogurt with Cherry-Almond Syrup Parfait	33
112.	Hash Browns	33
113.	Huevos Rancheros	33
114.	Leek & Spinach Frittata	33
115.	Maple Oatmeal	34
116.	Mediterranean Frittata	34
117.	Mushroom Crêpes	34
118.	Oat Porridge with Cherry & Coconut	35
119.	Oatmeal-Raisin Scones	35
120.	Oven-Poached Eggs	35
121.	Peanut Butter-Banana Muffins	35
122.	Pumpkin & Banana Waffles	36
123.	Quinoa & Beans Burgers	36
124.	Quinoa and Cauliflower Congee	36
125.	Raisin Bran Muffins	37
126.	Sautéed Veggies on Hot Bagels	37
127.	Savory Veggie Muffins	37
128.	Spicy Ginger Crepes	38
129.	Spinach Mushroom Omelet	38
130.	Strawberries and Cream Trifle	38
131.	Strawberry-Oat-Chocolate Chip Muffins	38
132.	Sweet Onion and Egg Pie	39
133.	Swiss Chard and Spinach with Egg	39
134.	Tomato Omelet	39
135.	Turkey Burgers	39

136.	Veggie Balls	40
137.	**White and Green Quiche**	40
138.	Yogurt Cheese and Fruit	40
139.	**Zucchini Bread**	40

LUNCH 41

140.	**Shrimp & Mango Salsa Lettuce Wraps**	41
142.	**Zucchini Pasta With Shrimp**	41
143.	**Sweet Potato Buns Sandwich**	42
144.	**Shrimp, Sausage & Veggie Skillet**	42
145.	**Sea Scallops With Spinach & Bacon**	42
146.	**Liver With Onion & Parsley One**	43
147.	**Egg & Avocado Wraps**	43
148.	**Prosciutto Wrapped Chicken**	43
149.	**Creamy Sweet Potato Pasta With Pancetta**	44
150.	**Roasted Beet Pasta With Kale & Pesto**	44
151.	**Veggies & Apple With Orange Sauce**	44
152.	**Cauliflower Rice With Prawns & Veggies**	45

Smoothies and Drinks 46

153.	**Almond Blueberry Smoothie**	46
154.	**Apple Cinnamon Water**	46
155.	**Beet and Cherry Smoothie**	46
156.	Time To Prepare:ten minutes Time to Cook: twenty minutes Yield:Servings 4	46
157.	**Blackberry Italian Drink**	46
158.	**Blueberry And Spinach Shake**	47
159.	**Blueberry Matcha Smoothie**	47
160.	**Blueberry Smoothie**	47
161.	**Carrot and Orange Turmeric Drink**	47
162.	**Chocolate Cherry Smoothie**	47
163.	**Cooked Iced Tea**	48
164.	**Cucumber Melon Smoothie**	48
165.	**Fig Smoothie**	48
166.	**Fresh Cranberry And Lime Juice**	48
167.	**Ginger Ale**	48
168.	**Golden Chai Latte**	49

169.	Hibiscus Tea	49
170.	Hot Peppermint Vanilla Latte	49
171.	Jamaican Hibiscus Tea	49
172.	Kiwi Strawberry Smoothie	49
173.	Mango and Ginger Infused Water	50
174.	Mixed Fruit & Nut Milkshake	50
175.	Peach And Raspberry Lemonade	50
176.	Peachy Keen Smoothie	50
177.	Pineapple and Greens Smoothie	50
178.	Pineapple Smoothie	51
179.	Pumpkin Pie Smoothie	51
180.	Raspberry Banana Smoothie	51
181.	Spicy Tomato Smoothie	51
182.	Sweet & Savoury Smoothie	52
183.	Triple Fruit Smoothie	52
184.	Tropical Pineapple Kiwi Smoothie	52
185.	Turmeric Delight	52
186.	Turmeric Tea	53
187.	Vanilla Blueberry Smoothie	53
188.	Voluptuous Vanilla Hot Drink	53
189.	White Hot Chocolate	53
190.	Zesty Citrus Smoothie	53
191.	Broccoli and Black Beans Stir Fry	54
192.	Cauliflower Broccoli Mash	54
193.	Citrus Couscous with Herb	54
194.	Crispy Corn	55
195.	Curry Wheatberry Rice	55
196.	Feta Cheese Salad	55
197.	Goat Cheese Salad	55
198.	Green, Red and Yellow Rice	56
199.	Lentil Salad	56
200.	Moroccan Style Couscous	56
201.	Onion and Orange Healthy Salad	56
202.	Quinoa Salad	57

203.	Rice with Pistachios	57
204.	Roasted Curried Cauliflower	57
205.	Roasted Portobellos With Rosemary	57
206.	Spiced Sweet Potato Bread	58
207.	Spicy Roasted Brussels Sprouts	58
208.	Stir-Fried Almond And Spinach	58
209.	Tender Farro	58
210.	Tomato Bulgur	59
211.	**Sauces And Dressings**	59
212.	Bean Potato Spread	59
213.	Creamy Avocado Dressing	59
214.	Creamy Raspberry Vinaigrette	60
215.	Cucumber and Dill Sauce	60
216.	Herby Raita	60
217.	Homemade Lemon Vinaigrette	60
218.	Honey Bean Dip	61
219.	Strawberry Poppy Seed Dressing	61
220.	Tomato and Mushroom Sauce	61
221.	Almonds and Blueberries Yogurt Snack	61
222.	Ants on a Log	62
223.	Apple Sauce Treat	62
224.	Avocado Hummus	62
225.	Baked Veggie Turmeric Nuggets	62
226.	Berry Energy bites	63
227.	Boiled Okra and Squash	63
228.	Bruschetta	63
229.	Buttered Banana Chickpea Cookies	63
230.	Carrot Sticks with Avocado Dip	64
231.	Grams Cashew Cheese	64
232.	Cereal Chia Chips	64
233.	Chia Cashew Cream	64
234.	Coconut Porridge	65
235.	Cucumber Rolls Hors D'oeuvres	65
236.	Delectable Cookies	65

237.	Easy Guacamole	65
238.	Energetic Oat Bars	66
239.	Flavorsome Almonds	66
240.	Ginger Flour Banana Ginger Bars	66
241.	Hummus Deviled Eggs	66
242.	Kale Chips	67
243.	Low Cholesterol-Low Calorie Blueberry Muffin	67
244.	Mini Pepper Nachos	67
245.	Olive and Tomato Balls	68
246.	Paleo Ginger Spiced Mixed Nuts	68
247.	Peanut Butter and Honey Oat Bars	68
248.	Roasted Beets	68
249.	Grams Salmon & Avocado Toast	69
250.	Grams Soft Flourless Cookies	69
251.	Grams Spicy Bean Dip	69
252.	Sweet Potato Muffins	69
253.	Tangy Turmeric Flavored Florets	70
254.	Tofu Pudding	70
255.	Turmeric Coconut Flour Muffins	70
256.	Spinach & Berries Smoothie	70
257.	Nutty Berries & Spinach Smoothie	71
258.	Veggies & Turmeric Smoothie	71
259.	Pineapple & Green Tea Smoothie	71
260.	Spiced Peach Smoothie	71
262.	Strawberry & Beet Smoothie	72
263.	Pineapple & Coconut Smoothie	72
264.	Pineapple & Mango Smoothie	72
265.	Berries, Watermelon & Avocado	72
266.	Apple, Strawberry & Beet Smoothie	72
267.	Spiced Banana Smoothie	73
268.	Papaya & Pineapple Smoothie	73
269.	Cherry & Pineapple Smoothie	73
270.	Pineapple, Mango & Coconut Smoothie	73
271.	Tangy Ginger & Radish Smoothie	73

272.	Strawberry & Kale Smoothie	74
273.	Almond Butter Smoothies	74
274.	Baby Kale Pineapple Smoothie	74
275.	Beet Smoothie	74
276.	Blackberry & Ginger Milkshake	74
277.	Blended Coconut Milk and Banana Breakfast Smoothie	75
278.	Blueberry Lime Juice	75
279.	Blueberry Pomegranate Smoothie	75
280.	Broccoli Smoothie	75
281.	Cherry Smoothie	75
282.	Chocolate Latte with Reishi	76
283.	Cucumber Kiwi Green Smoothie	76
284.	Dreamy Yummy Orange Cream Smoothie	76
285.	Flu Fighting Tonic	76
286.	Fresh Tropical Juice	76
287.	Ginger, Carrot, and Turmeric Smoothie	77
288.	Green Vanilla Smoothie	77
289.	Hot Apple Cider	77
290.	Instant Horchata	77
291.	Kale Smoothie	77
292.	Lemon Ginger Iced Tea	78
293.	Mango Tomato Smoothie	78
294.	Parsley Ginger Green Juice	78
295.	Peach Maple Smoothie	78
296.	Pineapple & Ginger Juice	78
297.	Pineapple- Ginger Smoothie	79
298.	Pink California Smoothie	79
299.	Grams Purple Fruit Smoothie	79
300.	Raspberry Smoothie	79
301.	Strawberry Oatmeal Smoothie	79
302.	Sweet Cranberry Juice	80
303.	Tropical Mango Coconut Smoothie	80
304.	Turmeric and Ginger Tonic	80
305.	Turmeric Hot Chocolate	80

306.	Vanilla Avocado Smoothie	80
307.	Vanilla Turmeric Orange Juice	81
308.	Wassail	81
309.	Wonderful Watermelon Drink	81
310.	Sides Beet Hummus	81
311.	Caramelized Pears and Onions	81
312.	Cilantro And Avocado Platter	82
314.	Creamy Polenta	82
315.	Cucumber Yogurt Salad with Mint	82
316.	Farro Salad with Arugula	83
317.	Fresh Strawberry Salsa	83
318.	Green Beans	83
319.	Hot Pink Coconut Slaw	83
320.	Mascarpone Couscous	84
321.	Mushroom Millet	84
322.	Parmesan Roasted Broccoli	84
323.	Red Cabbage with Cheese	84
324.	Roasted Carrots	85
325.	Roasted Parsnips	85
326.	Shoepeg Corn Salad	85
327.	Spicy Barley	85
328.	Spicy Wasabi Mayonnaise	86
329.	Stir-Fried Farros	86
330.	Thyme with Honey-Roasted Carrots	86
331.	Wheatberry Salad	86
332.	Balsamic Vinaigrette	86
333.	Cashew Ginger Dip	87
334.	Creamy Homemade Greek Dressing	87
335.	Creamy Siamese Dressing	87
336.	Dairy-Free Creamy Turmeric Dressing	87
337.	Homemade Ginger Dressing	88
338.	Homemade Ranch	88
339.	Soy with Honey and Ginger Glaze	88
340.	Tahini Dip	88

341.	Snacks Almond and Honey Homemade Bar	89
342.	Anti-Inflammatory Key Lime Pie	89
343.	Apple Crisp	89
344.	Avocado and Egg Sandwich	90
345.	Avocado with Tomatoes and Cucumber	90
346.	Berry Delight	90
347.	Blueberry & Chia Flax Seed Pudding	90
348.	Brownies Avocado	91
349.	Brussels Sprout Chips	91
350.	Candied Dates	91
351.	Cashew "Humus"	91
352.	Cauliflower Snacks	92
353.	Chewy Blackberry Leather	92
354.	Coco Cherry Bake-less Bars	92
355.	Cottage Cheese with Apple Sauce	92
356.	Cucumber Yogurt	93
357.	Dried Dates & Turmeric Truffles	93
358.	Grams Easy Peasy Ginger Date	93
359.	Energy Dates Balls	93
360.	Flourless & Flaky Muffin Munchies	94
361.	Ginger Turmeric ǁ Protein: Bars	94
362.	Hummus with Celery	94
363.	Lemony Ginger Cookies	95
364.	Mandarin Cottage Cheese	95
365.	Mushroom Chips	95
366.	Oven Crisp Sweet Potato	95
367.	Party-Time Chicken Nuggets	96
368.	Protein-Packed Croquettes	96
369.	Roasted Garlic Chickpeas	96
370.	Salt & Vinegar Kale Crisps	96
371.	Spiced Nuts	97
372.	Grams Spicy Roasted chickpeas	97
373.	Grams Sweet Sunup Seeds	97
374.	Toasted Pumpkin Seeds	97

375.	Turmeric Chickpea Cakes	98
376.	Turmeric Gummies	98
377.	Pineapple & Carrot Smoothie	98
378.	Cherry & Kale Smoothie	98
379.	Banana & Ginger Smoothie	99
380.	Pineapple, Kale & Ginger Smoothie	99
381.	Fruit & Veggie Smoothie	99
382.	Tangy Mango & Spinach Smoothie	99
383.	Kale & Avocado Smoothie	99
384.	Pineapple & Orange Smoothie	100
385.	Pineapple & watermelon Smoothie	100
386.	Cherry & Blueberry Smoothie	100
387.	Pear, Peach & Papaya Smoothie	100
388.	Cherry & Beet Smoothie	100
389.	Pineapple & Almond Smoothie	101
390.	Watermelon, Berries & Avocado Smoothie	101
391.	Nutty Banana & Ginger Smoothie	101
392.	Tangy Avocado & Ginger Smoothie	101
393.	Sweet Potato & Orange Smoothie	101
394.	Blueberry & Cucumber Smoothie	102

MEAT 103

395.	Beef with Mushroom & Broccoli	103
396.	Beef with Zucchini Noodles	103
397.	Spiced Ground Beef	103
398.	Ground Beef with Veggies	104
399.	Ground Beef with Greens & Tomatoes	104
400.	Ground Beef & Veggies Curry	104
401.	Curried Beef Meatballs	105
402.	Honey Glazed Beef	105
403.	Grilled Skirt Steak Coconut	105
404.	Lamb with Prunes	106
405.	Baked Lamb with Spinach	106
406.	Ground Lamb with Peas	106
407.	Broiled Lamb Shoulder	107

408.	Roasted Lamb Chops	107
409.	Lamb Burgers with Avocado Dip	107
410.	Baked Meatballs & Scallions	108
411.	Pork with Pineapple	108
412.	Pork Chili	108
413.	Glazed Pork chops with Peach	109
414.	Baked Pork & Mushroom Meatballs	109
415.	Beef with Carrot & Broccoli	109
416.	Citrus Beef with Bok Choy	110
417.	Beef with Asparagus & Bell Pepper	110
418.	Ground Beef with Cabbage	110
419.	Ground Beef with Cashews & Veggies	111
420.	Beef & Veggies Chili	111
421.	Spicy & Creamy Ground Beef Curry	111
422.	Beef Meatballs in Tomato Gravy	112
423.	Pan Grilled Flank Steak	112
424.	Spicy Lamb Curry	112
425.	Lamb with Zucchini & Couscous	113
426.	Ground Lamb with Harissa	113
427.	Roasted Leg of Lamb	113
428.	Pan-Seared Lamb Chops	114
429.	Grilled Lamb Chops	114
430.	Lamb & Pineapple Kebabs	114
431.	Fresh lime juice	115
432.	Spiced Pork One	115
433.	Ground Pork with Water Chestnuts	115
434.	Pork chops in Creamy Sauce	116

Soups and Stews 117

435.	Spring Pea Soup	117
436.	Bacon & Cheese Soup	117
437.	Broccoli Cheddar & Bacon Soup	117
438.	Brown Rice and Shitake Miso Soup with Scallion	118
439.	Butternut Squash Soup with Shrimp	118
440.	Carrot Broccoli Stew	118

441.	Cauliflower And Clam Chowder	118
442.	Celery Soup	119
443.	Cheesy Chicken Soup	119
444.	Chicken And Cauliflower Curry Stew	119
445.	Chicken Chili Blanco	120
446.	Chickpea Curry Soup	120
447.	Coconut Cashew Soup with Butternut Squash	120
448.	Cream of Mushroom Soup	121
449.	Creamy Broccoli Soup	121
450.	Creamy Leek Soup	121
451.	Creamy Pumpkin Puree Soup	122
452.	Creamy Turmeric Cauliflower Soup	122
453.	Detox Cabbage Soup	122
454.	French Caramelized Onion Soup	122
455.	Garlic Mushroom & Beef Soup	123
456.	Golden Chickpea And Vegetable Soup	123
457.	Green Blast Soup	123
458.	Hamburger & Tomato Soup	123
459.	Hearty Root Vegetable Soup	124
460.	Italian Beef Soup	124
461.	Sugars Italian Summer Squash Soup	124
462.	Lamb Stew	124
463.	Lebanese Lentil Soup	125
464.	Lemon Chicken Soup	125
465.	Minestrone Soup with Quinoa	125
466.	Mushroom And Thyme Soup	125
467.	Pork Stew	126
468.	Pumpkin, Coconut & Sage	126
469.	Red Lentil Dal	126
470.	Rich Onion And Beef Stew	126
471.	Russian Cabbage Soup	127
472.	Slow Cooker Lamb & Cauliflower Soup	127
473.	Sugars Spicy Cabbage Turmeric Coconut Soup	127
474.	Spicy Ramen Noodles	127

475.	Sweet Potato and Black Bean Chili	128
476.	Tex-Mex Chicken Soup	128
477.	Thai Winter Vegetable Soup	128
478.	Tomato Bisque Soup	128
479.	Tuscan Style Soup	129
480.	Vegetarian Garlic, Tomato & Onion Soup	129
481.	White Velvet Cauliflower Soup	129
482.	Sugars Zesty Broccoli Soup	129
483.	Carrot Soup	130
484.	Curried Carrot & Sweet Potato Soup	130
485.	Pumpkin Soup	130
486.	Butternut Squash Soup	131
487.	Cauliflower & Zucchini	131
488.	Kabocha Squash Soup	131
489.	Mixed Veggie Soup	132
490.	Tangy Mushroom Soup	132
491.	Tomatoes & Quinoa Soup	132
492.	Sweet Potato, Spinach & Lentil	133
493.	Barley, Beans & Veggie Soup	133
494.	Black Beans Soup	133
495.	Chicken & Veggies Soup	133
496.	Beef, Mushroom & Broccoli Soup	134
497.	Mixed Veggies Stew	134
498.	Chicken & Tomato Stew	134
499.	Beef & Squash Stew	135
500.	Haddock & Potato Stew	135
501.	Black-Eyed Beans Stew	135
502.	Lentil Stew	136
503.	Chilled Tomato & Bell Pepper Soup	136
504.	Chilled Spinach & Cucumber Soup	136
505.	Chilled Pineapple Soup	136
506.	Creamy Carrot Soup	137
507.	Chicken & Veggie Soup	137
508.	Roasted Veggies Soup	137

509.	Shrimp & Snow Peas Soup	137
510.	Spicy Leek Soup With Poached Eggs	138
511.	Sweet Potato Soup	138
512.	Beef And Veggie Soup	138
513.	Broccoli Soup with Gorgonzola Cheese	139
514.	Buffalo Sauce And Turkey Soup	139
515.	Cannellini Bean Soup	139
516.	Carrot, Ginger & Turmeric Soup	139
517.	Cauliflower, Coconut Milk, And Shrimp Soup	140
518.	Sugars Cheesy Broccoli Soup	140
519.	Cheesy Tomato And Basil Soup	140
520.	Chicken And Kale Soup	140
521.	Chicken Tortilla Soup	141
522.	Clear Clam Chowder	141
523.	Coconut Curried Ban-Apple Soup	141
524.	Creamy & Culture Tomato Sauce	142
525.	Creamy Celery And Chicken Broth	142
526.	Sugars Creamy Parsnip Soup	142
527.	Creamy Turkey Soup	142
528.	Crock-Pot Turkey Taco Soup	143
529.	Fennel and Pear Soup	143
530.	Sugars Garlic and Lentil Soup	143
531.	Garlicky Chicken Soup	143
532.	Greek Split Pea Soup	144
533.	Gut-Healing Bone Broth	144
534.	Harvest Stew	144
535.	Sugars Hungarian Lentil Soup	144
536.	Italian Modena Soup	145
537.	Kumara & Chickpea Soup	145
538.	Lamb Taco Soup	145
539.	Leek, Chicken and Spinach Soup	145
540.	Mediterranean Stew	146
541.	Moong Daal	146
542.	Onion, Kale and White Bean Soup	146

543.	Pumpkin And Sausage Soup	147
544.	Quick Miso Soup with Wilted Greens	147
545.	Ribollita	147
546.	Roasted Butternut Squash Apple Soup	148
547.	Saffron and Salmon Soup	148
548.	Spicy Asian-Style Soup	148
549.	Spicy Lime-Chicken "Tortilla-Less" Soup	149
550.	Spicy Seafood Stew	149
551.	Sweet Potato and Corn Soup	149
552.	Thai Chicken Noodle Soup	150
553.	Tomato And Basil Soup	150
554.	Turkey Meatball Soup	150
555.	Sugars Vegetable Beef Soup	151
556.	Wedding Soup	151
557.	Wholesome Cabbage Soup	151
558.	Zucchini And Chicken Broth	151
559.	Carrot & Ginger Soup	152
560.	Creamy Broccoli Soup	152
561.	Butternut Squash Soup	152
562.	Soup	153
563.	Cauliflower & Apple Soup	153
564.	Collard Greens Soup	153
565.	Citrus Acorn Squash Soup	154
566.	Butternut Squash & Lentil Soup	154
567.	Tomato & Lentil Soup	154
568.	Carrot & Lentil Soup	155
569.	Carrot Soup with Chickpeas	155
570.	Veggies & Quinoa Soup	155
571.	**Halibut, Quinoa & Veggies Soup**	156
572.	Butternut Squash & Chickpeas Stew	156
573.	Root Veggies Stew	156
574.	Chicken, Chickpeas & Olives Stew	157
575.	Baked Lamb Stew	157
576.	Adzuki Beans & Carrot Stew	157

577.	Creamy Chickpeas Stew	158
578.	Lentil & Quinoa Stew	158
579.	Chilled Peas Soup	158
580.	Chilled Fruit Soup	159
581.	Creamy Cauliflower Soup	159
582.	Green Veggie Soup	159
584.	Chicken & Asparagus Soup	160
585.	Zucchini & Squash Soup	160

SEAFOOD 161

586.	Shrimp with Fruit & Bell Pepper	161
587.	Shrimp with Asparagus	161
588.	Pan Fried Squid	161
589.	Scallops with Veggies	161
590.	Spicy Scallops	162
591.	Spicy Kingfish	162
592.	Spicy Salmon	162
593.	Salmon with Cabbage	163
594.	Basa with Mushroom & Bell Pepper	163
595.	Snapper with Carrot & Broccoli	163
596.	Steamed Snapper Parcel	164
597.	Broiled Sweet & Tangy Salmon	164
598.	Baked parsley Salmon	164
599.	Baked Crispy Cod	164
600.	Grilled Sweet & Tangy Salmon	165
601.	Grilled Spicy Salmon	165
602.	Rockfish Curry	165
603.	Lemony Shrimp	166
604.	Shrimp with Broccoli	166
605.	Prawns with Veggies	166
606.	Squid with Veggies	166
607.	Scallops with Broccoli	167
608.	Deep Fried Kingfish	167
609.	Gingered Tilapia	167
610.	Crispy Salmon	167

611.	Salmon with Vegetables	168
612.	Haddock with Swiss Chard	168
613.	Citrus Poached Salmon	168
614.	Broiled Spicy Salmon	168
615.	Baked Sweet Lemony Salmon	169
616.	Baked Walnut & Lemon Crusted Salmon	169
617.	Baked Cheesy Salmon	169
618.	Grilled Salmon with Peach & Onion	170
620.	Salmon in Spicy Yogurt Gravy	170
POULTRY		171
621.	Chicken with Bell Peppers & Carrot	171
622.	Chicken with Veggie Combo	171
623.	Chicken with Mango, Veggies & Cashews	171
624.	Chicken in Spicy Gravy	172
625.	Citrus Glazed Chicken	172
626.	Chicken with Chickpeas & Veggies	172
627.	Chicken Chili with Sweet Potato	173
628.	Chicken & Tomato Curry	173
629.	Ground Chicken & Peas Curry	173
630.	Ground Chicken with Basil	174
631.	Chicken & Cauliflower Rice Casserole	174
632.	Roasted Spatchcock Chicken	174
633.	Roasted Chicken Breast	175
634.	Grilled Chicken	175
635.	Grilled Chicken with Pineapple & Veggies	175
636.	Ground Turkey with Asparagus	176
637.	Turkey & Pumpkin Chili	176
639.	Grilled Turkey Breast	177
640.	Grilled Duck Breast & Peach	177
641.	Creamy Chicken with Broccoli & Spinach	177
642.	Chicken with Cabbage	178
643.	Chicken with Mixed Veggies & Almonds	178
644.	Chicken with Strawberries, Rhubarb & Zucchini	178
645.	Lemon Braised Chicken	179

646.	Herbed Chicken with Olives	179
647.	Chicken Chili with Zucchini	179
648.	Chicken Chili with Two Beans & Corn	180
649.	Chicken & Sweet Potato Curry	180
650.	Chicken Meatballs Curry	180
651.	Chicken &Veggie Casserole	181
653.	Roasted Chicken with Veggies & Orange	181
654.	Roasted Chicken Drumsticks	182
655.	Grilled Chicken Breast	182
656.	Ground Turkey with Veggies	182
657.	Ground Turkey with Peas & Potato	182
658.	Turkey & Veggies Chili	183
659.	Roasted Whole Turkey	183
660.	Duck with Bok Choy	183
SIDE DISHES		184
661.	Braised Onion & Cabbage	184
662.	Lemony Brussels Sprouts	184
663.	Curried Carrot & Leeks	184
664.	Pumpkin & Egg	184
665.	Kale With Cranberry	185
666.	Sweet & Sour Salsa	185
667.	Sautéed Garlic Broccolini	185
668.	Gingered Broccoli	185
669.	Broccoli with Coconut	186
670.	Gingered Asparagus	186
671.	Spiced Cauliflower	186
672.	Roasted Cauliflower	186
673.	Roasted Butternut Squash	187
674.	Enoki Mushroom & Spinach	187
675.	Garlicky Kale	187
676.	Garlicky Bok Choy	187
677.	Citrus Carrot	188
678.	Roasted Spicy Baby Carrot	188
679.	Spicy Cabbage	188

680.	Roasted Sweet Potato	188
681.	Roasted Summer Squash & Fennel Bulb	189
682.	Potato Mash	189
683.	Gingered Cauliflower Rice	189
684.	Simple Brown Rice	189
685.	Quinoa With Apricots	190
686.	Sautéed Spinach & Tomatoes	190
687.	Steamed Simple Asparagus	190
688.	Stir Fried Eggplant	190
689.	Garlicky Cauliflower Mash	190
690.	Pesto Coated Carrot Sticks	191
692.	Fried Avocado Slices	191
693.	Stir Fried Cauliflower Rice	191
694.	Spiced Broccoli	192
695.	Broccoli with Asparagus	192
696.	Spiced Brussels Sprout	192
697.	Cauliflower with Capers	192
698.	Roasted Spicy Cauliflower	193
699.	Spicy Button Mushrooms	193
700.	Spicy Spinach	193
701.	Spinach with Kale	193
702.	Turmeric Potato	194
703.	Roasted Honey Carrot	194
704.	Sweet & Citrus Glazed Carrot	194
705.	Cabbage with Apple	194
706.	Beetroot with Coconut	195
707.	Roasted Brussels Sprouts & Sweet Potato	195
708.	Creamy Sweet Potato Mash	195
709.	Spicy Cauliflower Rice	196
710.	Spicy Quinoa	196
SALAD VEGETARIAN And SNACK		197
711.	Roasted Veggies	197
712.	Grilled Veggie Skewers	197
713.	Three Mushrooms Medley	197

714.	Nutty Spinach	198
715.	Mixed Vegetables Stew	198
716.	Veggies Curry in Pumpkin Puree	198
717.	Stuffed Zucchini	199
718.	Veggies with Red Lentils	199
719.	Veggies with Chickpeas	199
720.	Red Kidney Beans with Tomato	200
721.	Spicy Three Beans Chili	200
722.	Lentils Chili	200
723.	Red Lentils Curry	201
724.	Vegetarian Balls in Gravy	201
725.	Quinoa with Asparagus	201
726.	Coconut Brown Rice	202
727.	Brown Rice Casserole	202
728.	Herbed Bulgur Pilaf	202
729.	Mango Salad	203
730.	Lemony Fruit Salad	203
731.	Wheat Berries & Mango Salad	203
732.	Berries & Watermelon Salad	203
733.	Pear & Jicama Salad	204
734.	Carrot & Almond Salad	204
735.	Beet, Carrot & Parsley Salad	204
736.	Greens & Seeds Salad	204
737.	Cucumber Salad	205
738.	Kale, Carrot & Radish Salad	205
739.	Citrus Mixed Veggie Salad	205
740.	Warm Chickpeas Salad	206
741.	Black Beans & Mango Salad	206
742.	Lentil & Beet Salad	206
743.	Nutty Chicken Salad	206
744.	Chicken, Bok Choy & Jicama Salad	207
745.	Chicken &Broccolini Salad	207
746.	Smoked Salmon & Veggie Salad	207
747.	Salmon, Spinach & Kale Salad	208

748.	Salmon & Beans Salad	208
749.	Parsnip Fries	208
750.	Sweet Potato Fries	208
751.	**Jicama Fries**	209
752.	Zucchini Chips	209
753.	Beet Greens Chips	209
754.	Plantain Chips	209
755.	Sweet & Tangy Seeds Crackers	210
756.	Beet Crackers	210
757.	Apple Leather	210
758.	Roasted Almonds	210
759.	Roasted Chickpeas	211
760.	Cucumber Bites	211
761.	Crispy Chicken Fingers	211
762.	Tuna & Sweet Potato Croquettes	212
763.	Turkey Burgers	212
764.	Salmon Burgers	212
765.	Veggie Balls	213
766.	Fennel Seeds Cookies	213
767.	Mango & Avocado Salad	213
768.	Berries & Fruit Salad	214
769.	Berries & Pineapple Salad	214
770.	Berries & Papaya Salad	214
771.	**Kiwi & Orange Salad**	214
772.	Apple, Carrot & Beet Salad	215
773.	Bok Choy & Carrot Salad	215
774.	Beet & Carrot Salad	215
775.	Kale Salad	215
776.	Green Beans Salad	216
777.	**Roasted Veggie Salad**	216
779.	Couscous & Chickpeas Salad	217
780.	Lentil & Apple Salad	217
781.	Creamy Chicken Salad	217
782.	Chicken Salad	217

783.	Chicken & Cabbage Salad	218
784.	Beef & Broccoli Salad	218
785.	Salmon, Orange & Beet Salad	218
786.	Salmon & Tomato Salad	219
787.	Grilled Veggies	219
788.	Broccolini & Bell Pepper	219
789.	Mushroom with Spinach	220
790.	Mixed Root Vegetables & Kale	220
791.	Veggie Curry	220
792.	Spicy Mixed Veggies	221
793.	Stuffed Bell Peppers	221
794.	Veggies with Green Lentils	221
795.	Spicy Black Beans	222
796.	Vegetables Chili	222
797.	Chickpeas Chili	222
798.	Grains Chili	223
799.	Red Lentils with Spinach	223
800.	Quinoa with Veggies	223
801.	Quinoa & Beans with Veggies	224
802.	Brown Rice & Cherries Pilaf	224
803.	Rice, Lentils & Veggie Casserole	224
804.	Okra Fries	225
805.	Potato Sticks	225
806.	Beet Chips	225
807.	Spinach Chips	225
809.	Fruit Crackers	226
810.	Quinoa & Seeds Crackers	226
812.	Roasted Pumpkin Seeds	227
813.	Spiced Popcorn	227
814.	Spinach Fritters	227
815.	Chicken Popcorn	227
816.	Quinoa & Veggie Croquettes	228
817.	Lamb Burgers	228
818.	Quinoa & Beans Burgers	228

819.	Coconut & Banana Cookies	228
820.	Almond Scones	229

DESSERT 230

821.	Raw Lime, Avocado & Coconut Pie	230
822.	Pudding Muffins	230
823.	Pineapple Sticks	230
824.	Grilled Peaches	231
825.	Stuffed Apples	231
826.	Citrus Strawberry Granita	231
827.	Chocolaty Cherry Ice-Cream	231
828.	Chocolate Sorbet	232
829.	Zesty Mousse	232
830.	Chocolaty Avocado Mousse	232
831.	Carrot Chia Pudding	232
832.	Pumpkin Custard	233
833.	Spiced Egg Custard	233
834.	Pumpkin Soufflé	233
835.	Cranberry & Apple Crisp	234
836.	Pumpkin Pie	234
837.	Cherry & Coconut Macaroons	234
838.	Zucchini Brownies	235
839.	Mini Upside-Down Cherry Cakes	235
840.	Chocolaty Pumpkin Cake	235
841.	Chocolate Mug Cake	236
842.	Cherry Crisp	236
843.	Almond Butter Balls Vegan	236
844.	Apricot Squares	236
845.	Avocado Brownies	237
846.	Avocado Choco Cake	237
847.	Banana & Avocado Mousse	237
848.	Banana Cinnamon	237
849.	Beet Pancakes	238
851.	Tea Cake	238
852.	Blueberry Energy Bites	238

853.	Blueberry Tarts	239
854.	Fiber Caramelized Pears	239
855.	Chocolate Bananas	239
856.	Chocolate Chip Cookies	239
857.	Chocolate Covered Strawberries	240
858.	Chocolate Mousse	240
859.	Citrus Cauliflower Cake	240
860.	Coconut and Chocolate Cream	240
861.	Coconut Muffins	241
862.	Comforting Baked Rice Pudding	241
863.	Creamy & Chilly Blueberry Bites	241
864.	Dark Chocolate Granola Bars	241
865.	Easy Peach Cobbler	242
866.	Fennel and Almond Bites	242
867.	Fried Pineapple Slice	242
868.	Grams Fruit Salad	242
869.	Glorious Blueberry Crumble	243
870.	Grilled Peaches	243
871.	Lemon Sorbet	243
872.	Lemonade Ice Pops	243
873.	Mediterranean Rolled Baklava With Walnuts	244
874.	No-Bake Carrot Cake Bites	244
875.	Paleo Raspberry Cream Pie	244
876.	Peanut Butter Cookies	245
877.	Pineapple Pie	245
878.	Pumpkin Ice Cream	245
879.	Raspberry Diluted Frozen Sorbet	245
880.	Raspberry Gummies	246
881.	Refreshing Raspberry Jelly	246
882.	Rum Butter Cookies	246
883.	Spiced Tea Pudding	246
884.	Strawberry Granita	247
885.	Strawberry Orange Sorbet	247
886.	Strawberry Soufflé	247

887.	The Most Elegant Parsley Soufflé Ever	247
888.	Tropical Popsicles	248
889.	Vanilla Cakes	248
890.	Watermelon Sorbet	248
891.	No-Bake Strawberry Cheesecake	248
892.	Blackberry & Apple Skillet Cake	249
893.	Black Forest Pudding	249
894.	Fried Pineapple Slices	249
895.	Baked Apples	250
897.	Pumpkin Ice-Cream	250
899.	Lemon Sorbet	251
900.	Chocolate & Coffee Mousse	251
901.	Chocolaty Chia Pudding	251
902.	Apple Chia Pudding	251
903.	Chocolate Custard	252
904.	Strawberry Soufflé	252
905.	Mango & Pineapple Crisp	252
906.	Cherry Cobbler	253
907.	No-Bake Lemony Cheesecake	253
908.	Banana Mug Cake	253
910.	Pineapple Upside-Down Cake	254
911.	**Fudge Brownies**	254
912.	Lemony Tarts	254
913.	Chocolaty Cherry Truffles	255
914.	Almond Cookies	255
915.	Apple Fritters	255
916.	Avocado Chia Parfait	255
917.	Avocado Chocolate Mousse	256
918.	Banana Bars	256
919.	Banana Cinnamon Cookies	256
920.	Berry Ice Pops	256
921.	Berry-Banana Yogurt	257
922.	Blueberry Crisp	257
923.	Blueberry Sour Cream Cake	257

924.	Café-Style Fudge	257
925.	Grams Choco Chia Cherry Cream	258
926.	Chocolate Cherry Chia Pudding	258
927.	Chocolate Chip Quinoa Granola Bars	258
928.	Chocolate Fudge Bites	258
929.	Cinnamon Apple Chips	259
930.	Citrus Strawberry Granita	259
931.	Coconut Butter Fudge	259
932.	Coffee Cream	259
933.	Cookie Dough Bites	260
934.	Creamy Frozen Yogurt	260
935.	Date Dough & Walnut Wafer	260
936.	Fall-Time Custard	260
937.	Flourless Sweet Potato Brownies	261
938.	Fruit Cobbler	261
939.	Glazed Banana	261
940.	Green Tea Pudding	261
941.	Hot Chocolate	262
942.	Lemon Vegan Cake	262
943.	Matcha and Blueberries Pudding	262
944.	Mint Chocolate Chip Ice-cream	262
945.	No-Bake Cheesecake	263
946.	Peanut Butter Balls	263
947.	Pineapple Cake	263
948.	Pistachioed Panna-Cotta Cocoa	263
949.	Pure Avocado Pudding	264
950.	Raspberry Gummies	264
951.	Raw Black Forest Brownies	264
952.	Roasted Bananas	264
953.	Pineapple	265
954.	Spicy Popper Mug Cake	265
955.	Strawberry Ice Cream	265
956.	Strawberry Shortcake	265
957.	Sweet Almond And Coconut Fat Bombs	266

958.	Tropical Fruit Crisp	266
959.	Turmeric Milkshake	266
960.	Watermelon and Avocado Cream	266
961.	Yummy Fruity Ice-Cream	267

SAUCES, DRESSINGS & CONDIMENTS 268

962.	Tomato Sauce (Ketchup)	268
963.	Beet Sauce	268
965.	Nutty Basil Sauce (Pesto)	269
966.	Veggie Sauce	269
967.	Moroccan Spice Rub	269
968.	Taco Seasoning	269
969.	Pumpkin Pie Spice	269
970.	Turmeric Paste	270
971.	Basic Mustard	270
972.	Cashew Cheese	270
973.	Worcestershire Sauce	270
974.	Hot Sauce	271
975.	Teriyaki Sauce	271
976.	Dressing Recipes Creamy Cashew	271
977.	Lemony Egg Dressing	271
978.	Sunflower Seeds Dressing	272
979.	Tahini Dressing	272
980.	Feta & Olives Dressing	272
981.	Sauces Sweet Potato Sauce	272
982.	Scallion Sauce	273
983.	Eggplant Sauce	273
984.	Cherry & Cranberry Sauce	273
985.	Avocado Sauce	273
986.	Condiments Curry Paste	274
987.	Garam Masala	274
988.	Adobo Seasoning	274
989.	Ginger-Garlic Paste	274
990.	Garlicky Harissa	275
992.	Mayonnaise	275

993.	**Fish Sauce**	275
994.	**Hoisin Sauce**	276
995.	**BBQ Sauce**	276
996.	**Lemony Dressing**	276
997.	**Lemony Avocado Dressing**	276
998.	**Sesame Dressing Such**	276
999.	**Lemony Tomato Dressing**	277
1000.	**Carrot Dressing**	277

Conclusion 278

Introduction

What is the Anti-Inflammatory Diet?

The anti-inflammatory diet is the best choice for your health if you have conditions that cause inflammation. Such conditions are asthma, chronic peptic ulcer, tuberculosis, rheumatoid arthritis, periodontitis, Crohn's disease, sinusitis, active hepatitis, etc. Along with medical treatment, proper nutrition is very important. An anti-inflammatory diet can help to reduce the pain from inflammation for a few notches. Such a diet isn't a panacea but a significant help in any treatment. Inflammation is a natural response of your body to infections, injuries, and illnesses. The classic symptoms of inflammation are redness, pain, heat, and swelling. Nevertheless, some diseases don't occur any symptoms. Such illnesses are diabetes, heart disease, cancer, etc. That's why we should care about our health permanently and an anti-inflammatory diet is one of the ways for it.

Inflammation is your immune system's response to injury or unwanted microbes in your body. It is a natural process and vital part of your body's healing process. When inflammation becomes systemic and chronic, however, it becomes a problem, and measures need to be taken. This type of inflammation serves no purpose, and can cause a lot of harm to the body.

This book has a LOT of recipes, and not every recipe might work for you. For example, if you're allergic to dairy or gluten, the recipes containing those ingredients will cause more harm than good. However, substitutions are possible for all of these, so you will be fine following this book as long as you keep an eye on the ingredients and use a bit of creativity where you have to! Once you understand the fundamentals of the diet, you will be fully equipped to create your own recipes from scratch!This is the most important information that you should know before starting a diet. Any diet is not a magic remedy for all diseases; it is a support for the body during a difficult time of treatment. Start your new healthy life from one small step and you will see the huge results within half a year. You can be sure that your body will be thankful to you by giving you a fresh look and energy for new achievements.

BreakFast

1. Quinoa Bread

Yield: 12 servings Preparation Time: 10 minutes Cooking Time: 1½ hours

Ingredients:

1¾ cups uncooked quinoa, soaked for overnight and rinsed • ¼ cup chia seeds, soaked in ½ cup of water for overnight • ½ teaspoon bicarbonate soda • Salt, to taste • ¼ cup extra virgin olive oil • ½ cup water • 1 tablespoon fresh lemon juice

Directions:

Preheat the oven to 320 degrees F. Line a loaf pan using a parchment paper. In a mixer, add all ingredients and pulse approximately 3 minutes. Place the amalgamation into prepared loaf pan evenly. Bake approximately 1½ hours. Remove from your oven and aside for around 30 minutes before removing from loaf pan.

2. Carrot Bread

Yield: 8 serving Preparation Time: 10 min Cooking Time: 60 minutes

Ingredients:

2 cups almond meal • 1 teaspoon organic baking powder • 1 tablespoon cumin seeds • Salt, to taste • 3 organic eggs • 2 tablespoons macadamia nut oil • 1 tablespoon using apple cider vinegar • 3 cups carrot, peeled and grated • ½-inch little bit of fresh ginger, peeled and grated • ¼ cup sultanas

Directions:

1. Preheat the oven to 350 degrees F. Line a loaf pan with parchment paper. 2. In a sizable bowl, mix together almond meal, baking powder, cumin seeds and salt. 3. In another bowl, add eggs, nut oil and vinegar and beat till well combined. 4. Add egg mixture into flour mixture and mix till well combined. 5. Fold in remaining ingredients. 6. Place the mix into prepared loaf pan evenly. 7. Bake for around 1 hour.

3. Blueberry Muffins

Yield: 10 servings Preparation Time: 10 minutes Cooking Time: 22-25 minutes

Ingredients:

2½ cups almond flour • 1 tablespoon coconut flour • ½ tsp baking soda • 3 tablespoons ground cinnamon, divided • Salt, to taste • 2 organic eggs • ¼ cup coconut milk • ¼ cup coconut oil • ¼ cup maple syrup • 1 tablespoon organic vanilla flavor • 1 cup fresh blueberries

Directions:

Preheat the oven to 350 degrees F. Grease 10 cups of a large muffin tin. 2. In a big bowl, mix together flours, baking soda, 2 tablespoons of cinnamon and salt. 3. In another bowl, add eggs, milk, oil, maple syrup and vanilla and beat till well combined. 4. Add egg mixture into flour mixture and mix till well combined. 5. Fold in blueberries. 6. Place a combination into prepared muffin cups evenly. 7. Sprinkle with cinnamon evenly. 8. Bake for approximately 22-25 minutes or till a toothpick inserted within the center is released clean.

4. Savory Bread

Yield: 8-10 servings Preparation Time: 10 minutes Cooking Time: twenty or so minutes

Ingredients:

½ cup plus 1tablespoon almond flour • 1 tsp. baking soda • 1 teaspoon ground turmeric • Salt, to taste • 2 large organic eggs • 2 organic egg whites • 1 cup raw cashew butter • 1 tablespoon water • 1 tablespoon apple cider vinegar

Directions:

1. Preheat the oven to 350 degrees F. Grease a loaf pan. 2. In a big pan, mix together flour, baking soda, turmeric and salt. 3. In another bowl, add eggs, egg whites and cashew butter and beat till smooth. 4. Gradually, add water and beat till well combined. 5. Add flour mixture and mix till well combined. 6. Stir in apple cider vinegar treatment. 7. Place a combination into prepared loaf pan evenly. 8. Bake for around twenty minutes or till a toothpick inserted within the center is released clean.

5. Crepes with Coconut Cream & Strawberry Sauce One

Preparation Time: quarter-hour Cooking Time: 8 minutes

Ingredients:

For Sauce: • 12-ounces frozen strawberries, thawed and liquid reserved • 1½ teaspoons tapioca starch • 1 tablespoon honey For Coconut cream: • 1 (13½-ounce) can chilled coconut milk • 1 teaspoon organic vanilla flavoring • 1 tablespoon organic honey For Crepes: • 2 tablespoons tapioca starch • 2 tablespoons coconut flour • ¼ cup almond milk • 2 organic eggs • Pinch of salt • Avocado oil, as required

Directions:

1. For sauce inside a bowl, mix together some reserved strawberry liquid and tapioca starch. 2. Add remaining ingredients and mmix well. 3. Transfer a combination inside a pan on medium-high heat. 4. Bring to a boil, stirring continuously. 5. Cook for about 2-3 minutes or till sauce becomes thick. 6. Remove from heat and aside, covered till serving. 7. For coconut cream, carefully, scoop your cream from your surface of can of coconut milk. 8. In a mixer, add coconut cream, vanilla flavoring and honey and pulse for around 6-8 minutes or till fluffy. 9. For crepes in a blender, add all ingredients and pulse till well combined and smooth. 10. Lightly, grease a substantial nonstick skillet with avocado oil as well as heat on medium-low heat. 11. Add a modest amount of mixture and tilt the pan to spread it evenly inside the skillet. 12. Cook approximately 1-2 minutes. 13. Carefully, change the side and cook for approximately 1-1½ minutes more. 14. Repeat with the remaining mixture. 15. Divide the coconut cream onto each crepe evenly and fold into quarter. 16. Place strawberry sauce ahead and serve.

6. Honey Pancakes Satisfying

Yield: 2 servings Preparation Time: 10 minutes Cooking Time: 5 minutes

Ingredients:

½ cup almond flour • 2 tablespoons coconut flour • 1 tablespoon ground flaxseeds • ¼ tsp baking soda • ½ tablespoon ground ginger • ½ tablespoon ground nutmeg • ½ tablespoon ground cinnamon • ½ teaspoon ground cloves • Pinch of salt • 2 tablespoons organic honey • ¾ cup organic egg whites • ½ teaspoon organic vanilla extract • Coconut oil, as required

Directions:

1. In a big bowl, mix together flours, flax seeds, baking soda, spices and salt. 2. In another bowl, add honey, egg whites and vanilla and beat till well combined. 3. Add egg mixture into flour mixture and mix till well combined. 4. Lightly, grease a big nonstick skillet with oil and heat on medium-low heat. 5. Add about ¼ cup of mixture and tilt the pan to spread it evenly inside skillet. 6. Cook for about 3-4 minutes. 7. Carefully, customize the side and cook approximately 1 minute more. 8. Repeat with the remaining mixture. 9. Serve along with your desired topping.

7. Zucchini Pancakes

Yield: 8 servings Preparation Time: 15 minutes Cooking Time: 6-10 min

Ingredients:

1 cup chickpea flour • 1½ cups water, divided • ¼ teaspoon cumin seeds • ¼ tsp cayenne • ¼ teaspoon ground turmeric • Salt, to taste • ½ cup zucchini, shredded • ½ cup red onion, chopped finely • 1 green chile, seeded and chopped finely • ¼ cup fresh cilantro, chopped

Directions:

1. In a large bowl, add flour and ¾ cup with the water and beat till smooth. 2. Add remaining water and beat till a thin 3. Fold inside onion, ginger, Serrano pepper and cilantro. 4. Lightly, grease a substantial nonstick skillet with oil and heat on medium-low heat. 5. Add about ¼ cup of mixture and tilt the pan to spread it evenly in the skillet. 6. Cook for around 4-6 minutes. 7. Carefully, alter the side and cook for approximately 2-4 minutes. 8. Repeat while using remaining mixture. 9. Serve together with your desired topping.

8. Blueberry & Cashew Waffles

Yield: 5 servings Preparation Time: quarter-hour Cooking Time: 4-5 minutes

Ingredients:

1 cup raw cashews • 3 tablespoons coconut flour • 1 tsp baking soda • Salt, to taste • ½ cup unswee10ed almond milk • 3 organic eggs • ¼ cup coconut oil, melted • 3 tablespoons organic honey • ½ teaspoon organic vanilla flavor • 1 cup fresh blueberries

Directions:

1. Preheat the waffle iron after which grease it. 2. In a mixer, add cashews and pulse till a flour like consis10cy forms. 3. Transfer the cashew flour in a big bowl. 4. Add almond flour, baking soda and salt and mix well. 5. In another bowl, add remaining ingredients and beat till well combined. 6. Add egg mixture into flour mixture and mix till well combined. 7. Fold in blueberries. 8. In preheated waffle iron, add required amount of mixture. 9. Cook for around 4-5 minutes. 10. Repeat with the remaining mixture.

9. Arugula & mushroom Frittata

Yield: 4-6 servings Preparation Time: quarter-hour Cooking Time: 23 minutes

Ingredients:

½ cup coconut milk • 12 large organic eggs • Salt, to taste • 2 tablespoons coconut oil, divided • 1 small red onion, chopped finely • 1 cup fresh mushrooms, sliced • 1 cup fresh arugula, chopped

Directions:

1. Preheat the oven to 375 degrees F. 2. In a bowl, add coconut milk, eggs and salt and beat well. Keep aside. 3. In an oven proof skillet, heat 1½ tablespoons of oil on medium-high heat. 4. Add onion and sauté for approximately 3 minutes. 5. Add mushrooms and cook for around 6-8 minutes. 6. Add arugula and cook for approximately 2-3 minutes. 7. Transfer the vegetable mixture in a bowl. 8. In exactly the same pan, heat remaining oil on medium-low heat. 9. Add egg mixture and tilt the pan to spread the amalgamation evenly. 10. Cook approximately 5 minutes. 11. Spread the vegetable mixture over cooked egg mixture evenly. 12. Immediately, transfer the skillet into oven. 13. Bake for about 5 minutes. 14. Remove from oven and carefully invert the frittata onto a plate. 15. Carefully, place within the skillet, cooked side up. 16. Bake for approximately 3-4 minutes more.

10. Baked Eggs with Spinach

Yield: 2 servings Preparation Time: 15 minutes Cooking Time: 22 minutes

Ingredients:

6 cups fresh baby spinach • 2-3 tablespoons water • 4 organic eggs • Salt and freshly ground black pepper, to taste • 2-3 tablespoons feta cheese, crumbled

Directions:

Preheat the oven to 400 degrees F. Lightly, grease 2 small baking dishes. In a substantial frying pan, add spinach and water on medium heat. Cook for approximately 3-4 minutes. Remove from heat and drain the excess water completely. Divide the spinach into prepared baking dishes evenly. Carefully, crack 2 eggs in each baking dish over spinach. Sprinkle with salt and black pepper and top with feta cheese evenly. Arrange the baking dishes onto a big cookie sheet. Bake for around 15-18 minutes.

11. Spiced Apple Omelet

Yield: 1 serving Preparation Time: 10 min Cooking Time: 10 min

Ingredients:

2 large organic eggs • 1/8 teaspoon organic vanilla flavor • Pinch of salt • 2 teaspoons coconut oil, divided • ½ of the large apple, cored and sliced thinly • ¼ teaspoon ground cinnamon • 1/8 teaspoon ground ginger • 1/8 teaspoon ground nutmeg

Directions:

1. In a bowl, add eggs, vanilla flavoring and salt and beat till fluffy. Keep aside. 2. In a nonstick frying pan, melt 1 teaspoon of coconut oil on medium-low heat. 3. Sprinkle the apple slices with spices evenly make in the pan inside a single layer. 4. Cook for around 4-5 minutes, flipping once inside middle way. 5. Add the rest of the oil in the skillet. 6. Add the egg mixture over apple slices evenly. 7. Tilt the pan to spread the egg mixture evenly. 8. Cook for approximately 3-4 minutes. 9. Transfer the omelet in a plate and serve.

12. Baked Oatmeal

Yield: 6 servings Preparation Time: 15 minutes Cooking Time: 32-37 minutes

Ingredients:

2¼ cups glu10-free rolled oats • 1½ teaspoons baking powder • 1½ teaspoons ground cinnamon • Salt, to taste • 1/3 cup maple syrup • 2½ cups unswee10ed almond milk • 2 teaspoons organic vanilla flavoring • 2½ cups carrots, peeled and shredded • 1½ teaspoons fresh ginger, grated finely • ½ cup walnuts, chopped • ¼ cup raisins

Directions: 1. Preheat the oven to 375 degrees F. Grease a 11x8-inch casserole dish. 2. In a large bowl, mix together oats, baking powder, cinnamon and salt. 3. In another bowl, add maple syrup, almond milk and vanilla extract. 4. Add oats mixture into almond milk mixture and mix till well combined. 5. Fold in carrots and ginger. 6. Transfer a combination into prepared casserole dish. 7. Top with raisins and walnuts evenly. 8. Bake for approximately 32-37 minutes.

13. Banana Porridge

Yield: 2-4 servings Preparation Time: 10 minutes Cooking Time: 5 minutes

Ingredients:

2 ripe bananas, peeled and mashed • ¾ cup almond meal • ¼ cup flax meal • ½ teaspoon ground ginger • 1 teaspoon ground cinnamon • 1/8 teaspoon ground nutmeg • 1/8 teaspoon ground cloves • Salt, to taste • 2 cups coconut milk

Directions:

1. In a pan, mix together all ingredients on medium-low heat. 2. Bring to some gentle simmer, stirring continuously. 3. Cook, stirring continuously for approximately 2-3 minutes or till desired consis10cy. 4. Serve using your desired topping.

14. Ham & Bell Pepper Muffins

Yield: 4 servings Preparation Time: 10 minutes Cooking Time: 18-twenty or so minutes

Ingredients:

8 organic eggs • Salt and freshly ground black pepper, to taste • 2 tablespoons water • 8-ounces cooked ham, crumbled • 1 cup red bell pepper, seeded and chopped • 1 cup onion, chopped

Directions:

1. Preheat the oven to 350 degrees F. Grease 8 cups of your muffin tray. 2. In a bowl, add eggs, salt, black pepper and water and beat till well combined. 3. Stir in ham, bell pepper and onion. 4. Transfer a combination in prepared muffin cups evenly. 5. Bake for about 18-20 min or till a toothpick inserted inside the center comes out clean.

15. Eggs In Avocado Cup

Yield: 2 servings Preparation Time: 10 minutes Cooking Time: 15-20 min

Ingredients:

2 ripe avocados, halved, pitted and scooped out about 2 tablespoons of flesh • 4 organic eggs • Salt and freshly ground black pepper, to taste • 1 tablespoon chives, minced

Directions:

1. Preheat the oven to 425 degrees F. 2. Arrange the avocado halves in a small baking dish. 3. In a smaller, bowl, break an egg after which carefully transfer into within an avocado half. 4. Repeat with remaining eggs. 5. Bake approximately 15-twenty minutes or till desired doneness. 6. Serve immediately with all the sprinkling of salt, black pepper and chives.

16. Veggie Poached Eggs

Yield: 4 servings Preparation Time: 10 min Cooking Time: quarter-hour

Ingredients:

2 tablespoons olive oil, divided • 1 pound zucchini, quartered and sliced thinly • 1 large red bell pepper, seeded and chopped • 1 medium onion, chopped • 1 teaspoon fresh rosemary, chopped finely • Sat, to taste • 4 large organic eggs • Freshly ground black pepper, to taste

Directions:

1. In a big skillet, heat 1 tablespoon of oil on medium-high heat. 2. Add zucchini, bell pepper and onion and sauté for approximately 5-8 minutes. 3. Stir in rosemary and salt. With a wooden spoon, create a large well inside the center of skillet by moving the veggie mixture on the sides. 4. Reduce the warmth to medium. Pour remaining oil inside well. 5. Carefully, crack the eggs within the well. Sprinkle the eggs with salt and black pepper. 6. Cook for approximately 1-2 minutes. Cover the skillet and cook approximately 1-2 minutes more. 7. For serving, carefully, scoop the veggie mixture in 4 serving plates. 8. Top with an egg and serve.

17. Apple Omelet

Yield: 1 serving Preparation Time: 10 min Cooking Time: 9 minutes

Ingredients:

2 teaspoons coconut oil, divided • ½ of enormous green apple, cored and sliced thinly • ¼ teaspoon ground cinnamon • 1/8 teaspoon ground nutmeg • 2 large organic eggs • 1/8 teaspoon organic vanilla extract • Pinch of salt • Maple syrup, if desired

Directions: 1. In a nonstick frying pan, heat 1 teaspoon of oil on medium-low heat. 2. Add apple slices and sprinkle with nutmeg and cinnamon. 3. Cook for approximately 4-5 minutes, turning once inside middle. 4. Meanwhile inside a bowl, add eggs, vanilla and salt and beat till fluffy. 5. Add remaining oil inside the pan and let it melt completely. 6. Place the egg mixture over apple slices evenly. 7. Cook for approximately 3-4 minutes or till desired doneness. 8. Carefully, turn the pan over a serving plate and immediately, fold the omelet. 9. Serve while using drizzling of maple syrup if you like.

18. No-Bake Veggie Fritatta

Yield: 4 servings Preparation Time: 10 minutes Cooking Time: 26 minutes

Ingredients:

2 tablespoons coconut oil • 1 large sweet potato, peeled and cut into thin slices • 1 red bell pepper, seeded and sliced • 2 zucchinis, sliced • 8 organic eggs • Salt and freshly ground black pepper, to taste • 2 tablespoons fresh parsley, chopped finely

Directions:

1. Preheat the oven to broiler. 2. In a substantial oven proof skillet, heat oil on medium-low heat. 3. Add sweet potato and cook approximately 7-8 minutes. 4. Add bell pepper and zucchini and cook for about 3-4 minutes. 5. Meanwhile in a bowl, add eggs, salt and black pepper and beat till well combined. 6. Pour egg mixture over veggies evenly. Immediately, decrease the heat to low. 7. Cook for about 10 minutes or till just done. 8. Transfer the skillet beneath the broiler and broil approximately 3-4 minutes or till top becomes golden brown. 9. Cut the frittata in desired size slices. Serve while using garnishing of parsley.

19. Almond Mascarpone Dumplings

Time To Prepare: ten minutes Time to Cook: ten minutes Yield: Servings 6

Ingredients:

¼ cup ground almonds ¼ cup honey 1 cup all-purpose unbleached flour 1 cup whole-wheat flour 1 tablespoon butter 1 teaspoon extra-virgin olive oil 2 teaspoons apple juice 3 ounces mascarpone cheese 4 egg whites

Directions:

Strain together both types of flour in a big container. Stir in the almonds. In a different container, whisk together the egg whites, cheese, oil, and juice on moderate speed using an electric mixer. Place the flour, and egg white mixture with a dough hook on moderate speed or using your hands until a dough forms. Boil 1 gallon water in a medium-size saucepot. Take a scoop of dough and use a second spoon to push it into the boiling water. Cook up to the dumpling floats to the top, minimum 5 to ten minutes. You can cook several dumplings at once — just take care not to crowd the pot. Take off using a slotted spoon and drain using paper towels. Warm a medium-size sauté pan on moderate to high heat. Put in the butter, then put the dumplings in the pan and cook until light brown. Set on serving plates and sprinkle with honey.

20. Almond Scones

Time To Prepare: ten minutes Time to Cook: twenty minutes Yield: Servings 6

Ingredients:

1 cup almonds ¼ cup arrowroot flour 1 tablespoon coconut flour 1 teaspoon ground turmeric Salt, to taste Freshly ground black pepper, to taste 1 egg ¼ cup essential olive oil 3 tablespoons raw honey 1 teaspoon vanilla flavoring 1 1/3 cups almond flour

Directions:

In a mixer, put almonds then pulse till chopped roughly Move the chopped almonds in a big container. Put flours and spices and mix thoroughly. In another container, put the rest of the ingredients and beat till well blended. Place the flour mixture into the egg mixture then mix till well blended. Position a plastic wrap over the cutting board. Put the dough over the cutting board. Use both your hands to pat into 1-inch thick circle. Chop the circle in 6 wedges. Set the scones onto a cookie sheet in a single layer. Bake for minimum fifteen-20 minutes.

21. Apple Bread

Time To Prepare: twenty-five minutes Time to Cook: 1 hour and ten minutes Yield: Servings 8

Ingredients:

¼ tsp. baking powder 1 cup peeled, chopped apples 1 packet yeast 1 tbsp. cinnamon mixed with 1 tablespoon sugar 1 tsp. Salt 1¾ cups all-purpose flour 1¾ cups whole-wheat flour 11/3 cups warm water 3 tbsp. sugar 3 tbsp. tender butter

Directions:

Mix yeast, ½ teaspoon sugar, and 1/3 cup water in a container. Allow to sit for five minutes. In a mixing container, put together remaining water, butter, remaining sugar, salt, and baking powder then mix. Mix in the all-purpose flour, then the yeast mixture using an electric mixer. Place the whole-wheat flour. Knead the dough hook for minimum ten minutes. Place the dough into an oiled container. Cover then rises in a warm place for minimum a couple of hours until doubled in bulk. Punch down dough, then form into a rectangle. Spread the apples on the dough and dust with the cinnamon sugar. Roll into a cylinder and put in an oiled loaf pan. Cover and allow it to rise in a warm for 90 minutes until doubled in size. Preheat your oven to 350°F. Uncover bread and bake for about fifty minutes.

22. Apple Oatmeal

Time To Prepare: ten minutes Time to Cook: five minutes Yield: Servings 2

Ingredients:

¼ cup fresh apple juice 1 chopped apple, (unpeeled or peeled) 1 cup of any non-fat milk, coconut milk or almond milk (not necessary) 1 cup water 1 teaspoon ground cinnamon 2/3 cups rolled oats

Directions:

Put the water, juice, and the apple in a deep pot. Bring to boil on moderate heat. Put in the oats and cinnamon. Bring to another boil. Reduce the heat temperature and allow it to simmer for about three minutes or until it is thick. Split the serving into two and serve with milk.

23. Bake Apple Turnover

Time To Prepare: thirty minutes Time to Cook: twenty-five minutes Yield: Servings 4

Ingredients:

½ cup palm sugar, crumbled using your hands to loosen granules ½ tsp. cinnamon powder 1 egg white, whisked in 1 frozen puff pastry, thawed 1 Tbsp. almond flour 2 Tbsp. water 4 apples, peeled, cored, diced into bite-sized pieces All-purpose flour, for rolling out the dough For the egg wash For the turnovers

Directions:

To make the filling: mix almond flour, cinnamon powder, and palm sugar until these resemble coarse meal. Toss in diced apples until thoroughly coated. Set aside. On a mildly floured surface, roll the puff pastry until ¼ inch thin. Cut into 8 pieces of 4" x 4" squares. Split prepared apples into 8 equivalent portions. Ladle on individual puff pastry squares. Fold in half diagonally. Push edges to secure. Put each filled pastry on a baking tray coated with parchment paper. Make sure there is ample space between pastries. Freeze for minimum twenty minutes, or till ready to bake. Preheat your oven to 400°F or 205°C for at ten minutes. Brush frozen pastries with egg wash. Bring in a hot oven, and cook for twelve to fifteen minutes, or until these turn golden brown all over. Take off the baking tray in your oven instantly. Cool slightly for easier handling. Put 1 apple turnover on a plate. Serve warm.

24. Banana Cashew Toast

Time To Prepare: ten minutes Time to Cook: 0 minutes Yield: Servings 3

Ingredients:

1 cup roasted cashews (unsalted) 2 ripe moderate-sized bananas 2 tsp. flax meals 2 tsp. honey 4 pieces oat bread Dash of salt Pinch of cinnamon

Directions:

Peel and slice the bananas into ½-inch pieces. Toast the bread. Use a food processor to puree the salt and cashews until they are smooth. Use the puree as a spread on the toasts. On top of the spread, position a layer of bananas. Put in flax meals and a dash of cinnamon on top of the bananas. Top the toast with honey.

25. Grams Banana-Oatmeal Vegan Pancakes

Time To Prepare: five minutes Time to Cook: five minutes Yield: Servings 12

Ingredients:

½ c. organic whole wheat flour ½ tsp. sea salt 1¼ c. old fashioned oats 1½ c. soymilk 2 ripe bananas 2 tsp. Baking powder

Directions:

To begin, heat griddle or frying pan on moderate heat. After this, place all ingredients, apart from for banana, into a blender and process until the desired smoothness is achieved. Put in the bananas to blender and blend until the desired smoothness is achieved. Lightly grease griddle with olive or coconut oil, then pour ¼ c. of batter onto griddle and cook for minimum two to three minutes, then flip and cook for approximately 2 minutes or maximum the pancake is golden brown and thoroughly cooked. Repeat process with remaining batter.

26. Beef Breakfast Casserole

Time To Prepare: ten minutes Time to Cook: thirty minutes Yield: Servings 5

Ingredients:

¼ cup cut black olives ½ cup Pico de Gallo 1 cup baby spinach 1 pound of ground beef, cooked 10 eggs Freshly ground black pepper

Directions:

Preheat your oven to 350 degrees Fahrenheit. Prepare a 9" glass pie plate with non-stick spray. Whisk the eggs until frothy. Sprinkle with salt and pepper. Layer the cooked ground beef, Pico de Gallo, and spinach in the pie plate. Slowly pour the eggs over the top. Top with black olives. Bake for minimum 30 minutes, until firm in the center. Cut into 5 pieces before you serve.

27. Blueberry-Bran Breakfast Sundae

Time To Prepare: ten minutes Time to Cook: 0 minutes Yield: Servings 2

Ingredients:

1/4 c. fresh blueberries 2 c. bran flakes 2 c. vanilla or lemon-flavored low-fat yogurt (if possible Greek yogurt) or flavor of choice. 2 tbsp. chopped pecans (or nuts of choice) 2 tbsp. cut almonds (or nuts of choice) 2 tbsp. dried cranberries (or dried or fresh fruit of choice)

Directions:

In a container, place 1 c. yogurt, and one c. bran flakes. Top with 1/8 c. fresh blueberries, followed by 1 tbsp. Each of cut almonds, chopped pecans, and dried cranberries. Repeat using the rest of the ingredients to make a second serving. Serve instantly.

28. Breakfast Pitas

Time To Prepare: 4 minutes Time to Cook: six minutes Yield: Servings 4

Ingredients:

1 c. raw spinach (cook if you prefer) 1 tsp. garlic powder 1 tsp. onion powder 2 c. bell peppers, chopped (any color) 2 tsp. extra virgin olive oil 4 whole-wheat pita pockets 8 egg whites

Directions:

Place the olive oil to a big sauté pan and place on moderate heat. When the oil is hot in shiny, throw in the bell pepper and sauté for approximately 3 minutes or until soft. Put in in the spinach now (if you wish it cooked) and sauté for approximately 1 to three minutes or just up to the sides begins to wilt. Put the egg whites into a small container, whisk well. Put in in spices; whisk well. Pour the egg mixture into the sauté pan and scramble everything together. Turn off the heat and stuff ½ to 1 c. mixture into a pita pocket before you serve.

29. Carrot Bread

Time To Prepare: ten minutes Time to Cook: 1 hour Yield: Servings 8

Ingredients:

¼ cup sultanas ½-inch piece of fresh ginger, peeled and grated 1 tablespoon apple cider vinegar 1 tablespoon cumin seeds 1 teaspoon organic baking powder 2 cups almond meal 2 tablespoons macadamia nut oil 3 cups carrot, peeled and grated 3 organic eggs Salt, to taste

Directions:

Set the oven to 35 F, then line a loaf pan using parchment paper. In a big container, put together the almond meal, baking powder, cumin seeds, and salt and mix. In another container, put in eggs, nut oil, and vinegar and beat till well blended. Place the egg mixture into the flour mixture and mix till well blended. Fold in rest of the ingredients. Put the mixture into prepared loaf pan equally. Bake for approximately 1 hour

30. Cauliflower and Chorizo

Time To Prepare: 55 minutes Time to Cook: forty minutes Yield: Servings 4

Ingredients:

½ teaspoon garlic powder 1 cauliflower head; florets separated 1 pound chorizo; chopped. 1 yellow onion; chopped. 12 ounces canned green chilies; chopped. 2 tablespoons green onions; chopped. 4 eggs; whisked Salt and black pepper to the taste.

Directions:

Heat a pan on moderate heat; put the chorizo and onion; stir and brown for a few minutes Put in green chilies, stir, cook for a few minutes and take off the heat. In your food processor, mix cauliflower with some salt and pepper and blend. Move this to a container, put in eggs, salt, pepper, and garlic powder and whisk everything. Put in chorizo mix as well, whisk again and move everything to a greased baking dish. Bake using your oven at 375F then bake at least forty minutes. Leave casserole to cool down for a few minutes, drizzle green onions on top, slice and serve

31. Cheesy Flax and Hemp Seeds Muffins

Time To Prepare: five minutes Time to Cook: thirty minutes Yield: Servings 2

Ingredients:

¼ cup almond meal ¼ cup cottage cheese, low-fat ¼ cup grated parmesan cheese ¼ cup raw hemp seeds ¼ cup scallion, cut thinly ¼ tsp baking powder 1 tbsp. olive oil 1/8 cup flax seeds meal 1/8 cup nutritional yeast flakes 3 organic eggs, beaten Salt, to taste

Directions:

Switch on the oven, then set it 360°F and allow it to preheat. In the meantime, take two ramekins, grease them with oil, and set aside until required. Take a medium container, put in flax seeds, hemp seeds, and almond meal, and then mix in salt and baking powder until combined. Crack eggs in a different container, put in yeast, cottage cheese, and parmesan, stir thoroughly until blended, and then stir this mixture into the almond meal mixture until blended. Fold in scallions, then spread the mixture between prepared ramekins and bake for thirty minutes until muffins are firm and the top is nicely golden brown. When finished, take out the muffins from the ramekins and allow them to cool to room temperature on a wire rack. For meal prepping, wrap each muffin using a paper towel and place in your fridge for maximum thirty-four days. When ready to eat, reheat muffins in the microwave until hot and then serve.

32. Grams Chicken Muffins

Time To Prepare: 1 hour ten minutes Time to Cook: thirty minutes Yield: Servings 3

Ingredients:

½ teaspoon garlic powder 2 tablespoons green onions; chopped. 3 tablespoons hot sauce mixed with 3 tablespoons melted coconut oil 3/4 pound chicken breast; boneless 6 eggs Salt and black pepper to the taste.

Directions:

Season chicken breast with pepper, salt, and garlic powder, place on a lined baking sheet, and bake in your oven at 425F for minimum twenty-five minutes. Move chicken breast to a container, shred using a fork, and mix with half of the hot sauce and melted coconut oil. Toss to coat and leave aside. In a container, mix eggs with salt, pepper, green onions, and the remaining hot sauce mixed with oil and whisk very well. Split this mix into a muffin tray, top each with shredded chicken, introduce in your oven at 350F then bake for minimum 30 minutes. Serve your muffins hot.

33. Cilantro Pancakes

Time To Prepare: ten minutes Time to Cook: 6-8 minutes Yield: Servings 6

Ingredients:

¼ teaspoon ground turmeric ½ cup almond flour ½ cup fresh cilantro, chopped ½ cup tapioca flour ½ of red onion, chopped ½ teaspoon chili powder 1 (½-inch) fresh ginger piece, grated finely 1 cup full-Fat coconut milk 1 Serrano pepper, minced Freshly ground black pepper, to taste Oil, as required Salt, to taste

Directions:

In a big container, put together the flours and spices then mix. Place the coconut milk and mix till well blended. Fold within the onion, ginger, Serrano pepper, and cilantro. Lightly, grease a sizable nonstick frying pan with oil and warmth on medium-low heat. Put in about ¼ cup of mixture and tilt the pan to spread it uniformly inside the frying pan. Cook for about four minutes from either side. Repeat with all the rest of the mixture. Serve together with your desired topping.

34. Cinnamon-Apple Granola with Greek Yogurt

Time To Prepare: five minutes Time to Cook: ten minutes Yield: Servings 2

Ingredients:

½ apple, peeled and diced ½ c. raw almonds, chopped (or raw nuts of choice) ½ c. raw walnuts, chopped (or raw nuts of choice) 1 cup Greek plain or vanilla yogurt (or flavor of choice) 1 tbsp. almond flour 1 tsp. ground cinnamon 1/16 tsp. vanilla extract 1/8 c. applesauce, unsweetened preferred 2 tbsp. vanilla Protein powder 2 tsp. almond butter 2 tsp. honey dash of sea salt

Directions:

In a mixing container, mix the chopped almonds, chopped walnuts (or preferred raw nuts), diced apple, vanilla Protein powder, almond flour, lucuma (opt), and cinnamon and salt in a container. Mix thoroughly. In a second container, mix the apple sauce, almond butter, honey, and vanilla extract. Mix thoroughly. Pour the container with the nuts into the container with the wet ingredients and blend together meticulously. Make sure all dry ingredients get coated. Put the granola mixture onto a parchment paperlined baking sheet and bake until the desired crunch is obtained roughly 8 to ten minutes. Take off from oven and allow to cool or eat hot. Put ½ cup each Greek yogurt into two bowls. Split the granola and drizzle over the yogurt in each container. Serve instantly.

35. Coco-Tapioca Bowl

Time To Prepare: ten minutes Time to Cook: twenty minutes Yield: Servings 2

Ingredients:

¼ cup maple syrup ¼ cup tapioca pearls, small sized ½ cup unsweetened coconut flakes, toasted 1 ½ tsp. lemon juice 1 can light coconut milk 2 cups water

Directions:

Put the tapioca in a deep cooking pan and pour over the 2 cups of water. Allow it to stand for minimum 30 minutes. Pour in the coconut milk and syrup and heat the deep cooking pan over moderate temperature. Bring to its boiling point while stirring continuously. Put in the lemon juice and stir and then decorate with coconut flakes.

36. Cranberry and Raisins Granola

Time To Prepare: fifteen minutes Time to Cook: twenty minutes Yield: Servings 4

Ingredients:

4 cups old-fashioned rolled oats 1 cup dried cranberries 1 cup golden raisins 2 tablespoons olive oil ½ cup almonds, slivered 2 tablespoons warm water 1 teaspoon vanilla extract 1 teaspoon cinnamon 6 tablespoons maple syrup 1/3 cup of honey 1/4 cup sesame seeds 1/4 teaspoon of salt 1/8 teaspoon nutmeg

Directions:

In a container, combine the sesame seeds, nutmeg, almonds, oats, salt, and cinnamon. In another container, combine the oil, water, vanilla, honey, and syrup. Slowly pour the mixture into the oats mixture. Toss to blend. Spread the mixture into a greased jelly-roll pan. Bake using your oven at 300°F for minimum 55 minutes. Stir and break the clumps every ten minutes. Once you get it from the oven, stir the cranberries and raisins. Allow cooling. This will last for a week when stored in an airtight container and up to a month when stored in your refrigerator.

37. Crepes with Coconut Cream & Strawberry Sauce

Time To Prepare: fifteen minutes Time to Cook: 8 minutes Yield: Servings 4

Ingredients:

For Sauce: 1 (13½-ounce) can chilled coconut milk 1 tablespoon honey 1 tablespoon organic honey 1 teaspoon organic vanilla flavoring 1½ teaspoons tapioca starch 12-ounces frozen strawberries, thawed and liquid reserved For the Coconut cream: For Crepes: ¼ cup almond milk 2 organic eggs 2 tablespoons coconut flour 2 tablespoons tapioca starch Avocado oil, as required Pinch of salt

Directions:

For sauce inside a container, combine some reserved strawberry liquid and tapioca starch. Put in rest of the ingredients and mix thoroughly. Move a combination inside a pan on moderate to high heat. Bring to its boiling point, stirring constantly. Cook for minimum 2-3 minutes, till the sauce, becomes thick. Turn off the heat and aside, covered till serving. For coconut cream, cautiously, scoop your cream from your surface of a can of coconut milk. In a mixer, put in coconut cream, vanilla flavoring, and honey and pulse for around 6-8 minutes or till fluffy. For crepes in a blender, put in all ingredients and pulse till well blended and smooth.Lightly, grease a substantial nonstick frying pan with avocado oil as well as heat on medium-low heat. Put in a modest amount of mixture and tilt the pan to spread it uniformly inside the frying pan. Cook roughly 1-2 minutes. Cautiously change the side and cook for roughly 1-1½ minutes more. Repeat with the rest of the mixture. Split the coconut cream onto each crepe uniformly and fold into four equivalent portions. Put strawberry sauce ahead before you serve.

38. Egg Muffins with Feta and Quinoa

Time To Prepare: fifteen minutes Time to Cook: thirty minutes Yield: Servings 6-12

Ingredients:

¼ cup Black olives, chopped ¼ cup Onion, chopped ¼ tsp. Salt 1 cup Feta cheese 1 cup Quinoa, cooked 1 cup Tomatoes, chopped 1 tbsp. Oregano, fresh chop 2 cups baby spinach, chopped 2 tsp. Olive oil 8 Eggs

Directions:

Heat oven to 350. Spray oil a muffin pan with twelve cups. Cook spinach, oregano, olives, onion, and tomatoes for 5 minutes in the olive oil on moderate heat. Beat eggs. Put in the cooked mix of veggies to the eggs with the cheese and salt. Ladle mix into muffin cups. Bake thirty minutes. These will remain fresh in your refrigerator for two days. To eat, just wrap in a paper towel and warm in the microwave for thirty seconds.

39. Fennel Seeds Cookies

Time To Prepare: ten minutes Time to Cook:twenty minutes Yield:Servings 5

Ingredients:

¼ cup coconut oil, softened ¼ teaspoon whole fennel seeds ½ teaspoon fresh ginger, grated finely 1 teaspoon vanilla extract 1/3 cup coconut flour 2 tablespoons raw honey Pinch freshly ground black pepper Pinch of ground cinnamon Pinch of salt

Directions:

Set the oven to 360°F. Coat a cookie sheet that has a parchment paper. In a substantial container, put in all together the ingredients and mix till a uniform dough form. Form a small balls in the mixture make onto a prepared cookie sheet inside a single layer. Using your fingers, softly push along the balls to form the cookies. Bake for minimum 9 minutes or till golden brown.

40. Fruity Muffins

Time To Prepare: ten minutes Time to Cook: 2-3 minutes Yield: Servings 8

Ingredients:

¼ cup brown rice flour ¼ cup extra-virgin olive oil ¼ cup raw sugar ½ cup almond meal ½ cup buckwheat flour ½ teaspoon ground ginger 1 big organic egg 1 cup rhubarb, cut finely 1 small apple, peeled, cored and chopped finely 1 tablespoon linseed meal 1 teaspoon organic vanilla extract 12 teaspoon ground cinnamon 2 tablespoons arrowroot flour 2 tablespoons crystallized ginger, chopped finely 2 tablespoons organic baking powder 7 tablespoons almond milk Pinch of salt

Directions:

Set the oven to 350F. Grease 8 cups of a big muffin tin. In a big container, combine almond meal, linseed meal, sugar, and crystalized ginger. In another container, put together flours, baking powder, spices, and salt, and mix. Sift the flour mixture into the container of almond meal mixture and mix thoroughly. In a third container, put in egg, milk, oil, and vanilla and beat till well blended. Put in egg mixture into the flour mixture and mix till well blended. Fold in apple and rhubarb. Put the mixture into prepared muffin cups equally. Bake for approximately 20-twenty-five minutes or till a toothpick inserted in the middle comes out clean

41. Grapefruit-Pomegranate Salad

Time To Prepare: ten minutes Time to Cook: 0 minutes Yield: Servings 6

Ingredients:

¼ cup Basic Vegetable Stock 1 pomegranate 2 ruby red grapefruits 3 ounces Parmesan cheese 6 cups mesclun leaves

Directions:

Peel the grapefruit using a knife, take off all the pith. (the white layer under the skin). Cut out every section with the knife, make sure that no pith remains. Shave Parmesan using a vegetable peeler to make curls. Peel the pomegranate using a paring knife; take off the berries/seeds. Toss the mesclun greens in the stock. To serve, mound the greens on plates and position the grapefruit sections, cheese, and pomegranate on top.

42. Ham and Veggie Frittata Muffins

Time To Prepare: ten minutes Time to Cook: twenty-five minutes Yield: Servings 12

Ingredients:

¼ cup coconut milk (canned) ½ yellow onion, finely diced 1 cup cherry tomatoes, halved 2 tablespoons coconut flour 4 tablespoons coconut oil 5 ounces thinly cut ham 8 big eggs 8 oz. frozen spinach, thawed and drained 8 oz. mushrooms, thinly cut Sea salt and pepper to taste

Directions:

Preheat your oven to 375 degrees Fahrenheit. In a moderate-sized frying pan, warm the coconut oil on moderate heat. Put in the onion and cook until tender. Put in the mushrooms, spinach, and cherry tomatoes. Sprinkle with salt and pepper. Cook until the mushrooms have become tender. About five minutes. Turn off the heat and save for later. In a huge container, beat the eggs with the coconut milk and coconut flour. Mix in the cooled the veggie mixture. Coat each cavity of a 12 cavity muffin tin with the thinly cut ham. Pour the egg mixture into each one and bake for about twenty minutes. Take out of the oven and let cool for approximately five minutes before transferring to a wire rack.

43. Honey Pancakes

Time To Prepare: ten minutes Time to Cook: five minutes Yield: Servings 2

Ingredients:

¼ tsp baking soda ½ cup almond flour ½ tablespoon ground cinnamon ½ tablespoon ground ginger ½ tablespoon ground nutmeg ½ teaspoon ground cloves ½ teaspoon organic vanilla extract ¾ cup organic egg whites 1 tablespoon ground flaxseeds 2 tablespoons coconut flour 2 tablespoons organic honey Coconut oil, as required Pinch of salt

Directions:

In a big container, combine flours, flax seeds, baking soda, spices, and salt. In another container, put in honey, egg whites and vanilla and beat till well blended. Place the egg mixture into the flour mixture then mix till well blended. Lightly, grease a big nonstick frying pan with oil and heat on medium-low heat. Put in about ¼ cup of mixture and tilt the pan to spread it uniformly inside the frying pan. Cook for approximately 3-4 minutes. Cautiously, customize the side and cook roughly one minute more. Repeat with the rest of the mixture. Serve together with your desired topping.

44. Kale Turmeric Scramble

Time To Prepare: five minutes Time to Cook: ten minutes Yield: Servings 1

Ingredients:

¼ tsp. Black pepper ½ cup Kale, shredded ½ cup Sprouts 1 tbsp. Garlic, minced 1 tbsp. Turmeric, ground 2 Eggs 2 tbsp. Olive oil

Directions: Beat the eggs and put in in the turmeric, black pepper, and garlic. Sauté the kale into the olive oil on moderate heat for 5 minutes, and then pour this egg mixture into the pan with the kale. Carry on cooking, frequently stirring, until the eggs are cooked to your preference. Top with raw sprouts before you serve.

45. Grams Mango Granola

Time To Prepare: ten minutes Time to Cook: thirty minutes Yield: Servings 4

Ingredients:

½ cup almonds, roughly chopped ½ cup dates, roughly chopped ½ cup nuts 1 cup dried mango, chopped 2 cups rolled oats 2 tbsp. coconut oil 2 tbsp. water 2 tsp. cinnamon 2/3 cup agave nectar 3 tbsp. sesame seeds

Directions: Set oven at 320F In a big container, put the oats, almonds, nuts, sesame seeds, dates, and cinnamon then mix thoroughly. In the meantime, heat a deep cooking pan on moderate heat, pour in the agave syrup, coconut oil, and water. Stir and allow it to cook for minimum 3 minutes or until the coconut oil has melted. Slowly pour the syrup mixture into the container with the oats and nuts and stir thoroughly, make sure that all the ingredients are coated with the syrup. Move the granola on a baking sheet coated with parchment paper and place in your oven to bake for about twenty minutes. After twenty minutes, take off the tray from the oven and lay the chopped dried mango on top. Put back in your oven then bake again for another five minutes. Allow the granola cool completely before you serve or placing it in an airtight container for storage. The shelf life of the granola will last up to 2-3 weeks.

46. Maple Toast and Eggs

Time To Prepare: 20 Minutes Time to Cook: 20 Minutes Yield: Servings 6

Ingredients:

¼ cup butter ½ cup maple syrup 12 bacon strips, diced 12 big eggs 12 slices white bread Salt and pepper to taste

Directions: Fry the bacon on a frying pan on moderate heat until the I Fat: has rendered. Take the bacon out and place it using paper towels to drain surplus Fat. Warm the maple syrup and butter until melted in a deep cooking pan. Set aside. Trim the edges of the bread and flatten the slices with a rolling pin. Brush one side with the syrup mixture and press the slices into greased muffin cups. Split the bacon into the muffin cups. Break one egg into each cup. Drizzle with salt and pepper to taste Cover using foil, then bake in your oven at 4000F for about twenty minutes or until the eggs have set

47. Mini Breakfast Pizza

Time To Prepare: 5 Minutes Time to Cook: 10 Minutes Yield: Servings 4

Ingredients:

4 eggs, beaten 2 English muffins, split and toasted ½ cup shredded Italian cheese Dried oregano leaves Cooking spray Salt and pepper to taste 1/3 cup commercial pizza sauce

Directions:

Preheat your oven to 4000F. Coat a frying pan with cooking spray then heat on medium flame. Flavour the eggs with salt and pepper to taste and pour into the frying pan. As the eggs start to set, pull the eggs across the pan with an inverted turner. Carry on cooking and folding the egg. Set aside. Spread pizza sauce uniformly on English muffin halves and top with eggs and cheese. Put on a baking sheet then bake for five minutes. Decorate using oregano last.

48. Nutty Oats Pudding

Time To Prepare: five minutes Time to Cook: 0 minutes Yield: Servings 3 -5

Ingredients:

¼ cup dry milk ¼ cup rolled oats ½ cup of water 1 ½ tablespoon natural peanut butter 1 tablespoon yogurt, fat-free 1 teaspoon peanuts, finely chopped

Directions: Using a microwaveable-safe container, put together peanut butter and dry milk. Whisk well. Put in in water to achieve a smooth consistency. Put in in oats. Cover container using plastic wrap. Create a small hole for the steam to escape. Put inside the microwave oven for a minute on high powder. Continue heating, this time on medium power for 90 seconds. Allow to sit for five minutes. To serve, spoon an equal amount of cereals in a container top with peanuts and yogurt.

49. Oatmeal-Applesauce Muffins

Time To Prepare: fifteen minutes Time to Cook: twenty-five minutes Yield: Servings 12

Ingredients:

Topping 1 tbsp. brown sugar 1 tbsp. unsalted butter, melted 1/4 cup rolled oats 1/8 tsp. cinnamon Muffins ½ c. brown sugar ½ c. unsweetened applesauce ½ tsp. Baking soda ½ tsp. Cinnamon ½ tsp. Salt ½ tsp. sugar 1 c. nonfat milk 1 c. old fashioned rolled oats (not instant) 1 c. whole wheat flour 1 tsp. Baking powder 2 egg whites raisins or nuts (opt.)

Directions: To begin, first, presoak the oats in milk for an hour, Set the oven to 400°F then grease a standard 12-cup muffin pan with cooking spray or use paper liners. In a mixing container, mix oat-milk mixture, applesauce, and egg whites. Blend well and save for later. In a different container, put together the whole wheat flour, brown sugar, baking powder, baking soda, salt, sugar, and cinnamon then mix. Slowly put wet ingredients to dry ingredients and blend until just blended, but do not over mix the batter as it will make the muffins firm. Put in raisins or nuts (opt.). Prepare topping: In a small container, whisk together the oats, brown sugar, and cinnamon. Put in in melted butter and toss lightly using a fork to coat ingredients. Fill each muffin cup 2/3 full of batter. Drizzle topping on the top of each batter-filled muffin cup. Tap the pan gently on the counter to even out the batter. Put muffin pan in preheated oven and cook for twenty to twenty-five minutes or until a toothpick put in the center of one of the muffins comes out clean. Remove from the oven and allow it to sit for five minutes before you serve.

50. Banana Breakfast

Time To Prepare: ten minutes Time to Cook: 0 minutes Yield: Servings 2

Ingredients:

½ cup cold milk 1 big cut Banana 2 tbsp. flaxseeds 2 tbsp. ground coconut 4 tbsp. sesame seeds 4 tbsp. sunflower seeds

Directions: Combine the milk and honey on your breakfast container. Use your coffee grinder to grind all the seeds. Put in the ground seeds to the honey and milk mixture. Put the cut bananas neatly on top. Drizzle the ground coconuts for added flavor.

51. Peaches with Honey Almond Ricotta

Time To Prepare: fifteen minutes Time to Cook: 0 minutes Yield: Servings 4-6

Ingredients:

¼ cup Almond extract ¼ cup Peaches, cut ½ cup Almonds, thin slices 1 cup Ricotta, skim milk 1 tsp. Honey Bread, whole grain bagel or toast Spread To Serve

Directions:

Combine the almond extract, honey, ricotta, and almonds. Spread one tablespoon of this mix on toasted bread and cover with peaches.

52. Poached Salmon Egg Toast

Time To Prepare: ten minutes Time to Cook: 4 minutes Yield: Servings 2

Ingredients:

¼ tsp. Black pepper ¼ tsp. Lemon juice 1 tbsp. Scallions, cut thin 1/8 tsp. Salt 2 Eggs, poached 2 tbs. Avocado, mashed 4 oz. Salmon, smoked Bread, two slices rye or whole-grain toasted

Directions:

Put in lemon juice to avocado with pepper and salt. Spread the mixed avocado over the toasted bread slices. Lay smoked salmon over toast and top with a poached egg. Top with cut scallions

53. Pumpkin Pancakes

Time To Prepare: twenty-five minutes Time to Cook: ten minutes Yield: Servings 6

Ingredients:

½ cup pumpkin puree 1 cup coconut cream 1 ounce egg white Protein 1 tablespoon chai masala 1 tablespoon swerve 1 teaspoon baking powder 1 teaspoon coconut oil 1 teaspoon vanilla extract 2 ounces flax seeds; ground 2 ounces hazelnut flour 3 eggs 5 drops stevia

Directions:

In a container, mix flax seeds with hazelnut flour, egg white Protein baking powder and chai masala and stir. In another container, mix coconut cream with vanilla extract, pumpkin puree, eggs, stevia, and swerve and stir thoroughly. Mix the 2 mixtures and stir thoroughly. Heat a pan with the oil on moderate to high heat; pour 1/6 of the batter, spread into a circle, cover, decrease the heat to low, cook for about three minutes on each side and move to a plate Repeat the process using the rest of the mixture and serve pumpkin pancakes immediately.

54. Quinoa & Veggie Croquettes

Time To Prepare: fifteen minutes Time to Cook: 9 minutes Yield: Servings 12-fifteen

Ingredients:

¼ cup fresh cilantro leaves, chopped ¼ teaspoon ground turmeric ½ cup frozen peas, thawed 1 cup cooked quinoa 1 tbsp. essential olive oil 1 teaspoon garam masala 2 big boiled potatoes, peeled and mashed 2 minced garlic cloves 2 teaspoons ground cumin Freshly ground black pepper, to taste Olive oil, for frying Salt, to taste

Directions:

In a frying pan, warm oil on moderate heat. Put in peas and garlic and sauté for approximately one minute. Move the pea mixture into a big container. Put in the remainder ingredients and mix till well blended. Make equal sized oblong shaped patties from your mixture. In a huge frying pan, heat oil on moderate to high heat. Put in croquettes and fry for approximately 4 minutes per side.

55. Quinoa Breakfast Bowl

Time To Prepare: thirty minutes Time to Cook: 0 minutes Yield: Servings 6

Ingredients:

¼ cup Greek yogurt, plain ½ tsp. Salt 1 cup Baby spinach, chopped 1 cup Feta cheese 1 Pint Cherry tomatoes, cut in halves 1 tsp. Black pepper 1 tsp. Garlic, minced 1 tsp. Olive oil 12 Eggs 2 cups Quinoa, cooked

Directions:

Mix together the eggs, salt, pepper, garlic, onion powder, and yogurt. Cook the spinach and tomatoes for 5 minutes in the olive oil on moderate heat. Pour in the egg mix and stir until eggs have set to your preferred doneness. Stir in quinoa and feta until they are hot. This will store in your refrigerator for two to three days.

56. Salmon Burgers

Time To Prepare: fifteen minutes Time to Cook: 8 minutes Yield: Servings 3

Ingredients:

½ of a medium onion, chopped 1 (6-oz. can) skinless, boneless salmon, drained 1 celery rib, chopped 1 tablespoon dried dill, crushed 1 tablespoon plus 1 teaspoon coconut flour 1 teaspoon lemon 2 big eggs 3 tablespoons coconut oil Freshly ground black pepper, to taste Salt, to taste

Directions:

In a substantial container, put in salmon and which has a fork, break it into little pieces. Put in rest of the ingredients excluding the for oil and mix till well blended. Make 6 equal sized small patties from the mixture. In a substantial frying pan, melt coconut oil on moderate to high heat. Cook the patties for about four minutes per side.

57. Savory Bread

Time To Prepare: ten minutes Time to Cook: 20 minutes Yield: Servings 8-10

Ingredients:

½ cup plus 1tablespoon almond flour 1 cup raw cashew butter 1 tablespoon apple cider vinegar 1 tablespoon water 1 teaspoon ground turmeric 1 tsp. baking soda 2 big organic eggs 2 organic egg whites Salt, to taste

Directions:

Set the oven to 350F. Grease a loaf pan. In a big pan, combine flour, baking soda, turmeric, and salt. In another container, put in eggs, egg whites, and cashew butter and beat till smooth. Slowly, put in water and beat till well blended. Put in flour mixture and mix till well blended. Mix in apple cider vinegar treatment. Put a combination into prepared loaf pan uniformly. Bake for around 20 minutes or till a toothpick inserted within the middle is released clean.

58. Shirataki Pasta with Avocado and Cream

Time To Prepare: ten minutes Time to Cook: six minutes Yield: Servings 2

Ingredients:

½ of an avocado ½ packet of shirataki noodles, cooked ½ tsp cracked black pepper ½ tsp dried basil ½ tsp salt 1/8 cup heavy cream

Directions:

Put a medium pot half full with water on moderate heat, bring it to boil, then put in noodles and cook for a couple of minutes. Then drain the noodles and set aside until required. Put avocado in a container, purée it using a fork, Mash avocado in a container, move it to a blender, put in rest of the ingredients, and pulse until the desired smoothness is achieved. Take a frying pan, place it on moderate heat and when hot, put in noodles in it, pour in the avocado mixture, stir thoroughly and cook for a couple of minutes until hot. Serve straight away.

59. Spicy Marble Eggs

Time To Prepare: fifteen minutes Time to Cook: 2 hours Yield: Servings 12

Ingredients:

1 dried cinnamon stick, whole 1 thumb-sized fresh ginger, unpeeled, crushed 1 tsp. dried Szechuan peppercorns 1 tsp. salt 2 dried bay leaves 2 oolong black tea bags 3 dried star anise, whole 3 Tbsp. brown sugar 3 Tbsp. light soy sauce 4 cups of water 4 Tbsp. dark soy sauce 6 medium-boiled eggs, unpeeled, cooled For the Marinade

Directions:

Use the back of a spoon to crack eggshells in places to create a spider web effect. Do not peel. Set aside until needed. Pour marinade into big Dutch oven set using high heat. Put lid partly on. Bring water to a rolling boil, approximately five minutes. Turn off heat. Close the lid. Steep ingredients for about ten minutes. Use a slotted spoon to fish out and discard solids. Cool marinade completely to room proceeding. Put eggs into an airtight non-reactive container just small enough to tightly fit all these in. Pour in marinade. Eggs must be completely immersed in liquid. Discard leftover marinade, if any. Coat container rim with generous layers of saran wrap. Secure container lid. Chill eggs for one day before you use. Extract eggs and drain each piece well before you use, but keep the rest immersed in the marinade.

60. Spinach Mushroom Omelet

Time To Prepare: three minutes Time to Cook: fifteen minutes Yield: Servings 2

Ingredients:

¼ cup Red onion, diced ½ Spinach, fresh, chopped ½ tsp. Salt 1 Green onion, diced 1 oz. Feta cheese 1 tbsp. Olive oil 3 Egg 5 Mushrooms, button, cut

Directions:

Sauté the mushrooms, onions, and spinach for four minutes and set them aside. Beat eggs meticulously and pour into the frying pan. Cook for three to four minutes until edges start to turn brown. Drizzle all other ingredients onto half of the omelet and fold the other half over. Cook the omelet for a minute on each side.

61. Strawberry Yogurt treat

Time To Prepare: ten minutes Time to Cook: 0 minutes Yield: Servings 2

Ingredients:

1 cup cut strawberries 4 cups 0% Fat plain yogurt 4 tbsp. honey 8 tbsp. of flax meal 8 tbsp. walnuts (chopped)

Directions:

Distribute 2 cups of the yogurt into your serving bowls. Neatly layer the flax meal and the walnut in the center. Put in a sprinkle of half of the honey before covering with the final layer of yogurt. Put in the honey on top of the yogurt to put in color when you serve.

62. Sun-Dried Tomato Garlic Bruschetta

Time To Prepare: ten minutes Time to Cook: five minutes Yield: Servings 6

Ingredients:

1 garlic clove, peeled 1 tsp. chives, minced 1 tsp. olive oil 2 slices sourdough bread, toasted 2 tsp. sun-dried tomatoes in olive oil, minced

Directions:

Vigorously rub garlic clove on 1 side of each of the toasted bread slices Spread equivalent portions of sun-dried tomatoes on the garlic side of bread. Drizzle chives and sprinkle olive oil on top. Pop both slices into oven toaster, and cook until well thoroughly heated. Put bruschetta on a plate. Serve warm

63. Sweetened Brown Rice

Time To Prepare: ten minutes Time to Cook: 45-60 minutes Yield: Servings 8

Ingredients:

¼ teaspoon nutmeg 1 cup brown rice 1 tablespoon honey 1½ cups soy milk 1½ cups water Fresh fruit (not necessary)

Directions:

Put all the ingredients excluding the fresh fruit in a medium-size deep cooking pan; put the mixture to a slow simmer then cover using a tight-fitting lid. Simmer for minimum 45-60 minutes, up to the rice is soft and done. Serve in bowls, topped with your favorite fresh fruit.

64. Tomato and Avocado Omelet

Time To Prepare: five minutes Time to Cook: five minutes Yield: Servings 1

Ingredients:

¼ avocado, diced 1 tablespoon cilantro, chopped 2 eggs 4 cherry tomatoes, halved Pinch of salt Squeeze of lime juice

Directions:

Put together the avocado, tomatoes, cilantro, lime juice, and salt in a small container, then mix thoroughly and save for later. Warm a moderate-sized nonstick frying pan on moderate heat. Whisk the eggs until frothy and put in to the pan. Move the eggs around gently using a rubber spatula until they start to set. Spread the avocado mixture over half of the omelet. Turn off the heat, and slide the omelet onto a plate as you fold it in half. Serve instantly.

65. Tuna & Sweet Potato Croquettes

Time To Prepare: fifteen minutes Time to Cook: twelve minutes Yield: Servings 8

Ingredients:

¼ cup almond flour ¼ cup tapioca flour ¼ teaspoon garam masala ¼ teaspoon ground turmeric ¼ teaspoon red chili powder ½ big onion, chopped ½ teaspoon ground coriander 1 (1-inch piece fresh ginger, minced 1 cup sweet potato, peeled and mashed 1 egg 1 Serrano pepper, seeded and minced 1 tablespoon coconut oil 2 (5 oz.) cans tuna 3 garlic cloves, minced Freshly ground black pepper, to taste Olive oil, as required Salt, to taste

Directions: In a frying pan, warm the coconut oil on moderate heat. Put onion, ginger, garlic, and Serrano pepper and sauté for roughly 5-6 minutes. Mix in spices and sauté roughly one minute more. Move the onion mixture in a container. Put in tuna and sweet potato and mix till well blended. Make equal sized oblong shaped patties in the mixture. Position the croquettes inside a baking sheet in a very single layer and place in your fridge for overnight. In a shallow dish, beat the egg. In another shallow dish, combine both flours. In a big frying pan, heat the enough oil. Put in croquettes in batches and shallow fry for about two to three minutes per side.

66. Vegan-Friendly Banana Bread

Time To Prepare: fifteen minutes Time to Cook: forty minutes Yield: Servings 4-6

Ingredients:

2 ripe bananas, mashed 3 tbsp. chia seeds 6 tbsp. water ½ cup tender vegan butter ½ cup maple syrup 2 cups flour 2 tsp. baking powder 1 tsp. cinnamon powder 1 tsp. allspice ½ tsp. salt 1/3 cup brewed coffee

Directions: Set oven at 350F. Bring the chia seeds in a small container then soak it with 6 tbsp. of water. Stir thoroughly and save for later. In a mixing container, mix using a hand mixer the vegan butter and maple syrup until it turns fluffy. Put in the chia seeds together with the mashed bananas. Mix thoroughly and then put in the coffee. In the meantime, sift all the dry ingredients (flour, baking powder, cinnamon powder, all spice, and salt) and then progressively put in into the container with the wet ingredients. Mix the ingredients well and then pour over a baking pan coated with parchment paper. Put in your oven to bake for minimum 30-40 minutes, or until the toothpick comes out clean after inserting in the bread. Let the bread cool before you serve

67. Weekend Breakfast Salad

Time To Prepare: thirty minutes Time to Cook: 0 minutes Yield: Servings 4

Ingredients:

½ cup Cucumber, chopped ½ cup Dill, chopped 1 cup Almonds, chopped 1 cup Quinoa, cooked and cooled 1 Large Avocado, cut thin 1 Large Tomato, cut in wedges 1 Lemon 10 cups Arugula 2 tbsp. Olive oil 4 Eggs, hard-boiled

Directions:

Mix together the quinoa, cucumber, tomatoes, and arugula. Toss these ingredients lightly with olive oil, salt, and pepper. Split the salad into 4 plates and position the egg and avocado on top. Top each salad with almonds and herbs. Sprinkle with juice from the lemon.

68. Whole Grain Blueberry Scones

Time To Prepare: ten minutes Time to Cook: twenty-five minutes Yield: Servings 8

Ingredients:

¼ cup maple syrup ½ teaspoon sea salt 1 cup blueberries 1 teaspoon vanilla extract 2 cups of whole-wheat flour 2 tablespoons of coconut milk 2½ teaspoons baking powder 6 tablespoons of olive oil

Directions:

Set the oven 400°F. Place parchment paper on your baking sheet. Put in the syrup, flour, salt, and baking powder in a container. Mix well by whisking together. Pour the olive oil into a container with the dry ingredients. Work the oil into your flour mix. Mix the vanilla extract and coconut milk into the dry ingredients container. Fold in the blueberries gently. Your dough must be sticky and thick. Put some flour on your hand then mold the dough into a circle. Use a knife to make triangle slices. Place them over the baking sheet. Maintain an 8-inch gap. Bake for about twenty-five minutes. Set aside on the baking sheet for cooling when finished.

69. Yummy Steak Muffins

Time To Prepare:ten minutes Time to Cook: twenty minutes Yield:Servings 4

Ingredients:

¼ teaspoon of sea salt 1 cup of finely diced onion 1 cup red bell pepper, diced 2 Tablespoons of water 8 free-range eggs 8 ounce thin steak, cooked and finely chopped Dash of freshly ground black pepper

Directions:

Set the oven to 350°F Take 8 muffin tins and line then using parchment paper liners. Get a big container and crack all the eggs in it. Beat well the eggs. Blend in all the rest of the ingredients. Ladle the batter into the position muffin tins. Fill three-fourth of each tin. Place the muffin tins in the preheated oven for approximately twenty minutes, until the muffins are baked and set in the center. Enjoy!

70. Zucchini Pancakes

Time To Prepare: fifteen minutes Time to Cook: 6-10 min Yield: Servings 8

Ingredients:

¼ cup fresh cilantro, chopped ¼ teaspoon cumin seeds ¼ teaspoon ground turmeric ¼ tsp cayenne ½ cup red onion, chopped finely ½ cup zucchini, shredded 1 cup chickpea flour 1 green chile, seeded and chopped finely 1½ cups water, divided Salt, to taste

Directions: In a big container, put in flour and ¾ cup with the water and beat till smooth. Put in remaining water and beat till a thin Fold inside the onion, ginger, Serrano pepper, and cilantro. Lightly, grease a substantial nonstick frying pan with oil and heat on medium-low heat. Put in about ¼ cup of mixture and tilt the pan to spread it uniformly in the frying pan. Cook for around 4-6 minutes. Cautiously, alter the side and cook for roughly 2-4 minutes. Repeat while using the rest of the mixture. Serve with your desired topping.

71. Cherry & Apple Bowl

Yield: 2-3 servings Preparation Time: 10 minutes

Ingredients:

• 1½ cups almond milk • ½ cup pumpkin puree • 2 tablespoon organic honey • 2 tablespoon almond butter • 1 teaspoon organic vanilla flavor • 1 scoop Protein powder • 1 teaspoon ground cinnamon • 1/8 teaspoon ground ginger • 1/8 teaspoon cloves • ¼ teaspoon ground nutmeg • Pinch of salt • ¼ cup chia seeds

Directions: In a blender, add all ingredients except chia seeds and pulse till smooth. Transfer the amalgamation in a large bowl. Add chia seeds and stir to blend well. Refrigerate for overnight.

72. Healthy Bread

Yield: 8-12 servings Preparation Time: quarter-hour Cooking Time: 30-40 minutes

Ingredients: •

1 cup sorghum flour • Pinch of salt • ½ cup carrot juicing remains • ½ cup apple juice remains • 2 tablespoons ginger juice remains • 2 organic eggs • ¼ cup coconut butter • ½ cup coconut sugar • 1 teaspoon organic vanilla extract

Directions: Preheat the oven to 350 degrees F. Lightly, grease a loaf pan. In a sizable bowl, mix together flour, salt, carrot juice remains, apple juice remains and carrot juice remains. In another bowl, add remaining ingredients and beat till fluffy. Add egg mixture into flour mixture and mix till well combined. Place the mixture into prepared loaf pan evenly. Bake for around 30-40 minutes.

73. Fruity Muffins

Yield: 8 servings Preparation Time: 10 minutes Cooking Time: 2-3 minutes

Ingredients:

½ cup almond meal • 1 tablespoon linseed meal • ¼ cup raw sugar • 2 tablespoons crystalized ginger, chopped finely • ½ cup buckwheat flour • ¼ cup brown rice flour • 2 tablespoons arrowroot flour • 2 tablespoons organic baking powder • ½ teaspoon ground ginger • 12 teaspoon ground cinnamon • Pinch of salt • 1 large organic egg • 7 tablespoons almond milk • ¼ cup extra-virgin organic olive oil • 1 teaspoon organic vanilla flavoring • 1 small apple, peeled, cored and chopped finely • 1 cup rhubarb, sliced finely

Directions: 1. Preheat the oven to 350 degrees F. Grease 8 cups of a large muffin tin. 2. In a large bowl, mix together almond meal, linseed meal, sugar and crystalized ginger. 3. In another bowl, mix together flours, baking powder, spices and salt. 4. Sift the flour mixture into bowl of almond meal mixture and mix well. 5. In one third bowl, add egg, milk, oil and vanilla and beat till well combined. 6. Add egg mixture into flour mixture and mix till well combined. 7. Fold in apple and rhubarb. 8. Place a combination into prepared muffin cups evenly. 9. Bake for approximately 20-25 minutes or till a toothpick inserted in the center comes out clean.

74. Gingered Carrot & Coconut

Yield: 12 servings Preparation Time: fifteen minutes Cooking Time: 20-22 minutes

Ingredients:

2 cups blanched almond flour • ½ cup unswee10ed coconut shreds • 1 tsp baking soda • ½ teaspoon allspice • ½ teaspoon ground ginger • Pinch of ground cloves • Salt, to taste • 3 organic eggs • ½ cup organic honey • ½ cup coconut oil • 1 cup carrot, peeled and grated • 2 tablespoons fresh ginger, peeled and grated • ¾ cup raisins, soaked in water for quarter-hour and drained

Directions: Preheat the oven to 350 degrees F. Grease 12 cups of a large muffin tin. 2. In a sizable bowl, mix together flour, coconut shreds, baking soda, spices and salt. 3. In another bowl, add eggs, honey, and oil and beat till well combined. 4. Add egg mixture into flour mixture and mix till well combined. 5. Fold in carrot, ginger and raisins. 6. Place the mix into prepared muffin cups evenly. 7. Bake approximately 20-22 minutes or till a toothpick inserted inside center arrives clean.

75. Savory Veggie Muffins

Yield: 5 servings Preparation Time: quarter-hour Cooking Time: 18-23 minutes

Ingredients:

¾ cup almond meal • ½ tsp baking soda • ¼ cup whey Protein concentrate powder • 2 teaspoons fresh dill, chopped • Salt, to taste • 4 large organic eggs • 1½ tablespoons nutritional yeast • 2 teaspoons apple cider vinegar • 3 tablespoons fresh lemon juice • 2 tablespoons coconut oil, melted • 1 cup coconut butter, sof1oed • 1 bunch scallion, chopped • 2 medium carrots, peeled and grated • ½ cup fresh parsley, chopped

Directions:

1. Preheat the oven to 350 degrees F. Grease 10 cups of your large muffin tin. 2. In a large bowl, mix together flour, baking soda, Protein powder and salt. 3. In another bowl, add eggs, nutritional yeast, vinegar, lemon juice and oil and beat till well combined. 4. Add coconut butter and beat till mixture becomes smooth. 5. Add egg mixture into flour mixture and mix till well combined. 6. Fold in scallion, carts and parsley. 7. Place the amalgamation into prepared muffin cups evenly. 8. Bake for about 18-23 minutes or till a toothpick inserted inside center comes out clean.

76. Spicy Ginger Crepes

Yield: 8 servings Preparation Time: fifteen minutes Cooking Time: 20-30 seconds

Ingredients:

1 1/3 cups chickpea flour • ½ teaspoon red chili powder • Salt, to taste • 1 (1-inch) fresh ginger piece, grated finely • 1 cup fresh cilantro leaves, chopped • 1 green chili, seeded and chopped finely • 1 cup water • Cooking spray, as required

Directions: 1. In a sizable bowl, mix together flour, chili powder and salt. 2. Add ginger, cilantro and chili and mix well. 3. Add water and mix till an even mixture forms. 4. Keep aside, covered for approximately ½-120 minutes. 5. Lightly, grease a substantial nonstick skillet with cooking spray and heat on medium-high heat. 6. Add desired volume of mixture and tilt the pan to spread it evenly inside skillet. 7. Cook approximately 10-15 seconds per side. 8. Repeat while using remaining mixture.

77. Cilantro Pancakes

Yield: 6 servings Preparation Time: 10 minutes Cooking Time: 6-8 minutes

Ingredients:

• ½ cup tapioca flour • ½ cup almond flour • ½ teaspoon chili powder • ¼ teaspoon ground turmeric • Salt and freshly ground black pepper, to taste • 1 cup full- Fat coconut milk • ½ of red onion, chopped • 1 (½-inch) fresh ginger piece, grated finely • 1 Serrano pepper, minced • ½ cup fresh cilantro, chopped • Oil, as required

Directions: 1. In a big bowl, mix together flours and spices. 2. Add coconut milk and mix till well combined. 3. Fold within the onion, ginger, Serrano pepper and cilantro. 4. Lightly, grease a sizable nonstick skillet with oil and warmth on medium-low heat. 5. Add about ¼ cup of mixture and tilt the pan to spread it evenly inside the skillet. 6. Cook for around 3-4 minutes from either side. 7. Repeat with all the remaining mixture. 8. Serve along with your desired topping.

78. Pumpkin & Banana Waffles

Yield: 4 servings Preparation Time: fifteen minutes Cooking Time: 5 minutes

Ingredients:

½ cup almond flour • ½ cup coconut flour • 1 tsp baking soda • 1½ teaspoons ground cinnamon • ¾ teaspoon ground ginger • ½ teaspoon ground cloves • ½ teaspoon ground nutmeg • Salt, to taste • 2 tablespoons olive oil • 5 large organic eggs • ¾ cup almond milk • ½ cup pumpkin puree • 2 medium bananas, peeled and sliced

Directions: 1. Preheat the waffle iron and after that grease it. 2. In a sizable bowl, mix together flours, baking soda and spices. 3. In a blender, add remaining ingredients and pulse till smooth. 4. Add flour mixture and pulse till 5. In preheated waffle iron, add required quantity of mixture. 6. Cook approximately 4-5 minutes. 7. Repeat using the remaining mixture. Nutritional Information per Serving:

79. Zucchini Quiche

Yield: 2 servings Preparation Time: 15 minutes Cooking Time: 40 minutes

Ingredients:

5 organic eggs • Salt and freshly ground black pepper, to taste • 1 carrot, peeled and grated • 1 small zucchini, shredded

Directions:

1. Preheat the oven to 350 degrees F. Lightly, grease a tiny baking dish. 2. In a substantial bowl, add eggs, salt and black pepper and beat well. 3. Add carrot and zucchini and stir to mix. 4. Transfer the mixture into prepared baking dish evenly. 5. Bake for about 40 minutes.

80. Kale & Bell Pepper Frittata

Yield: 3 servings Preparation Time: quarter-hour Cooking Time: 17 minutes

Ingredients:

1-2 tablespoons coconut oil • ½-1 teaspoon ground turmeric • 1 small red bell pepper, seeded and chopped • 1 cup fresh kale, trimmed and chopped • ¼ cup chives, chopped • 6 organic eggs • Salt, to taste

Directions:

1. In a certain skillet, melt the coconut oil on medium-low heat. 2. Sprinkle turmeric inside oil and immediately, stir in bell pepper and kale. 3. Sauté for around 2 minutes and lower heat to low. 4. Meanwhile inside a bowl, add eggs and salt and beat well. 5. Add bea10 eggs inside the skillet over bell pepper mixture evenly. 6. Cover and cook for about 10-quarter-hour

81. Tomato Omelet

Yield: 2 servings Preparation Time: 10 min Cooking Time: 2-3 minutes

Ingredients:

4 large organic eggs • Salt, to taste • 1 tbsp organic olive oil • 1/8 teaspoon ground turmeric • ¼ teaspoon brown mustard seeds • 2 scallions, chopped finely • ¼ cup plum tomato, chopped • Pinch of freshly ground black pepper

Directions:

1. In a bowl, add eggs and salt and beat well. Keep aside. 2. In a cast iron skillet, heat coconut oil on medium-high heat. 3. Add turmeric and mustard seeds and sauté for around half a minute. 4. Add scallion and sauté for around thirty seconds. 5. Add tomato and cook approximately 1 minute. 6. Add the egg mixture inside the skillet evenly and cook for approximately 2 minutes. 7. Carefully, tilt the pan and cook for approximately 2 minutes more. 8. Transfer the omelet in to a plate and cut into 2 wedges. 9. Serve hot using the sprinkling of black pepper.

82. Kale Scramble

Yield: 1 serving Preparation Time: 10 min Cooking Time: 6 minutes

Ingredients:

2 organic eggs • 1 tablespoon coconut oil • 1 cup fresh kale, trimmed and chopped • 1 ½ teaspoon ground turmeric • 1 teaspoon garlic powder • Salt and freshly ground black pepper, to taste

Directions:

1. In a bowl, add eggs and beat well. Keep aside. 2. In a skillet, melt coconut oil on medium heat. 3. Add kale and cook approximately 2 minutes. 4. Add eggs and remaining ingredients and cook, stirring and cook approximately 3-4 minutes or till desired doneness.

83. Oats & Seeds Granola

Yield: 10-12 servings Preparation Time: 15 minutes Cooking Time: 50 minutes

Ingredients:

2 cups oats • 1 cup pumpkin seeds • 1 cup sunflower seeds • 1 cup buckwheat • 1½ cups dates, pitted and chopped • 1 cup fresh apple puree • 1/3 cup coconut oil • 1 fresh ginger piece, grated finely • ¼ cup raw cacao powder

Directions:

1. Preheat the oven to 355 degrees F. Grease a large baking dish. 2. In a substantial bowl, mix together oats, seeds and buckwheat. 3. In a pan, mix together dates, apple puree and coconut oil on medium-low heat. 4. Simmer approximately 5 minutes or till dates becomes soft. 5. Stir in ginger and take off from heat. 6. Keep aside to chill slightly. 7. In a blender, add date mixture and cacao powder and pulse till smooth. 8. Add the date mixture inside bowl with oat mixture and stir to mix well. 9. Transfer the mix into prepared baking dish evenly. 10. Bake for about 15 minutes. 11. Remove from oven and stir well. 12. Bake approximately thirty minutes, stirring after every 5-10 minutes. 13. This granola might be preserved in the airtight container.

84. Millet Porridge

Yield: 4 servings Preparation Time: fifteen minutes Cooking Time: 6-10 minutes

Ingredients:

1tablespoon coconut oil • 1 teaspoon ground ginger • 2 teaspoons ground cinnamon • ½ teaspoon ground cloves • 1½ cups millet, grounded • 1½ cups water • 4 cups coconut milk

Directions:

1. In a pan, melt coconut oil on medium-low heat. 2. Add spices and sauté approximately half a minute. 3. Stir in millet with all the spice mixture. 4. Stir in water and coconut milk and convey to your boil. 5. Reduce the heat to low and cover the pan partially. 6. Simmer, beating occasionally for approximately 10-quarter-hour or till desired thickness. 7. Serve using your desired topping.

85. Baked Simple Eggs

Yield: 12 servings Preparation Time: 5 minutes Cooking Time: 8-12 minutes

Ingredients:

12 large organic eggs • Salt and freshly ground black pepper, to taste

Directions:

1. Preheat the oven to 350 degrees F. Grease a 12 cups whoopie pie pan. 2. In a little, bowl, break an egg then carefully transfer into prepared cup of whoopie pie pan. 3. Repeat with remaining eggs. 4. Bake for about 8-12 minutes or till desired doneness. 5. Serve immediately using the sprinkling of salt and black pepper.

86. Eggs In Mushrooms Caps

Yield: 2 servings Preparation Time: 10 minutes Cooking Time: 20-30 minutes

Ingredients:

4 large Portobello mushrooms, stemmed, scrapped the gills and wiped clean • 4 prosciutto slices • Freshly ground black pepper, to taste • 4 organic eggs • 2 tablespoons fresh parsley, chopped finely

Directions:

1. Preheat the oven to 375 degrees F. Lightly, grease a baking dish. 2. Arrange a prosciutto slice in each egg. 3. In a smaller, bowl, break an egg and after that carefully transfer into mushroom cap. 4. Repeat with remaining eggs. 5. Sprinkle with black pepper and parsley. 6. Bake for around 20-half an hour or till desired doneness.

87. Baked Veggie Omelet Definitely

Yield: 4 servings Preparation Time: 15 minutes Cooking Time: 20-25 minutes

Ingredients:

6 large organic eggs • Salt and freshly ground black pepper, to taste • ½ cup coconut milk • ½ of onion, chopped • ¼ cup red bell pepper, seeded and chopped • ¼ cup fresh mushrooms, sliced • 1 tablespoon chives, minced

Directions:

1. Preheat the oven to 350 degrees F. Lightly, grease a pie dish. 2. In a bowl, add eggs, salt, black pepper and coconut oil and beat till well combined. 3. In another bowl, mix together onion, bell pepper and mushrooms. 4. Transfer the egg mixture in prepared pie dish evenly. 5. Top with vegetable mixture evenly. Sprinkle with chives evenly. 6. Bake approximately 20-25 minutes.

88. Smoked Salmon Scramble

Yield: 1 serving Preparation Time: 10 minutes Cooking Time: 5 minutes

Ingredients:

2 organic eggs • 1 organic egg yolk • 1 tablespoon fresh dill, chopped finely • 1/8 teaspoon red pepper flakes, crushed • 1/8 teaspoon garlic powder • Salt and freshly ground black pepper, to taste • 2 smoked salmon pieces, chopped • 1 tablespoon organic olive oil

Directions:

1. In a bowl, add all ingredients except salmon and oil and beat till well combined. 2. Stir in chopped salmon. 3. In a little frying pan, heat oil on medium-low heat. 4. Add egg mixture and cook, stirring continuously approximately 3-5 minutes or till done completely. 5. Serve immediately.

89. Almond Pancakes with Coconut Flakes

Time To Prepare: 5 minutes Time to Cook: ten minutes Yield: Servings 6

Ingredients:

¼ cup coconut flakes, sweetened ¼ cup of water ¼ tsp. coconut oil ½ cup unsweetened applesauce 1 cup almond flour, finely milled 1 overripe banana, mashed 2 eggs, yolks, and whites separated 2 Tbsp. blanched almond flakes Dash of cinnamon powder Garnish Pinch of sea salt Pure maple syrup, use sparingly

Directions:

Whisk egg whites until tender peaks form. Except for egg whites and coconut oil, mix rest of the ingredients in a different container. Mix until batter comes together. Lightly fold in egg whites. Ensure that you do not over mix, or the pancake will become dense and chewy. Pour oil into a nonstick frying pan set on moderate heat. Wait for the oil to heat up before dropping in roughly ½ cup of batter. Cook until each side are set, and bubbles form in the middle. Turn on the other side then cook for an extra two minutes. Move flapjacks to a plate. Repeat step until all batter is cooked. Pour in more oil into the frying pan only if required. This recipe should yield between four to 6 moderate-sized pancakes. Stack pancakes. Pour the desired amount of pure maple syrup on top. Decorate each stack with cinnamon-flavored almond-coconut flakes just before you serve. For the decorate, set the oven to 350°F for minimum ten minutes before use. Coat a baking sheet using parchment paper. Set aside. Mix almond and coconut flakes together in a container. Spread mixture uniformly on a readied baking sheet. Bake for 7 to ten minutes until flakes turn golden brown. Stir almond and coconut flakes once midway through roasting to stop over-browning. Take away the baking sheet from the oven. Cool almond and coconut flakes for minimum ten minutes before drizzling in cinnamon powder and salt. Toss to blend. Set aside.

90. Breakfast Frittata

Time To Prepare: ten minutes Time to Cook: forty minutes Yield: Servings 4

Ingredients:

¼ cup water ½ tsp. cracked black pepper ½ tsp. ground turmeric 1 onion, chopped 1 tbsp. minced garlic 125g firm tofu 4 big eggs 450g baby spinach 450g button mushrooms 6 egg whites Kosher salt to taste

Directions:

Set the oven to 350F. Sauté the mushrooms in a little bit of extra virgin olive oil in a big non-stick ovenproof pan on moderate heat. Put in the onions once the mushrooms start turning golden and cook for about three minutes until the onions become tender. Mix in the garlic then cook for minimum half a minute until aromatic before you put in the spinach. Pour in water, cover, and cook until the spinach becomes wilted for approximately 2 minutes. Take off the lid and carry on cooking up to the water evaporates. Now, mix the eggs, egg whites, tofu, pepper, turmeric, and salt in a container. When all the liquid has vaporized, pour in the egg mixture, allow to cook for approximately 2 minutes until the edges start setting, then move to the oven and bake for approximately twenty-five minutes or until cooked. Remove from the oven then allow it to sit for minimum five minutes before cutting it into four equivalent portions and serving. Enjoy!

91. Apple Bruschetta with Almonds and Blackberries

Time To Prepare: twenty minutes Time to Cook: thirty minutes Yield: Servings 5

Ingredients:

¼ cup blackberries, thawed, lightly mashed ½ tsp. fresh lemon juice 1 apple, cut into ¼-inch thick half-moons 1/8 cup almond slivers, toasted Sea salt

Directions:

 Sprinkle lemon juice on apple slices. Place these on a tray coated with parchment paper. Spread a small number of mashed berries on top of each slice. Top these off with the desired amount of almond slivers. Drizzle sea salt on "bruschetta" just before you serve.

92. Apple, Ginger, and Rhubarb Muffins

Time To Prepare: fifteen minutes Time to Cook: twenty-five minutes Yield: Servings 4

Ingredients:

¼ cup brown rice flour ¼ cup extra virgin olive oil ½ cup buckwheat flour ½ cup thoroughly ground almonds ½ tsp. ground cinnamon ½ tsp. ground ginger 1 big egg 1 cup finely chopped rhubarb 1 small apple, peeled and finely diced 1 tbsp. linseed meal 1 tsp. pure vanilla extract 1/3 cup almond/ rice milk 1/8 cup unrefined raw sugar 2 tbsp. arrowroot flour 2 tbsp. crystallized ginger, finely chopped 2 tsp. gluten-free baking powder A pinch of fine sea salt

Directions:

Set the oven to 350Fgrease an eight-cup muffin tin and line with paper cases. Mix the almond four, linseed meal, ginger and sugar in a mixing container. Sieve this mixture over the other flours, spices and baking powder and use a whisk to blend well. Mix in the apple and rhubarb in the flour mixture until uniformly coated. In a different container, whisk the milk, vanilla, and egg then pour it into the dry mixture. Stir until just blended – do not overwork the batter as this can yield very tough muffins. Scoop the mixture into the position muffin tin and top with a few slices of rhubarb. Bake for minimum twenty-five minutes, till they start turning golden or when an inserted toothpick emerges clean. Remove from the oven and allow it to sit for minimum five minutes before transferring the muffins to a wire rack for further cooling. Serve warm with a glass of squeezed juice. Enjoy!

93. Baked French Toast Casserole

Time To Prepare: twenty minutes Time to Cook: forty-five minutes Yield: Servings 12

Ingredients:

½ lb. blueberries ½ lb. raspberries ¾ cup strawberries 1 cup of egg white liquid 1 lb. French bread 1 teaspoon of vanilla extract 1/3 cup maple syrup 1½ cups of rice milk, 6 eggs

Directions:

Cut the bread into little cubes. Keep them in a greased casserole dish. Put in all the berries. Only leave a few for the topping. Mix together the egg whites, eggs, rice milk, and maple syrup in a container. Mix well. Place the egg mixture on the top of the bread. Push the bread down. All pieces must be soaked well. Put in berries on the top. Fill up the holes, if any. Place in your fridge covered for a couple of hours at least. Take out the casserole half an hour before you bake. Set the oven to 350 degrees F. Now, bake your casserole uncovered for half an hourBake for another fifteen minutes covered with a foil. Let it rest for 15 minutes. Serve it warm with maple syrup.

94. Banana Pancakes

Time To Prepare: five minutes Time to Cook:fifteen minutes Yield:Servings 2

Ingredients:

½ Teaspoon Sea Salt 1 Banana, Ripe 1 Cup Rolled Oats 1 Egg White 1 Tablespoon Coconut Oil, Divided 1 Teaspoon Vanilla Extract, Pure 2 Eggs 2 Teaspoons Ground Cinnamon

Directions:

Prepare your food processor, grinding your oats until they make a coarse flour. Put in your cinnamon, egg whites, eggs, banana, vanilla, and salt. Blend until it becomes a smooth batter, and then heat a small frying pan on moderate heat. Heat a half a tablespoon of coconut oil, and then pour your batter in. Cook for a couple of minutes per side, and carry on till all of your batter has been used.

95. Barley Breakfast Bowl with Lemon Yogurt Sauce

Time To Prepare: ten minutes Time to Cook: 0 minutes Yield: Servings 2

Ingredients:

¼ c. cut almonds, toasted ¼ c. fresh mint or parsley, chopped ¼ tsp. fresh ground black pepper ¼ tsp. kosher salt ½ tsp. Sea salt 1 c. Greek plain yogurt 1 c. mung bean sprouts (or preferred variety) 1 small avocado – peeled/pitted, and flesh diced or cut 1 tsp. Fresh lemon juice 1 tsp. lemon zest, finely grated 1/3 c. Cotija cheese or queso fresco - crumbled 1½ c. cooked barley, keep warm Fresh ground black pepper, to taste Lemon Yogurt Sauce Sea salt, to taste

Directions:

First, prepare the Lemon Yogurt Sauce: Mix the plain yogurt, lemon zest and juice, fresh mint or parsley, and salt & pepper in a container and stir to combine well. Cover and place in your fridge until ready to serve. After this, prepare the barley container: In a small mixing container, mix the barley, bean sprouts, cheese, almonds, and salt. Stir to mix thoroughly. Split barley mixture into 2 serving bowls. Top each barley container with 2 tbsp. lemon yogurt sauce and avocado. Place a pinch of salt and pepper to taste, serve, and enjoy!

96. Blueberry & Cashew Waffles

Time To Prepare: fifteen minutes Time to Cook:4-5 minutes Yield: Servings 5

Ingredients:

¼ cup coconut oil, melted ½ cup unsweetened almond milk ½ teaspoon organic vanilla flavor 1 cup fresh blueberries 1 cup raw cashews 1 tsp baking soda 3 organic eggs 3 tablespoons coconut flour 3 tablespoons organic honey Salt, to taste

Directions:

Preheat the waffle iron after which grease it. In a mixer, put in cashews and pulse till flour-like consistency forms. Move the cashew flour in a big container. Put in almond flour, baking soda and salt and mix thoroughly. In another container, put the rest of the ingredients and beat till well blended. Place the egg mixture into the flour mixture then mix till well blended. Fold in blueberries. In preheated waffle iron, put in the required amount of mixture. Cook for about five minutes. Repeat with the rest of the mixture.

97. Breakfast ArrozHot

Time To Prepare: twenty minutes Time to Cook: thirty minutes Yield: Servings 5

Ingredients:

¼ cup raisins ½ cup frozen peas, thawed 1 garlic clove, minced 1 white onion, minced 1½ cups brown rice, cooked 6 eggs, white only For the filling oil, for greasing

Directions:

To make the filling, spray a small amount of oil into a frying pan set on moderate heat. Put in in onion and garlic. Stir-fry until former is limp and transparent. Stir-fry while breaking up clumps, approximately 2 minutes. Put in in rest of the ingredients. Stir-fry for one more minute. Turn down the heat, and let filling cook for ten to fifteen minutes, or until juices are greatly reduced. Stir frequently. Turn off heat. Split into 6 equivalent portions. For the eggs, spray a small amount of oil into a smaller frying pan set on moderate heat. Cook eggs. Discard yolk. Move to holding the plate. To serve, place 1 portion of rice on a plate, 1 portion of filling, and 1 egg white. Serve warm.

98. Breakfast Sausage and Mushroom Casserole

Time To Prepare: twenty minutes Time to Cook: forty-five minutes Yield: Servings 4

Ingredients:

1 ½ tsp. of sea salt, divided 1 medium onion, finely diced 1 red bell pepper, roasted 2 Tablespoons of organic ghee 3/4 tsp. of ground black pepper, divided 450g of Italian sausage, cooked and crumbled 6 free-range eggs 600g of sweet potatoes 8 ounces of white mushrooms, cut Three-fourth cup of coconut milk

Directions: Peel and shred the sweet potatoes. Take a container, fill it with ice-cold water, and soak the sweet potatoes in it. Set aside. Peel the roasted bell pepper, remove its seeds and finely dice it. Set the oven 375°F. Get a casserole baking dish and grease it with the organic ghee. Place a frying pan using moderate heat and cook the mushrooms in it. Cook until the mushrooms are crunchy and brown. Take the mushrooms out and mix them with the crumbled sausage. Now sauté the onions in the same frying pan. Cook up to the onions are tender and golden. This should take approximately four – five minutes. Take the onions out and mix them in the sausage-mushroom mixture.Put in the diced bell pepper to the same mixture. Mix thoroughly and set aside for a while. Now drain the soaked shredded potatoes, put them on a paper towel, and pat dry. Bring the sweet potatoes in a container and put in about a teaspoon of salt and half a teaspoon of ground black pepper to it. Mix thoroughly and save for later. Now take a big container and crack the eggs in it. Break the eggs and then mix in the coconut milk. Mix in the rest of the black pepper and salt. Take the greased casserole dish and spread the seasoned sweet potatoes uniformly in the base of the dish. After this, spread the sausage mixture uniformly in the dish. To finish, spread the egg mixture. Now cover the casserole dish using a piece of aluminium foil. Bake for 20 - thirty minutes. To check if the casserole is baked properly, insert a tester in the center of the casserole, and it should come out clean. Uncover the casserole dish and bake it again, uncovered for 5 - ten minutes, until the casserole is a little golden on the top. Let it cool for approximately ten minutes. Enjoy!

99. Carrot Cake Overnight Oats

Time To Prepare: five minutes + overnight   Time to Cook: 0 minutes   Yield: Servings 1

Ingredients:

½ cup Raisins 1 cup Coconut or almond milk 1 Large Carrot, peel, and shred 1 tbsp. Chia seeds 1 tsp. Cinnamon, ground 1 tsp. Vanilla 2 tbsp. Cream cheese, low fat, at room temperature 2 tbsp. Honey

Directions:

Mix together all of the listed ingredients and store them in a safe fridge container overnight. Eat cold in the morning. If you choose to warm this, just microwave for a minute and stir thoroughly before eating.

100.   Cheddar and Chive Souffles

Time To Prepare: ten minutes   Time to Cook: twenty-five minutes   Yield: Servings 8

Ingredients:

¼ cup chopped chives ¼ tsp cayenne pepper ½ cup almond flour ½ cup baking powder ½ tsp cracked black pepper ½ tsp xanthan gum ¾ cup heavy cream 1 tsp ground mustard 1 tsp salt 2 cups shredded cheddar cheese 6 organic eggs, separated

Directions:

Switch on the oven, then set its temperature to 350°F and allow it to preheat. Take a medium container, put in flour in it, put in rest of the ingredients, apart from for baking powder and eggs, and whisk until blended. Separate egg yolks and egg whites between two bowls, put in egg yolks in the flour mixture and whisk until blended. Put in baking powder into the egg whites and beat using an electric mixer until stiff peaks form and then stir egg whites into the flour mixture until thoroughly combined. Split the batter uniformly between eight ramekins and then bake for about twenty-five minutes until done. Serve straight away or store in your fridge until ready to eat.

101.   Cherry Chia Oats

Time To Prepare: ten minutes   Time to Cook:twenty minutes   Yield:Servings 2

Ingredients:

¼ Cup Whole Milk Yogurt, Plain ¼ Teaspoon Vanilla Extract, Pure 1 ¼ Cup Almond Milk 1 Cup Quick Cook Oats 2 Tablespoons Almond Butter 2 Tablespoons Chia Seeds 8 Cherries, Fresh, Pitted & Halved

Directions:

Combine all the ingredients until they're blended well. Seal in two jars and place in your fridge for twenty-five minutes before you serve.

102.   Choco-Banana Oats

Time To Prepare: five minutes   Time to Cook: 8 minutes   Yield: Servings 2

Ingredients:

¼ tsp. almond extract ¼ tsp. Vanilla ¾ cup water 1/3 cup toasted walnuts, chopped 1/8 tsp. cinnamon 1/8 tsp. salt 2 cups almond milk 2 cups oats 2 ripe bananas, cut 2 tbsp. agave nectar 2 tbsp. cocoa powder, unsweetened 2 tbsp. vegan chocolate chips, semisweet

Directions:

In a big deep cooking pan, pour the almond milk, water, bananas, vanilla, and almond extract. Put in the salt, stir, and heat over high temperature. Combine the oats in the pan together with the unsweetened cocoa powder, 1 tbsp. agave nectar and reduce the temperature to moderate. Cook for 7-8 minutes, or until the oats are cooked to your preference. Stir regularly. Scoop the cooked oats into serving bowls and decorate with the chopped walnuts, chocolate chips, and sprinkle with the remaining agave nectar.

103. Cinnamon Pancakes with Coconut

Time To Prepare: five minutes Time to Cook: eighteen minutes Yield: Servings 2

Ingredients:

¼ cup shredded coconut and more for decorationing ½ tbsp. erythritol ½ tbsp. olive oil 1 tbsp. almond flour 1 tsp cinnamon 1/8 tsp salt 2 organic eggs 2oz cream cheese 4 tbsp. stevia

Directions:

Crack eggs in a container, beat until fluffy and then beat in flour and cream cheese until the desired smoothness is achieved. Put in rest of the ingredients and then stir until well blended. Take a frying pan, place it on moderate heat, grease it with oil, then pour in half of the batter and cook for three to four minutes per side until the pancake has cooked and nicely golden brown. Move pancake to a plate and cook another pancake similarly by using the rest of the batter. Drizzle coconut on top of cooked pancakes before you serve.

104. Coconut & Banana Cookies

Time To Prepare: fifteen minutes Time to Cook: twenty-five minutes Yield: Servings 7

Ingredients:

½ tsp. ground cinnamon ½ tsp. ground turmeric 2 cups unsweetened coconut, shredded 3 medium bananas, peeled Freshly ground black pepper Pinch of salt, to taste

Directions:

Set the oven to 350°F. Coat a cookie sheet a mildly greased parchment paper. In a mixer, put all together ingredients and pulse till a dough-like mixture forms. Make small balls through the mixture and set onto a prepared cookie sheet in a single layer. Using your fingers, press along the balls to form the cookies. Bake for minimum fifteen-twenty minutes or till golden brown.

105. Cornmeal Grits

Time To Prepare: five minutes Time to Cook: fifteen minutes Yield: Servings 4

Ingredients:

1 cup polenta meal 1 teaspoon salt 2 tablespoons butter 4 cups water

Directions:

Put water and salt in a deep cooking pan then place it to its boiling point. Slowly put in polenta and continuously stir on moderate to low heat until it has become thick, approximately fifteen minutes. Mix in butter. Serve instantly for tender grits or pour into a greased loaf pan and allow to cool. Once cool, grits can be cut and fried or grilled.

106. Cream Cheese Salmon

Toast Time To Prepare: fifteen minutes Time to Cook: five minutes Yield: Servings 2

Ingredients:

½ cup Arugula or spinach, chopped ½ tsp. Basil flakes 1 tbsp. Red onion, chopped fine 2 oz. Smoked salmon 2 tbsp. Cream cheese, low-fat Whole grain or rye toast, two slices

Directions:

Toast the wheat bread. Mix cream cheese and basil and spread this mixture on the toast. Put in salmon, arugula, and onion.

107. Edamame Omelet

Time To Prepare: five minutes Time to Cook: five minutes Yield: Servings 2

Ingredients:

½ cup shelled edamame ½ cup shredded regular or soy Cheddar cheese 1 bunch scallions, cut into 1-inch pieces 1 tbsp. low-sodium soy sauce, or to taste 1 tsp. minced garlic 3 big eggs or ¾ cup egg substitute 3 tbsp. olive oil, divided Snips of fresh cilantro, for decoration

Directions:

Warm 2 tablespoons oil in a small frying pan on moderate heat and sauté the garlic and scallion for approximately 2 minutes. Put in the edamame and soy sauce and sauté one minute more. Remove from the frying pan and save for later. Warm the other 1 tablespoon oil in the same frying pan. Whisk the eggs until combined and pour into the hot oil. Spread the shredded cheese on top. Lift up the omelet's edges, tipping the frying pan back and forth to cook the uncooked eggs. Once the top looks firm, drizzle the scallion mixture over one half of the omelet and fold the other half over the top. Lift the omelet out of the frying pan. Split it in half, drizzle with the cilantro, before you serve.

108. Fantastic Spaghetti Squash with Cheese and Basil Pesto

Time To Prepare: ten minutes Time to Cook: thirty-five minutes Yield: Servings 2

Ingredients:

¼ cup ricotta cheese, unsweetened ½ tbsp. olive oil 1 cup cooked spaghetti squash, drained 1/8 cup basil pesto 2oz fresh mozzarella cheese, cubed Freshly cracked black pepper, to taste Salt, to taste

Directions:

Switch on the oven, then set its temperature to 375 °F and allow it to preheat. In the meantime, take a medium container, put in spaghetti squash in it and then sprinkle with salt and black pepper. Take a casserole dish, grease it with oil, put in squash mixture in it, top it with ricotta cheese and mozzarella cheese and bake for about ten minutes until cooked. When finished, remove the casserole dish from the oven, sprinkle pesto on top and serve instantly.

109. Flaxseed Porridge with Cinnamon

Time To Prepare: ten minutes Time to Cook: five minutes Yield: Servings 4

Ingredients:

½ cup shredded coconut 1 cup heavy cream 1 tbsp. unsalted butter 1 tsp cinnamon 1½ tsp stevia 2 cups of water 2 tbsp. flaxseed meal 2 tbsp. flaxseed oatmeal

Directions: Take a medium pot, place it using low heat, put in all the ingredients in it, stir until combined and bring the mixture to boil. When the mixture has boiled, remove the pot from heat, stir it well and split it uniformly between four bowls. Let porridge rest for about ten minutes until slightly become thick and then serve.

110. Gingerbread Oatmeal Breakfast

Time To Prepare: ten minutes Time to Cook: 0 minutes Yield: Servings 4

Ingredients:

¼ tsp ground allspice ¼ tsp ground cardamom ¼ tsp ground coriander ¼ tsp ground ginger 1 ½ tbsp. ground cinnamon 1 cup steel-cut oats 1 tsp ground cloves 1/8 tsp nutmeg 4 cups drinking water Fresh mixed berries Organic Maple syrup, to taste

Directions:

Cook the oats based on the package instructions. When it comes to its boiling point, decrease the heat and simmer. Mix in all the spices and carry on cooking until cooked to desired doneness. Serve in four serving bowls and sprinkle with maple syrup and top with fresh berries. Enjoy!

111. Greek Yogurt with Cherry-Almond Syrup Parfait

Time To Prepare: twenty-five minutes Time to Cook: five minutes Yield: Servings 2

Ingredients:

1 c. fresh black or red cherries, pitted 1 tsp. fresh-squeezed lemon juice 2 c. Greek plain yogurt, stir to loosen 2 tbsp. almond syrup 2 tbsp. coconut palm sugar 2 tbsp. cut almonds, to decorate 4 tbsp. granola of choice, to decorate (opt.)

Directions:

Put a deep cooking pan on moderate to high heat and mix cherries, almond syrup, sugar, lemon juice, and 1 tbsp. of water. Stir to blend, then place it to simmer, continuously stirring until sugar is dissolved. Continue to simmer for further five minutes, until liquid begins to turn into a syrupy mixture, but the cherries are still holding firm. Put the mixture to a container and allow to cool for five minutes at room temperature, then bring it in your fridge to chill until it is completely cold. Put 1 cup of Greek yogurt into 2 serving bowls and spoon ½ of the cherries and their syrupy juices over the yogurt. Decorate using cut almonds or granola, if you wish. Serve instantly.

112. Hash Browns

Time To Prepare: fifteen minutes Time to Cook: fifteen minutes Yield: Servings 4

Ingredients:

1 pound Russet potatoes, peeled, processed using a grater 3 Tbsp. olive oil Pinch of black pepper, to taste Pinch of sea salt

Directions:

Coat a microwave safe-dish using paper towels. Spread shredded potatoes on top. Microwave veggies on the maximum heat setting for a couple of minutes. Turn off the heat. Pour 1 tablespoon of oil into a non-stick frying pan set on moderate heat. Cooking in batches, place a generous pinch of potatoes into the hot oil. Push down using the back of a spatula. Cook for about three minutes every side, or until brown and crunchy. Drain over paper towels. Repeat step for remaining potatoes. Put in more oil as required. Sprinkle with salt and pepper and serve.

113. Huevos Rancheros

Time To Prepare: five minutes Time to Cook: five minutes Yield: Servings 2

Ingredients:

(2) 8-inch whole wheat tortillas 1-ounce slice of cheddar cheese 2 hard-boiled eggs, cut 2 slices of Canadian bacon or ham 2 tbsp. salsa

Directions:

Prepare the hardboiled eggs. Put one tortilla on a plate, top with a slice of Canadian bacon or ham, the cut egg, and a slice of cheddar cheese. Roll the tortilla up. Repeat with the rest of the ingredients to prepare the second burrito. Serve instantly with 1 tbsp. Salsa.

114. Leek & Spinach Frittata

Time To Prepare: ten minutes Time to Cook:fifteen minutes Yield:Servings 4

Ingredients:

½ Teaspoon Bail, Dried ½ Teaspoon Garlic Powder 1 Cup Baby Spinach, Fresh & Packed 1 Cup Cremini Mushrooms, Sliced 2 Leeks, Chopped Fine 2 Tablespoons Avocado Oil 8 Eggs Sea Salt & Black Pepper to Taste

Directions:

Set the oven to 400°F then get an ovenproof frying pan. Put it on moderate to high heat, sautéing your leeks in your avocado oil until tender. It should take roughly five minutes Get out a container, and whisk the eggs with your garlic, basil, and salt. Put in them to the frying pan with your leeks, cooking for 5 minutes. You'll need to stir regularly. Mix in your mushrooms and spinach, seasoning with pepper. Put the frying pan in your oven then bake for about ten minutes. Serve warm.

115. Maple Oatmeal

Time To Prepare:five minutes Time to Cook:twenty minutes Yield:Servings 4

Ingredients:

¼ cup Coconut flakes, unsweetened ½ cup Milk, almond or coconut ½ cup Pecans, chopped ½ cup Walnuts, chopped 1 tsp. Cinnamon 1 tsp. Maple flavoring 3 tbsp. Sunflower seeds 4 tbsp. Chia seeds

Directions:

Pulse the sunflower seeds, walnuts, and pecans in a food processor to crumble. Or you can just put the nuts in a sturdy plastic bag, wrap the bag using a towel, lay it on a sturdy surface, and beat the towel with a hammer until the nuts are crumbled. Combine the crushed nuts with the remaining ingredients and pour them into a big pot. Simmer this mixture using low heat for thirty minutes. Stir frequently, so the mix does not cling to the bottom. Serve decorated with fresh fruit or a drizzle of cinnamon if you wish.

116. Mediterranean Frittata

Time To Prepare:five minutes Time to Cook:twenty minutes Yield:Servings 6

Ingredients:

¼ cup Black olives, chopped ¼ cup Feta cheese, crumbled ¼ cup Green olives, chopped ¼ cup Milk, almond or coconut ¼ cup Tomatoes, diced ¼ tsp. Black pepper 1 tsp. Oregano 1 tsp. Sea salt 6 Eggs Oil, spray or olive

Directions:

Heat oven to 400. Oil one eight by eight-inch baking dish. Beat the milk into the eggs, and then put in other ingredients. Pour all of this mixture into the baking dish and bake for 20 minutes

117. Mushroom Crêpes

Time To Prepare: 1 hour thirty minutes Time to Cook: thirty minutes Yield: Servings 6

Ingredients:

2 eggs ½ cup all-purpose flour For the filling 3 tablespoons all-purpose flour 2 cups of cremini mushrooms, cut ½ cup Parmesan cheese, grated ¾ cup milk 3 garlic cloves, minced 2 tablespoons of parsley (chopped) 6 slices of deli-cut cooked lean ham Freshly ground pepper 1/4 teaspoon salt 1/4 teaspoon of salt 3/4 cup milk 3/4 cup chicken broth 1/8 teaspoon cayenne 1/8 teaspoon nutmeg

Directions:

Put and mix the salt and flour in a container. In another container, whisk the eggs and milk. Slowly mix the two mixtures until the desired smoothness is achieved. Leave for fifteen minutes. Spray a frying pan using non-stick cooking spray and put on moderate heat. Mix the batter a little. Put in 1/4 of the batter into the frying pan. Tilt the frying pan to make a thin and even crêpe. Cook for a couple of minutes or until the bottom is golden and the top is set. Flip and cook for twenty seconds. Move to a plate. Repeat the steps with the rest of the batter. Loosely cover the cooked crêpes using plastic wrap. For the filling. Combine all ingredients for filling in a deep cooking pan on moderate heat – flour, milk, cayenne, nutmeg, and pepper. Constantly whisk until thick or around seven minutes. Take off the stove. Mix in a tablespoon of parsley and cheese. Loosely cover to keep warm. Spray a frying pan using non-stick cooking spray and put on moderate heat. Cook the garlic and mushrooms. Sprinkle with salt. Cook for about six minutes or until the mushrooms are tender. Put in 2 tablespoons of sherry. Cook for about 2 minutes. Take off the stove. Put in the remaining parsley and stir. Place the crêpes side by side on a flat surface. Spread a tablespoon of the sauce and 2 tablespoons of the cooked mushrooms. Roll up the crêpes and move them to a greased baking dish. Put all the sauce on top. Bake using your oven at 450°F for fifteen minutes.

118. Oat Porridge with Cherry & Coconut

Time To Prepare: ten minutes Time to Cook: 0 minutes Yield: Servings 3

Ingredients:

1 ½ cups regular oats 3 cups coconut milk 3 tbsp. raw cacao 4 tbsp. chia seed A pinch of stevia, optional Coconut shavings Dark chocolate shavings Fresh or frozen tart cherries Maple syrup, to taste (not necessary)

Directions:

Mix the oats, milk, stevia, and cacao in a moderate-sized deep cooking pan on moderate heat and bring to its boiling point. Reduce the heat, then simmer until the oats are cooked to desired doneness. Split the porridge among 3 serving bowls and top with dark chocolate and coconut shavings, cherries, and a little sprinkle of maple syrup.

119. Oatmeal-Raisin Scones

Time To Prepare:ten minutes Time to Cook: fifteen minutes Yield:Servings 6

Ingredients:

½ cup all-purpose flour ½ teaspoon salt ½ teaspoon vanilla 1 cup raisins 1 egg white 1½ cups rolled oats 11/8teaspoons baking powder 2 eggs or ½ cup egg substitute 2 tablespoons granulated sugar 2 tablespoons wheat germ 2/3 cup buttermilk 3 tablespoons sugar 6 tablespoons cold unsalted butter

Directions:

Preheat your oven to 400°F. Coat a baking pan w/ parchment paper or spray lightly with oil. Grind half of the oats into flour in a food processor. Mix remaining oats, oat flour, all-purpose flour, wheat germ, sugar, salt, baking powder, and butter in a food processor using a metal blade. Process until mixture looks like cornmeal. In a huge container, put together eggs, buttermilk, and vanilla then whisk. Mix in raisins using a spatula or wooden spoon. Place the dry ingredients and fold in using a spatula. Drop scones into rounds onto the readied baking sheet. Brush scones with egg white and dust with granulated sugar. Bake for fifteen minutes

120. Oven-Poached Eggs

Time To Prepare: 2minutes Time to Cook: 11minutes Yield: Servings 4

Ingredients:

2 cups of ice cubes 2 cups water, chilled 6 eggs, at room temperature Ice bath Water

Directions:

Set the oven to 350°F. Put 2 cups of water into a deep roasting tin, and place it into the lowest rack of the oven. Put one egg into each cup of cupcake/muffin tins, together with one tablespoon of water. Cautiously place muffin tins into the middle rack of the oven. Bake eggs for about forty-five minutes. Remove the heat instantly. Take off the muffin tins from the oven and set on a cake rack to cool before extracting eggs. Pour ice bath ingredients into a big heat-resistant container. Bring the eggs into an ice bath to stop the cooking process. After ten minutes, drain eggs well. Use as required.

121. Peanut Butter-Banana Muffins

Time To Prepare: fifteen minutes Time to Cook: twenty-five minutes Yield: Servings 12

Ingredients:

½ tsp. Baking soda ½ tsp. salt ¾ c. light brown sugar 1 c. low-fat buttermilk 1 c. mashed banana (about 3 bananas) 1 c. old-fashioned oats 1 tsp. Baking powder 1½ c. all-purpose flour 2 big eggs 2 tbsp. Applesauce 6 tbsp. creamy peanut butter

Directions: Bring a small nonstick frying pan on moderate heat and spray lightly with cooking spray. Put in in the bell pepper and onion and sauté for one to two minutes, or until both are soft and the onion translucent. In a small container, crack in eggs and whisk. Put in in milk; whisk until well-mixed. Pour eggs into the pan and cook, regularly stirring until eggs are scrambled to your preference. To serve, spoon half the egg mixture into each tortilla, wrap, before you serve. Try serving with a side of fresh fruit for a complete meal.

122. Pumpkin & Banana Waffles

Time To Prepare: fifteen minutes Time to Cook: five minutes Yield: Servings 4

Ingredients:

½ cup almond flour ½ cup coconut flour ½ cup pumpkin puree ½ teaspoon ground cloves ½ teaspoon ground nutmeg ¾ cup almond milk ¾ teaspoon ground ginger 1 tsp baking soda 1½ teaspoons ground cinnamon 2 medium bananas, peeled and cut 2 tablespoons olive oil 5 big organic eggs Salt, to taste

Directions:

Preheat the waffle iron, and after that, grease it. In a sizable container, combine flours, baking soda, and spices. In a blender, put the rest of the ingredients and pulse till smooth. Put in flour mixture and pulse till In preheated waffle iron, put in the required quantity of mixture. Cook roughly 4-5 minutes. Repeat using the rest of the mixture

123. Quinoa & Beans Burgers

Time To Prepare: fifteen minutes Time to Cook: 55 minutes Yield: Servings 12

Ingredients:

½ cup dry quinoa ½ cup fresh cilantro, chopped ½ teaspoon fresh ginger, grated finely ½ teaspoon ground turmeric 1 (fifteen oz.) can black beans, drained 1 cup cooked corn kernels 1 small boiled potato, peeled 1 small onion, chopped 1 teaspoon chili flakes 1 teaspoon flax meal 1 teaspoon garlic, minced 1 teaspoon ground cumin 1 teaspoon paprika 1½ cups water Freshly ground black pepper, to taste Salt, to taste

Directions:

In a pan, put in water and quinoa on high heat and provide to its boiling point. Reduce the heat to moderate and simmer for around fifteen-twenty or so minutes. Drain surplus water. Set the oven to 375°F. Coat a sizable baking sheet that has a parchment paper. In a sizable container, put in quinoa and rest of the ingredients. Use a fork to mix till well blended. Make equal-sized patties from the mixture. Position the patties onto the readied baking sheet in the single layer. Bake for around 20-twenty-five minutes. Cautiously, alter the side and cook for approximately 8-ten minutes

124. Quinoa and Cauliflower Congee

Time To Prepare: ten minutes Time to Cook: 1 hour Yield: Servings 8

Ingredients:

¼ cup loosely packed cilantro leaves, torn ¼ cup loosely packed spearmint leaves, torn ¼ cup packed basil leaves, torn 1 cauliflower head, minced 1 lime, cut into wedges 1 tablespoon fish sauce 1 tablespoon fresh ginger, grated 1 tablespoon olive oil 2 garlic cloves, grated 2 leeks, minced 2 onions, minced 2 red chili, minced 2 tablespoons brown rice 2 tablespoons red quinoa 4 eggs, soft-boiled 6 cups of water For Garnish Pinch of white pepper

Directions:

Put olive oil into a huge frying pan on moderate heat. Sauté shallots, garlic, and ginger until limp and aromatic; pour into a slow cooker set at moderate heat. Except for decorationes, pour rest of the ingredients into slow cooker; stir. Place the lid on. Cook for around six hours. Turn off heat. Taste; tweak seasoning if required. Ladle congee into separate bowls. Decorate using basil leaves, cilantro leaves, red chilli, and spearmint leaves. Put in 1 piece of soft-boiled egg on top of each; serve with a wedge of lime on the side. Slice egg just before eating so yolk runs into congee. Squeeze lime juice into congee just before eating.

125. Raisin Bran Muffins

Time To Prepare: fifteen minutes Time to Cook: thirty minutes Yield: Servings 36

Ingredients:

½ cup vegetable oil 1 cup boiling water 1 cup bran flakes 1 cup sugar 1 teaspoon salt 1½ cups raisins 2 cups buttermilk 2 eggs, beaten 2½ cups All-Bran cereal 2½ cups all-purpose flour 2½ teaspoons baking soda

Directions:

Set the to 400°F. Grease a muffin tin. Place the boiling water over 1 cup All-Bran, and allow it to sit for about ten minutes. Put the baking soda, flour, and salt in a mixing container then mix, set aside. Mix the oil into the bran and water mixture, then put the rest of the bran, sugar, eggs, and buttermilk. Place the flour mixture to the bran mixture and mix to blend. Mix in the raisins and bran flakes then fill the muffin cups ¾ full with the batter. Bake muffins for about twenty minutes

126. Sautéed Veggies on Hot Bagels

Time To Prepare: ten minutes Time to Cook: 16 minutes Yield: Servings 2

Ingredients:

½ onion, cut thin 1 clove of garlic, chopped 1 tbsp. olive oil 1 yellow squash, diced 1 zucchini, cut thin 2 pcs. tomatoes, cut 2 pcs. vegan bagels salt and pepper to taste vegan butter for spread

Directions:

Heat the olive oil on the medium temperature in a cast-iron frying pan. Reduce the heat to moderate-low and sauté the onions for about ten minutes or until the onions start to brown. Turn the heat again to moderate and then put in the diced squash and zucchini to the pan and cook for five minutes. Put in the clove of garlic and cook for one more minute. Throw in the tomato slices to the pan and cook for a minute. Flavor it with pepper and salt and remove the heat. Toast the bagels and cut in half. Spread the bagels lightly with butter and serve with the sautéed veggies on top.

127. Savory Veggie Muffins

Time To Prepare: fifteen minutes Time to Cook: 18-23 minutes Yield: Servings 5

Ingredients:

¼ cup concentrate powder ½ cup fresh parsley, chopped ½ tsp baking soda ¾ cup almond meal 1 bunch scallion, chopped 1 cup coconut butter, softened 1½ tablespoons nutritional yeast 2 medium carrots, peeled and grated 2 tablespoons coconut oil, melted 2 teaspoons apple cider vinegar 2 teaspoons fresh dill, chopped 3 tablespoons fresh lemon juice 4 big organic eggs Salt, to taste

Directions:

Set the oven to 350F. Grease 10 cups of your big muffin tin. In a big container, combine flour, baking soda | Protein: powder, and salt. In another container, put in eggs, nutritional yeast, vinegar, lemon juice, and oil and beat till well blended. Put in coconut butter and beat till the mixture becomes smooth. Put egg mixture into the flour mixture and mix till well blended. Fold in scallion, carts, and parsley. Put the amalgamation into prepared muffin cups uniformly. Bake for approximately 18-23 minutes or till a toothpick inserted inside center comes out clean.

128. Spicy Ginger Crepes

Time To Prepare: fifteen minutes Time to Cook: 20 Minutes Yield: Servings 8

Ingredients:

½ teaspoon red chili powder 1 (1-inch) fresh ginger piece, grated finely 1 1/3 cups chickpea flour 1 cup fresh cilantro leaves, chopped 1 cup water 1 green chili, seeded and chopped finely Cooking spray, as required Salt, to taste

Directions: In a sizable container, combine flour, chili powder, and salt. Put in ginger, cilantro, and chili and mix thoroughly. Put in water and mix till a uniform mixture form. Keep aside, covered for roughly ½-2 hours. Lightly, grease a substantial nonstick frying pan with cooking spray and heat on moderate to high heat. Put in the desired volume of the mixture and tilt the pan to spread it uniformly inside the frying pan. Cook roughly 10-fifteen seconds per side. Repeat while using the rest of the mixture

129. Spinach Mushroom Omelet

Time To Prepare: three minutes Time to Cook: fifteen minutes Yield: Servings 2

Ingredients:

¼ Red onion, diced 1 ½ cup Spinach, fresh, chopped 1 Green onion, diced 1 oz. Feta cheese 2 tbsp. Olive oil, 3 Eggs 5 Mushrooms, button, cut

Directions:

Sauté the mushrooms, onions, and spinach for 3 minutes in one tablespoon of olive oil and set aside. Beat the eggs thoroughly and cook them in the other tablespoon of olive oil for three to four minutes until edges start to brown. Drizzle all the other ingredients onto half of the omelet and fold the other half over the sautéed ingredients. Cook for a minute on each side.

130. Strawberries and Cream Trifle

Time To Prepare: 10 Minutes Time to Cook: 45 Minutes Yield: Servings 12

Ingredients:

1 ½ cups condensed milk 1 angel food cake, cubed 12 ounces frozen whipped cream, thawed 3 pints fresh strawberries, hulled and cut 6 ounces packaged cream cheese, softened

Directions: In a container, put together the cream cheese, sweetened condensed milk, and whip in until the desired smoothness is achieved. In a trifle container, place a layer of angel food cake cubes. Put in a layer of strawberries and cream on top. Repeat the layers. Bring it in your fridge to cool for minimum thirty-five minutes.

131. Strawberry-Oat-Chocolate Chip Muffins

Time To Prepare: ten minutes Time to Cook: 23 minutes Yield: Servings 12

Ingredients:

¼ tsp. salt ½ c. unsweetened vanilla almond milk ½ tsp. Baking powder ¾ tsp. Baking soda 1 c. rolled oats 1 egg 1 egg white 1 heaping cup bananas (approximately two to three big very ripe bananas) 1 tbsp. extra virgin olive oil 1 tbsp. honey or agave nectar 1 tsp. vanilla 1/3 c. mini chocolate chips 1/3 c. nonfat plain Greek yogurt 1¼ c. whole wheat pastry flour 12 thin slices of strawberries (about 3-4 strawberries) for decoration, if you wish 2/3 c. diced strawberries

Directions: Set the oven to 350°F and mildly grease a standard 12-cup muffin pan or grease with paper liners. In a large-sized mixing container, mix flour, oats, baking powder, baking soda, and salt. Stir to blend. Set aside the 2 tbsp. of the mixture. In a different huge mixing container, mix together the mashed banana, olive oil, honey, and vanilla. After this, beat in the egg and egg white and beat until blended. Now put in in Greek yogurt and almond milk and beat using an electric mixer on low until the desired smoothness is achieved. Slowly put wet ingredients to dry ingredients and blend until just blended, but do not over mix the batter as it will make the muffins firm. Fill each muffin cup 2/3 full of batter. Lightly tap the pan on the counter to even out the batter. Put a thin slice of strawberry onto each muffin, if you wish. Place the pan in your oven, then cook for eighteen to 23 minutes, up to a toothpick place in the center of the muffins, and comes out clean. Remove from the oven and allow it to sit for five to ten minutes in the pan before placing on a cooling rack

132. Sweet Onion and Egg Pie

Time To Prepare: 20 Minutes Time to Cook: 35 Minutes Yield: Servings 10

Ingredients:

1 cup vaporized milk 1 tablespoons butter 11 frozen deep-dish pie crust 2 sweet onions, halved and cut 6 eggs Salt and pepper to taste

Directions:

Preheat your oven 4000F. Melt the butter in a non-stick frying pan. Sauté the onions on moderate to low heat until super soft. Put the onions in a container. Put in in eggs and vaporized milk. Sprinkle with salt and pepper to taste. Pour the egg and onion mixture into the commercial pie crust. Bake using your oven for a little more than half an hour.

133. Swiss Chard and Spinach with Egg

Time To Prepare: five minutes Time to Cook: ten minutes Yield: Servings 4

Ingredients:

1 tsp. olive oil 20 pieces spinach leaves 20 pieces Swiss chard leaves 4 egg whites 4 pieces of rice bread 4 tbsp. parsley (fresh) Sea salt, ground pepper, and dried mint

Directions:

Bring to its boiling point 2 cups of water in a pan just below the boiling point. Open an egg, separate the whites from the yolks. Place the whites in a small container. Lower the container towards the heated water, and gently pour the egg into the pan. Do the same with the other eggs. Poach the eggs for about four minutes. Next, gently take the eggs, one by one and move them into a plate. Do the same with the rest of the 2 eggs. Cut the parsley and sauté the leaves in a pan for about six minutes. Toast the bread while doing this. When finished, make a layer of the sautéed greens and the chopped parsley on top of the toasted rice bread. Place the poached eggs above the bed of greens. Drizzle each serving with ground pepper, sea salt, and dried mint.

134. Tomato Omelet

Time To Prepare: two minutes Time to Cook: 8 minutes Yield: Servings 1

Ingredients:

¼ cup Cheese, any type, shredded ½ cup Basil, fresh ½ cup Cherry tomatoes ½ tsp. Salt 1 tsp. Black pepper 2 Eggs 2 tbsp. Olive oil

Directions: Chop the tomatoes into four equivalent portions. Fry the tomatoes for around three hours. Set the tomatoes off to the side. Put in the salt and pepper to the eggs in a small container and beat together well. Pour the mix of beaten egg into the pan and use a spatula to gently work around the edges under the omelet, letting the eggs fry unmoved for 3 minutes. When just the center third of the egg mix is still runny, put in on the basil, tomatoes, and cheese. Fold over half of the omelet onto the other half. Cook two more minutes before you serve.

135. Turkey Burgers

Time To Prepare: fifteen minutes Time to Cook: 8 minutes Yield: Servings 5

Ingredients:

1 ripe pear, peeled, cored and chopped roughly 1 teaspoon fresh ginger, grated finely 1 teaspoon fresh rosemary, minced 1 teaspoon fresh sage, minced 1-2 tablespoons coconut oil 1-pound lean ground turkey 2 minced garlic cloves Freshly ground black pepper, to taste Salt, to taste

Directions:

In a blender, put in pear and pulse till smooth. Move the pear mixture in a big container with rest of the ingredients except for oil and mix till well blended. Make small equal sized 10 patties from the mixture. In a heavy-bottomed frying pan, heat oil on moderate heat. Put in the patties and cook for about five minutes. Flip the inside and cook for roughly 2-3 minutes.

136. Veggie Balls

Time To Prepare: fifteen minutes Time to Cook: twenty-five minutes Yield: Servings 5-6

Ingredients:

¼ tsp. ground turmeric ½ teaspoon granulated garlic 1 cup fresh kale leaves, trimmed and chopped 1 medium shallot, chopped finely 1 tsp. ground cumin 2 medium sweet potatoes, cubed into ½-inch size 2 tablespoons coconut milk Freshly ground black pepper, to taste Ground flax seeds, as required Salt, to taste

Directions:

Set the oven to 400°F. Coat a baking sheet using parchment paper. In a pan of water, position a steamer basket. Bring the sweet potato in a steamer basket and steam roughly 10-fifteen minutes. In a sizable container, put the sweet potato. Put in coconut milk and purée well. Put in rest of the ingredients except for flax seeds and mix till well blended. Make approximately 1½-2-inch balls from your mixture. Position the balls onto the readied baking sheet inside a single layer. Drizzle with flax seeds. Bake for around 20-twenty-five minutes.

137. White and Green Quiche

Time To Prepare: ten minutes Time to Cook: forty minutes Yield: Servings 3

Ingredients:

1 ½ cups of coconut milk 1 ½ teaspoon of baking powder 1 small sized onion, finely chopped 3 cloves of garlic, minced 3 cups of fresh spinach, chopped 5 white mushrooms, cut fifteen big free-range eggs Ghee, as required to grease the dish Ground black pepper to taste Sea salt to taste

Directions: Set the oven to 350°F. Get a baking dish then grease it with the organic ghee. Break all the eggs in a huge container then whisk well. Mix in coconut milk. Beat well While you are whisking the eggs, start putting in the rest of the ingredients in it. When all the ingredients are completely mixed, pour all of it into the readied baking dish. Bake for minimum forty minutes, up to the quiche is set in the center. Enjoy!

138. Yogurt Cheese and Fruit

Time To Prepare: ten minutes Time to Cook: 0 minutes Yield: Servings 6

Ingredients:

¼ cup dried cranberries or raisins ¼ cup honey ½ cup orange juice ½ cup water 1 fresh Golden Delicious apple 1 fresh pear 1 teaspoon fresh lemon juice 3 cups plain nonfat yogurt

Directions: Prepare the yogurt cheese the day before by lining a colander or strainer with cheesecloth. Scoop the yogurt into the cheesecloth, put the strainer over a pot or container to catch the whey, and place in your fridge for minimum 8 hours before you serve. In a huge mixing container, combine the juices and water. Chop the apple then pear into wedges, put the wedges in the juice mixture, allow it to sit for minimum five minutes. Strain off the liquid. When the yogurt is firm, remove from fridge, slice, and place on plates. Position the fruit wedges around the yogurt. Sprinkle with honey and drizzle with cranberries or raisins just before you serve.

139. Zucchini Bread

Time To Prepare: ten minutes Time to Cook: 60 minutes Yield: Servings 16

Ingredients:

¼ teaspoon baking powder 1 cup canola oil 1 cup chopped pecans 1 cup raisins 1 tablespoon cinnamon 1 teaspoon baking soda 1 teaspoon salt 1½ cups 100% whole-wheat flour 1½ cups all-purpose flour 2 cups grated zucchini 2 cups sugar 3 eggs, beaten, or ¾ cup of egg substitute

Directions: Preheat your oven to 350°F. Oil 2 loaf pans and save for later. Put and mix the flour, salt, baking soda, baking powder, and cinnamon in a container. Combine the eggs, oil, and sugar in a different container. Put in the zucchini and dry ingredients alternately until fully blended into a smooth batter. Fold in the pecans and raisins and scrape the batter into the loaf pans. Bake for 60 minutes, cool on a rack, and wrap when cool

LUNCH

140. Shrimp & Mango Salsa Lettuce Wraps

Yield: 6 servings Preparation Time: 20 min Cooking Time: 3 minutes

Ingredients:

For Salsa: • 1 mango, peeled, pitted and chopped • ¼ cup red onion, chopped finely • ½ cup red bell pepper, seeded and chopped finely • ¼ cup fresh cilantro, chopped • 1 jalapeño pepper, seeded and chopped finely • 2 tablespoons fresh lime juice • Salt and freshly ground black pepper, to taste • For Shrimp Wraps: • 1 teaspoon organic olive oil • 2 pounds large shrimp, peeled, deveined and chopped • ½ teaspoon ground cumin • 1 tablespoon red chili powder • Salt and freshly ground black pepper, to taste • 2 heads butter lettuce, leaves separated

Directions:

1. For salsa in a large bowl, mix together all ingredients. Keep aside. 2. In a big skillet, heat oil on medium heat. 3. Add shrimp and seasoning and cook for approximately 2-3 minutes. 4. Remove from heat and cool slightly. 5. Divide shrimp mixture over lettuce leaves evenly. 6. Top with mango salsa evenly and serve.

141. Bacon Wrapped Asparagus

Yield: 6 servings Preparation Time: 10 min Cooking Time: 25-a half-hour

Ingredients:

10 bacon slices, cut in half • 1 pound fresh asparagus, trimmed • 1 tablespoon extra virgin olive oil • 1 tablespoon balsamic vinegar • Freshly ground black pepper, to taste • 1 lemon, sliced

Directions:

1. Preheat the oven to 400 degrees F. Line a substantial baking dish with foil paper. 2. Wrap one bacon slice around each asparagus piece. 3. Arrange asparagus in prepared baking dish. 4. Drizzle with oil and vinegar and sprinkle with black pepper. 5. Bake approximately fifteen minutes. Change the inside and bake for 10-fifteen minutes more. 6. Serve immediately with lemon slices.

142. Zucchini Pasta With Shrimp

Yield: 4-6 servings Preparation Time: 15 minutes Cooking Time: 21 minutes

Ingredients:

2 tablespoons ghee or coconut oil • 1 tablespoon extra virgin olive oil • 3 garlic cloves, minced • 1 pound shrimp, peeled and deveined • 4 large zucchinis, spiralized with blade C • Salt and freshly ground black pepper, to taste • 4-6 fresh basil, eaves, chopped

Directions:

In a big skillet, heat ghee and essential olive oil on medium heat. 2. Add garlic and sauté approximately 1 minute. 3. Add shrimp and cook for approximately 2-3 minutes. 4. Add zucchini, tossing occasionally and cook approximately 2-3 minutes. 5. Stir in salt and black pepper and take off from heat. 6. Serve while using garnishing of basil leaves.

143. Sweet Potato Buns Sandwich

Yield: 1 serving Preparation Time: fifteen minutes Cooking Time: 19 minutes

Ingredients:

For Sweet Potato Buns: • 1½ tablespoons extra virgin olive oil, divided • 1 large sweet potato, peeled and spiralized with blade C • 2 teaspoons garlic powder • Salt and freshly ground black pepper, to taste • 1 large organic egg • 1 organic egg white • For Sandwich: • 1½-ounce salmon piece • Salt and freshly ground black pepper, to taste • 1 teaspoon fresh lime juice • 1 tomato slice • 1 onion slice • ½ of an avocado, peeled, pitted and chopped • 2 teaspoons fresh cilantro, chopped • 1 large bit of fresh kale • 1 bacon piece

Directions:

1. For buns in a sizable skillet, heat ½ tablespoon of oil on medium heat. 2. Add sweet potato and sprinkle with garlic powder, salt and black pepper. 3. Cook for 5-7 minutes. Transfer the sweet potato mixture in to a bowl. 4. Add egg and egg white and mix well. Now, transfer a combination into 2 (6-ounce) ramekins, midway full. 5. Cover the ramekins with wax paper. Now, place a over noodles to press firmly down. Refrigerate for about 15-20 minutes. 6. Preheat the grill to medium heat. Grease the grill grate. 7. Meanwhile in a very bowl, add salmon, salt, black pepper and lime juice and toss to coat well. 8. In a substantial skillet, heat remaining oil on medium-low heat. Carefully, transfer the sweet potato patties into skillet. Cook for 3-4 minutes. Change the medial side and cook for two-3 minutes more. 9. Place salmon, onion and tomato slices over grill. 10. Grill tomato slice for 1 minute. Grill onion slice for approximately 2 minutes. 11. Grill the salmon for approximately 4-5 minutes or till desired doneness. 12. In a bowl, add avocado and cilantro and mash well. 13. In a plate, place one sweet potato bun. Place onion slice, salmon, tomato, bacon and kale over bun. 14. Spread avocado mash around the bottom side of another bun. Place the bun, avocado mash side downwards over kale. 15. Secure having a toothpick and serve.

144. Shrimp, Sausage & Veggie Skillet

Yield: 4 servings Preparation Time: 15 minutes Cooking Time: 13 minutes

Ingredients:

3 tablespoons organic olive oil, divided • 1 pound shrimp, peeled and deveined • 2 teaspoons old bay seasoning • ½ of medium yellow onion, chopped • ¾ cup green peppers, seeded and chopped • ¾ cup green peppers, seeded and chopped • 1 zucchini, chopped • 6-ounces cooked sausage, chopped • 2 garlic cloves, minced • ¼ cup chicken broth • Pinch of red pepper flakes, crushed • Salt and freshly ground black pepper, to taste

Directions: 1. In a sizable skillet, heat 1 tablespoon of oil on medium-high heat. 2. Add shrimp and cook for around 3-4 minutes. Transfer the shrimp into a bowl. 3. In the identical skillet, heat remaining oil on medium heat. 4. Add onion and sweet peppers and sauté for about 4-5 minutes. 5. Add zucchini and sausage and cook for approximately 2 minutes. 6. Add garlic and cooled shrimp and cook for approximately 1 minute. 7. Add broth and stir to combine well. Stir in red pepper flakes, salt and black pepper and cook for approximately 1 minute. 8. Serve hot.

145. Sea Scallops With Spinach & Bacon

Yield: 4 servings Preparation Time: quarter-hour Cooking Time: 21 minutes

Ingredients:

3 bacon slices • 1½ pound jumbo sea scallops • Salt and freshly ground black pepper, to taste • 1 cup onion, chopped • 6 garlic cloves, minced • 12-ounces fresh baby spinach

Directions: 1. Heat a sizable nonstick skillet on medium-high heat. 2. Add bacon and cook approximately 8-10 min. 3. Transfer the bacon in to a bowl, reserving 1 tablespoon of bacon Fat within the skillet. 4. Chop the bacon and keep aside. 5. Add scallops and sprinkle with salt and black pepper. 6. Immediately, boost the heat to high heat. 7. Cook for about 5 minutes, turning once after 2½ minutes. 8. Transfer the scallops into another bowl. Cover having a foil paper to ensure that they're warm. 9. In exactly the same skillet, add onion and garlic minimizing the temperature to medium-high. 10. Sauté onion and garlic for around 3 minutes. 11. Add spinach and cook approximately 2-3 minutes. Season with salt and black pepper and remove from heat. 12. Divide the spinach among serving plates. Top with scallops and bacon evenly. Serve immediately.

146. Liver With Onion & Parsley One

Yield: 2-4 servings Preparation Time: 10 minutes Cooking Time: 26 minutes

Ingredients:

3 tablespoons coconut oil, divided • 2 large o ions, sliced • Salt, to taste • 1 pound grass-fed beef liver, cut into ½-inch thick slices • Freshly ground black pepper, to taste • ½ cup fresh parsley, chopped • 2 tablespoons freshly squeezed lemon juice

Directions:

1. In a sizable skillet, heat 1 tablespoon of oil on high heat. 2. Add onion plus some salt and sauté for about 5 minutes. 3. Reduce the warmth to medium. Sauté the onion for 10-15 minutes. 4. Transfer the onion right into a plate. 5. In exactly the same skillet, heat another 1vtablespoon of oil on medium-high heat. 6. Add liver and sprinkle with salt and black pepper. Cook for approximately 1-1½ minutes or till browned. 7. Flip along side it and cook for approximately 1-1½ minutes or till browned. 8. Transfer the liver right into a plate. 9. In the same skillet, heat remaining oil on medium heat. 10. Add cooked onion, parsley and lemon juice and stir well. Cook for about 2-3 minutes. 11. Place onion mixture over liver and serve immediately.

147. Egg & Avocado Wraps

Yield: 5 servings Preparation Time: 20 minutes

Ingredients:

1 ripe avocado, peeled, pitted and chopped • 1 tablespoon freshly squeezed lemon juice • 1 tablespoon fresh parsley, chopped • 2 tablespoons celery stalk, chopped • 4 organic hard-boiled eggs, peeled and chopped finely • Salt and freshly ground black pepper, to taste • 4-5 endive bulbs • 2 cooked bacon slices, chopped

Directions:

1. In a bowl, add avocado and freshly squeezed lemon juice and mash till smooth and creamy. 2. Add parsley, celery, eggs, salt and black pepper and stir to mix well. 3. Separate the endive leaves. Divide the avocado mixture over endive leaves evenly. 4. Top with bacon evenly and serve immediately.

148. Prosciutto Wrapped Chicken

Yield: 8 servings Preparation Time: 10 min Cooking Time: 26 minutes

Ingredients:

3 tablespoons plus 1 teaspoon coconut oil, melted and divided • 2 garlic cloves, minced • 1 teaspoon fresh lemon zest, grated finely • 1 tablespoon fresh lemon juice • Salt, to taste • 8 grass-fed skinless, boneless chicken thighs • 8 sprigs fresh rosemary • 8 prosciutto slices

Directions:

Preheat the oven to 400 degrees F. Arrange a big baking rack onto a big baking dish. 2. In a substantial bowl, add 3 tablespoon of coconut oil, garlic, lemon zest, fresh lemon juice and salt and mix till well combined. 3. Add chicken thighs and cot with mixture generously. Keep aside approximately 10 min. 4. Remove chicken thighs from mixture. Place 1 rosemary sprig within the center of each and every thigh and then then fold each thigh in half. 5. Wrap a prosciutto slice around each thighs tightly. 6. In a sizable skillet, heat remaining oil on medium-high heat. 7. Add thighs and cook approximately 3 minutes per side. 8. Now, transfer thighs in prepared baking dish in the single layer. 9. Bake for approximately 18-twenty minutes.

149. Creamy Sweet Potato Pasta With Pancetta

Yield: 4 servings Preparation Time: 15 minutes Cooking Time: 21 minutes

Ingredients:

For Creamy Sauce: • 4-5 cups cauliflower florets • 1 small shallot, minced • 1 large garlic herb, chopped • Pinch of red pepper flakes, crushed • 1 cup chicken broth • 1 tablespoon nutritional yeast • Sat, to taste • For Pancetta: • 8 pancetta slices, cubed • For Sweet Potato Pasta: • 1 tablespoon extra-virgin olive oil • 3 medium sweet potato, peeled and spiralized with blade C • 3 cups leeks, chopped • Salt and freshly ground black pepper, to taste • 1 tablespoon fresh parsley, chopped

Directions:

1. In a pan of salted boiling water, add broccoli florets and cook for around 7-8 minutes. Drain well. 2. Meanwhile in heat a large nonstick skillet on medium heat. 3. Add pancetta slices and cook approximately 5-7 minutes. 4. Transfer pancetta into a bowl. 5. In the identical skillet, add shallot, garlic and red pepper flakes and sauté for around 2 minutes. 6. Transfer the shallot mixture into a higher speed blender. 7. Add cauliflower and remaining sauce ingredients and pulse till smooth and creamy. 8. In the identical skillet, heat extra virgin olive oil on medium heat. 9. Add sweet potato and leeks and cook, tossing occasionally for approximately 8-10 min. 10. Stir in sauce and cook for about 1 minute. 11. Serve this creamy pasta with all the topping of pancetta and parsley.

150. Roasted Beet Pasta With Kale & Pesto

Yield: 3 servings Preparation Time: quarter-hour Cooking Time: 21 minutes

Ingredients:

For Pesto: • 3 cups fresh basil leaves • 1 large garlic oil • ¼ cup organic olive oil • ¼ cup pine nuts, chopped • Salt and freshly ground black pepper, to taste • For Beet Pasta: • 2 medium beets, trimmed, peeled and spiralized with blade C • Olive oil cooking spray, as required • Salt and freshly ground black pepper, to taste For Kale: • 2 cups fresh baby kale

Directions:

1. Preheat the oven to 425 degrees F. Lightly, grease a large baking sheet. 2. In a mixer, add all pesto ingredients and pulse till smooth. Keep aside. 3. Place beet pasta in prepared baking sheet. 4. Drizzle with cooking spray and sprinkle with salt and black pepper and gently, toss to coat well. 5. Roast for around 5-10 minutes or till desired doneness. 6. Transfer the pasta in a sizable bowl. 7. Add kale and pesto and gently, toss to coat well.

151. Veggies & Apple With Orange Sauce

Yield: 4 servings Preparation Time: quarter-hour Cooking Time: 16 minutes

Ingredients:

For Sauce: • 1 (1-inch) fresh ginger, minced • 2 garlic cloves, minced • 1 tablespoon fresh orange zest, grated finely • ½ cup fresh orange juice • 2 tablespoons white wine vinegar • 2 tablespoons coconut aminos • 1 tablespoon red boat fish sauce • For Veggies & Apple: • 1 tablespoon extra virgin olive oil • 1 cup carrot, peeled and julienned • 1 head broccoli, cut into florets • 1 cup celery, chopped • 1 cup onion, chopped • 2 apples, cored and sliced

Directions:

In a sizable bowl, mix together all sauce ingredients. Keep aside. 2. In a big skillet, heat oil on medium-high heat. 3. Add carrot and broccoli and stir fry for about 4-5 minutes. 4. Add celery and onion and stir fry for approximately 4-5 minutes. 5. Pour sauce and stir to combine. Cook approximately 2-3 minutes. 6. Stir in apple slices and cook for about 2-3 minutes more. 7. Serve hot.

152. Cauliflower Rice With Prawns & Veggies

Yield: 4 servings Preparation Time: 15 minutes Cooking Time: 21 minutes

Ingredients:

2 tablespoons coconut oil, divided • 14 prawns, peeled and deveined • 2 organic eggs, bea10 • 1 brown onion, chopped • 1 garlic cloves, minced • 1 small fresh red chili, chopped • ½ pound grass-fed ground chicken • 1 cauliflower head, cut into florets, processed like rice consis10cy • ¼ of red cabbage, chopped • ½ cup green peas, shelled • 1 head small broccoli, cut into small florets • 1 large carrot, peeled and chopped finely • 1 small red bell pepper, seeded and chopped • 2 bokchoy, sliced thinly • 3 tablespoons coconut aminos • Salt and freshly ground black pepper, to taste

Directions:

1. In a substantial skillet, heat ½ tablespoon of oil on medium-high heat. 2. Add prawns and cook approximately 3-4 minutes. Transfer in a large bowl. 3. In exactly the same skillet, heat ½ tablespoon of oil on medium heat. 4. Add bea10 eggs and with the back of spoon, spread the eggs. Cook for around 2 minutes. 5. Remove eggs from skillet and cut into strips. 6. In the identical skillet, heat remaining oil on high heat. Add onion, garlic and red chili and sauté for about 4-5 minutes. 7. Add chicken and cook for about 4-5 minutes. 8. Add cauliflower rice and remaining veggies except bokchoy and coconut aminos and cook for around 2-3 minutes. 9. Add bokchoy, coconut aminos, cooked eggs, prawns, salt and black pepper and cook for 2 minutes more.

Smoothies and Drinks

153. Almond Blueberry Smoothie

Time To Prepare: ten minutes Time to Cook: 0 minutes Yield: Servings 1

Ingredients:

1 banana 1 cup frozen blueberries 1 tbsp. almond butter 1/2 cup almond milk Water, as required

Directions:

Put in everything to a blender jug. Cover the jug firmly. Blend until the desired smoothness is achieved. Serve and enjoy!

154. Apple Cinnamon Water

Time To Prepare: five minutes Time to Cook: five minutes Yield: Servings 4

Ingredients:

1 whole apple, diced 5 cinnamon sticks Water to cover contents

Directions:

Put ingredients in the steamer basket. Put in pot. Put in water cover contents. Secure the lid. Cook on HIGH pressure five minutes. When done, depressurize swiftly. Remove steamer basket. Discard cooked produce. Let flavored water cool. Chill completely before you serve

155. Beet and Cherry Smoothie

Time To Prepare: five minutes Time to Cook: 0 minutes Yield: Servings 4

Ingredients:

½ cup frozen cherries, pitted ½ teaspoon frozen banana 1 tablespoon almond butter 10-ounce almond milk, unsweetened 2 small beets, peeled and slice into four

Directions: Put in all ingredients in a blender. Blend until the desired smoothness is achieved.

Berry Shrub

156. Time To Prepare:ten minutes Time to Cook: twenty minutes Yield:Servings 4

Ingredients:

½ a cup of chopped fresh oregano 1 cup of dried elderberries 2 cups of apple cider vinegar 2 cups of honey 2 cups of water

Directions: Put in listed ingredients to the instant pot. Secure the lid. Cook on HIGH pressure twenty minutes. When done, depressurize naturally. Pour ingredients through a sieve into a jar. Let cool down. Chill.

157. Blackberry Italian Drink

Time To Prepare:five minutes Time to Cook: fifteen minutes Yield:Servings 4

Ingredients:

1 bottle sparkling water 1 cup blackberries 1 lemon, cut 2 tbsp. honey

Directions: Put in 1 cup (non-carbonated) water to the instant pot. Put in blackberries to the instant pot. Secure the lid. Cook on HIGH pressure ten minutes. When done, depressurize naturally. Mash the berries in the instant pot. Move to dish. Let cool. As blackberries cook, in a separate small deep cooking pan with a heavy bottom. Put in honey. Simmer five minutes. Cool down. To make the drink. Ladle 1 teaspoon honey. Pour in fruit mixture. Put in carbonated water. Stir.

158. Blueberry And Spinach Shake

Time To Prepare: five minutes Time to Cook: 0 minutes Yield: Servings 2

Ingredients:

1 cup of low-fat Greek yogurt (not necessary) 1 cup of organic blueberries (or washed if non-organic) 1/2 cup of spinach ice cubes to the desired concentration

Directions:

Put in ingredients together in a blender until the desired smoothness is achieved and then serve in a tall glass. Drizzle a few fresh berries on top if you prefer!

159. Blueberry Matcha Smoothie

Time To Prepare: five minutes Time to Cook: 0 minutes Yield: Servings 2

Ingredients:

¼ Teaspoon Ground Cinnamon ¼ Teaspoon Ground Ginger 1 Banana 1 Tablespoon Chia Seeds 1 Tablespoon Matcha Powder 2 Cups Almond Milk 2 Cups Blueberries, Frozen 2 Tablespoons Protein Powder, Optional A Pinch Sea Salt

Directions:

Blend all ingredients until the desired smoothness is achieved.

160. Blueberry Smoothie

Time To Prepare: ten minutes Time to Cook: 0 minutes Yield: Servings 1

Ingredients:

1 banana, peeled 1 tbsp. almond butter 1 tsp. maca powder 1/2 cup almond milk, unsweetened 1/2 cup blueberries 1/2 cup water 1/4 tsp. ground cinnamon 2 handfuls baby spinach

Directions:

In your blender, combine the spinach with the banana, blueberries, almond butter, cinnamon, maca powder, water, and milk. Pulse thoroughly, pour into a glass, before you serve. Enjoy!

161. Carrot and Orange Turmeric Drink

Time To Prepare: five minutes Time to Cook: 0 minutes Yield: Servings 2

Ingredients:

1 cup orange juice 1 tbsp. lemon juice 1/2 inch ginger slice 1/4 tsp. turmeric powder 2 carrots, peeled, chopped 2 tbsp. sugar

Directions:

In a blender, put in orange juice, sugar, turmeric powder, carrots, and lemon juice. Blend well. Serve!

162. Chocolate Cherry Smoothie

Time To Prepare: five minutes Time to Cook: 0 minutes Yield: Servings 2

Ingredients:

2 cups almond milk, unsweetened 2 dates, pitted, chopped or 2 teaspoons pure maple syrup 2 scoops protein powder or 4 tablespoons almond butter (not necessary) 4 cups pitted, frozen cherries 4 tablespoons cocoa or cacao powder Cacao nibs Granola Hemp hearts To serve: Optional

Directions: Combine all ingredients into a blender and blend until the desired smoothness is achieved. Pour into 2 tall glasses and serve topped with optional ingredients.

163. Cooked Iced Tea

Time To Prepare: two minutes Time to Cook: 4 minutes Yield: Servings 4

Ingredients:

2 tbsp. honey 4 regular tea bags 6 cups water

Directions:

Put in ingredients to the instant pot. Secure the lid. Cook on HIGH pressure 4 minutes. When done, depressurize naturally. Allow to cool to room temperature. Serve over ice.

164. Cucumber Melon Smoothie

Time To Prepare: five minutes Time to Cook: 0 minutes Yield: Servings 2

Ingredients:

1 ½ cups of chopped honeydew 1 cup of chilled coconut water 1 cup of seedless cucumber, diced 2 tbsp. of fresh mint 6 to 8 ice cubes

Directions:

Mix the smoothie ingredients in your high-speed blender. Pulse the ingredients a few times to cut them up. Combine the mixture on the highest speed setting for thirty to 60 seconds. Pour into glasses and serve.

165. Fig Smoothie

Time To Prepare: five minutes Time to Cook: 0 minutes Yield: Servings 2

Ingredients:

1 Banana 1 Cup Almond Milk 1 Cup Whole Milk Yogurt, Plain 1 Tablespoon Almond Butter 1 Teaspoon Flaxseed, Ground 1 Teaspoon Honey, Raw 3-4 Ice Cubes 7 Figs, Halved (Fresh or Frozen)

Directions:

Blend all together ingredients until the desired smoothness is achieved, and serve instantly.

166. Fresh Cranberry And Lime Juice

Time To Prepare: five minutes Time to Cook: 0 minutes Yield: Servings 2

Ingredients:

1/2½ cups of mixed berries (frozen are fine) 1/2½ cups of spinach 2 limes, juiced 4 cups of cranberries

Directions:

Mix all the ingredients with water in a juicer until pureed and serve instantly over ice.

167. Ginger Ale

Time To Prepare: five minutes Time to Cook: thirty minutes Yield: Servings 4

Ingredients:

1 pound fresh ginger, unpeeled, diced 1 quart carbonated water 1 tbsp. honey Ice for serving Juice and rind of 2 lemons Lime wedges

Directions:

Put ginger and lemon juice in a food processor. Pulse to smooth consistency. Move puree to the instant pot. Mix in honey. Put in lemon peel to the instant pot. Secure the lid. Cook on HIGH pressure thirty minutes. When done, depressurize naturally. Strain and chill. Serve over ice

168. Golden Chai Latte

Time To Prepare: five minutes Time to Cook: ten minutes Yield: Servings 2

Ingredients:

¼ teaspoon ground cinnamon ½ cup water ½ tablespoon maple syrup ½ tablespoon turmeric powder 1 ¼ cups cashew milk or any other non-dairy milk of your choice 1 teaspoon loose leaf chai tea 1/8 teaspoon ground nutmeg A pinch ground cardamom

Directions:

Put in water and 1-cup milk into a deep cooking pan. Put the deep cooking pan on moderate heat. Put in chai leaves in a tea strainer (the type that that has a lid and you can close). Lower the strainer in the deep cooking pan. Put in spices. When it just comes to a light boil, remove the heat. Allow it to cool for five minutes. Take out the tea strainer and discard the leaves. Put in maple syrup and stir. Pour into glasses. Sprinkle remaining cashew milk on top. Decorate using cinnamon and nutmeg before you serve

169. Hibiscus Tea

Time To Prepare: five minutes Time to Cook: ten minutes Yield: Servings 4

Ingredients:

1 tbsp. honey 1 tsp fresh ginger, grated 10 cups water 2 cup dried hibiscus petals Rind from 1 pineapple

Directions:

Wash hibiscus leaves meticulously with cold water. Take away the dust. Put in water, honey, and ginger to the instant pot. Stir. Mix in hibiscus petals and pineapple rind. Secure the lid. Cook on HIGH pressure ten minutes. When done, depressurize naturally. Remove pineapple rind. Pass liquid through a fine-mesh strainer. Cool thoroughly. Chill before you serve.

170. Hot Peppermint Vanilla Latte

Time To Prepare: five minutes Time to Cook: five minutes Yield: Servings 4

Ingredients:

¼ cup honey 1 tsp vanilla 2 cups coffee 23 drops peppermint oil 4 cups almond milk

Directions:

Put in listed ingredients to the instant pot. Secure the lid. Cook on HIGH pressure five minutes. When done, depressurize naturally. Serve warm.

171. Jamaican Hibiscus Tea

Time To Prepare: five minutes Time to Cook: five minutes Yield: Servings 4

Ingredients:

½ tsp ginger, minced 1 cup dried hibiscus flowers 1 tbsp. honey 8 cups water Ice as required Juice of 1 lime

Directions: Put in hibiscus flowers, water, honey, and ginger to the instant pot. Secure the lid. Cook on HIGH pressure five minutes. When done, depressurize naturally. Cool thoroughly. Move to glass decanter. Mix in lime Juice. Pour over ice.

172. Kiwi Strawberry Smoothie

Time To Prepare: ten minutes Time to Cook: 0 minutes Yield: Servings 1

Ingredients:

¼ cup Chia seed powder ½ cup Strawberries, fresh or frozen, chopped 1 Banana, diced 1 cup Milk, almond or coconut 1 Kiwi, peeled and chopped 1 tsp. Basil, ground 1 tsp. Turmeric, ground

Directions: Drink instantly after all the ingredients have been thoroughly combined.

173. Mango and Ginger Infused Water

Time To Prepare: five minutes Time to Cook: five minutes Yield: Servings 4

Ingredients:

1 cup fresh mango, chopped 2-inch piece ginger, peeled, cubed Water to cover ingredients

Directions:

Put ingredients in the mesh steamer basket. Put basket in the instant pot. Put in water to immerse contents. Secure the lid. Cook on HIGH pressure five minutes. When done, depressurize swiftly. Remove steamer basket. Discard cooked produce. Let flavored water cool. Chill completely and serve

174. Mixed Fruit & Nut Milkshake

Time To Prepare: five minutes Time to Cook: 0 minutes Yield: Servings 2

Ingredients:

1 tbsp. of honey 1/2 cup of almond milk 1½ grapefruit; peeled and chopped 1/2 ½ inch piece of ginger, minced 12 strawberries 2 tbsp. of chopped almonds juice of 1 orange

Directions:

Put everything but the strawberries in a blender until the desired smoothness is achieved. Put in in the strawberries and blend until pureed, serving in a tall glass.

175. Peach And Raspberry Lemonade

Time To Prepare: five minutes Time to Cook: five minutes Yield: Servings 4

Ingredients:

½ cup fresh raspberries 1 cup fresh peaches, chopped Water to cover ingredients Zest and juice of 1 lemon

Directions:

Put ingredients in mesh basket for instant pot. Put in pot. Put in water to barely cover the fruit. Secure the lid. Cook on HIGH pressure five minutes. When done, depressurize swiftly. Remove steamer basket. Discard cooked produce. Let flavored water cool. Chill completely before you serve.

176. Peachy Keen Smoothie

Time To Prepare: five minutes Time to Cook: 0 minutes Yield: Servings 2

Ingredients:

1 ½ cups of frozen peaches 1 cup of almond milk 1 small frozen banana 2 tbsp. of raw hemp seeds 6 to 8 ice cubes Pinch of ground ginger

Directions: Mix the smoothie ingredients in your high-speed blender. Pulse the ingredients a few times to cut them up. Combine the mixture on the highest speed setting for thirty to 60 seconds. Pour into glasses and serve.

177. Pineapple and Greens Smoothie

Time To Prepare: five minutes Time to Cook: 0 minutes Yield: Servings 2

Ingredients:

¾ cup of almond milk 1 cup of chopped spinach 1 cup of frozen pineapple 1 small frozen banana 1 tbsp. of honey 2 tbsp. Of chia seeds

Directions: Mix the smoothie ingredients in your high-speed blender. Pulse the ingredients a few times to cut them up. Combine the mixture on the highest speed setting for thirty to 60 seconds. Pour into glasses and serve.

178. Pineapple Smoothie

Time To Prepare: ten minutes Time to Cook: 0 minutes Yield: Servings 2

Ingredients:

1 1/2 cups pineapple chunks 1 cup coconut water 1 orange, peeled and slice into quarters 1 tbsp. fresh grated ginger 1 tsp. chia seeds 1 tsp. turmeric powder A pinch black pepper

Directions:

In your blender, combine the coconut water with the orange, pineapple, ginger, chia seeds, turmeric, and black pepper. Pulse thoroughly, pour into a glass. Makes for a great breakfast

179. Pumpkin Pie Smoothie

Time To Prepare: five minutes Time to Cook: 0 minutes Yield: Servings 2

Ingredients:

½ Cup Pumpkin, Canned & Unsweetened 1 Banana 1 Cup Almond Milk 1 Teaspoon Ground Cinnamon 1 Teaspoon Ground Nutmeg 1 Teaspoon Maple Syrup, Pure 1 Teaspoon Vanilla Extract Pure 2 Tablespoons Almond Butter, Heaping 2-3 Ice Cubes

Directions:

Blend all ingredients together until the desired smoothness is achieved.

180. Raspberry Banana Smoothie

Time To Prepare: ten minutes Time to Cook: 0 minutes Yield: Servings 1

Ingredients:

1 banana 1 cup almond milk 1 cup frozen raspberries 1 cup raspberry yogurt 1 tbsp. flaxseed meal 1/4 cup Concord grape juice 1/4 cup rolled oats 16 whole almonds

Directions:

Put in everything to a blender jug. Cover the jug firmly. Blend until the desired smoothness is achieved and then serve. Enjoy!

181. Spicy Tomato Smoothie

Time To Prepare: five minutes Time to Cook: 0 minutes Yield: Servings 2

Ingredients:

¼ cup chopped red onion 1 jalapeño, cut, deseed if you wish 1 small bunch cilantro, chopped 1 small cucumber 2 big carrots, chopped 2 cloves garlic, peeled 6 small vine tomatoes Juice of 2 limes

Directions:

Combine all ingredients into a blender and blend until the desired smoothness is achieved. Pour into 2 tall glasses before you serve.

182. Sweet & Savoury Smoothie

Time To Prepare: five minutes Time to Cook: 0 minutes Yield: Servings 2

Ingredients:

1 apple, peeled and cut 1 banana, peeled and cut 1 cup of almond or soy milk 1 cup of fresh pineapple, peeled and cut 1 tbsp. of lemon juice 1/2 tbsp. of ginger, grated 1/4 tsp of ground turmeric 2 cups of carrots, peeled and cut 2 cups of filtered water.

Directions:

Blend carrots and water to make a pureed carrot juice. Pour into a Mason jar or sealable container, cover, and store in the refrigerator. When done, put in the rest of the smoothie ingredients to a blender or juicer until the desired smoothness is achieved. Put in the carrot juice in at the end, blending meticulously until the desired smoothness is achieved. Serve with or without ice.

183. Triple Fruit Smoothie

Time To Prepare: ten minutes Time to Cook: 0 minutes Yield: Servings 1

Ingredients:

1 banana, peeled and chopped 1 container (8 oz.) peach yogurt 1 cup ice cubes 1 cup strawberries 1 kiwi, cut 1/2 cup blueberries 1/2 cup orange juice

Directions:

Put in everything to a blender jug. Cover the jug firmly. Blend until the desired smoothness is achieved. Serve and enjoy!

184. Tropical Pineapple Kiwi Smoothie

Time To Prepare: five minutes Time to Cook: 0 minutes Yield: Servings 2

Ingredients:

1 ½ cup of frozen pineapple 1 cup of canned full-fat coconut milk 1 ripe kiwi; peeled and chopped 1 tsp of spirulina powder 3 tsp of lime juice 6 to 8 ice cubes

Directions:

Mix the smoothie ingredients in your high-speed blender. Pulse the ingredients a few times to cut them up. Combine the mixture on the highest speed setting. Pour into glasses and serve

185. Turmeric Delight

Time To Prepare: five minutes Time to Cook: 0 minutes Yield: Servings 2

Ingredients:

¼ Teaspoon Ginger ½ Teaspoon Cinnamon 1 Banana, Sliced 1 Tablespoon Lemon Juice, Fresh 1 Teaspoon Turmeric 2 Cups Yogurt, Plain & Whole Milk 2 Teaspoons Honey, Raw

Directions:

Combine all ingredients into a blender then blend until the desired smoothness is achieved.

186. Turmeric Tea

Time To Prepare: five minutes Time to Cook: fifteen minutes Yield: Servings 2

Ingredients:

½ teaspoon ground ginger ½ teaspoon turmeric powder ½ tsp ground cinnamon 2 cups water 2 lemon juices 2 tablespoons honey

Directions:

Put in water into a deep cooking pan. Put the deep cooking pan on moderate heat. When it starts to boil, put in turmeric, cinnamon, and ginger and stir slowly. Remove the heat. Cover and allow the mixture to steep for 12 – fifteen minutes. Put in honey and lemon juice. Stir and pour into mugs. Serve.

187. Vanilla Blueberry Smoothie

Time To Prepare: five minutes Time to Cook: 0 minutes Yield: Servings 1

Ingredients:

1 cup fresh blueberries 1 tbsp. flaxseed oil 2 cups hemp milk 2 tbsp. hemp protein powder Handful of ice/ 1 cup frozen blueberries

Directions:

Mix milk and fresh blueberries plus ice (or frozen blueberries) in a blender. Blend for a minute, move to a glass, and mix in flaxseed oil.

188. Voluptuous Vanilla Hot Drink

Time To Prepare: ten minutes Time to Cook: 0 minutes Yield: Servings 1

Ingredients:

1 scoop of hemp protein 1/2 Tbsp. ground cinnamon (or more to taste) 1/2 Tbsp. vanilla extract 3 cups unsweetened almond milk (or 1 1/2 cup full-fat coconut milk + 1 1/2 cups water) Stevia to taste

Directions:

Put the almond milk into a pitcher. Put ground cinnamon, hemp, vanilla extract in a small deep cooking pan on moderate to high heat. Heat until the pure liquid stevia is just melted and then pour the pure liquid stevia mixture into the pitcher. Stir until the pure liquid stevia is well blended with the almond milk. Bring the pitcher in your refrigerator and let it cool for minimum two hours. Stir thoroughly before you serve.

189. White Hot Chocolate

Time To Prepare: five minutes Time to Cook: six minutes Yield: Servings 2

Ingredients:

¼ cup cocoa powder/butter 2 - 2½ Tbsp honey 2 tsp vanilla extract 3 cups coconut milk Pinch of sea salt

Directions: Put in milk, cocoa powder/butter, honey, vanilla extract, and salt to the instant pot. Secure the lid. Cook on LOW pressure six minutes. Depressurize swiftly. Use a hand blender to blend contents 25 seconds. Serve hot.

190. Zesty Citrus Smoothie

Time To Prepare: five minutes Time to Cook: 0 minutes Yield: Servings 1

Ingredients:

1 cup almond milk 1 med orange peeled, cleaned, and cut into sections 1 tbsp. flaxseed oil 2 tsp hemp protein powder half cup lemon juice Handful of ice

Directions: Mix milk, lemon juice, orange, and ice in a blender. Blend for a minute, move to a glass, and mix in flaxseed oil.

191. Broccoli and Black Beans Stir Fry

Time To Prepare: ten minutesTime to Cook:fifteen minutes Yield: Servings 4

Ingredients:

1 tablespoon sesame oil 2 cloves garlic, thoroughly minced 2 cups cooked black beans 2 teaspoons ginger, finely chopped 4 cups broccoli florets 4 teaspoons sesame seeds A big pinch red chili flakes A pinch turmeric powder Lime juice to taste (not necessary) Salt to taste

Directions:

Pour enough water to immerse the bottom of the deep cooking pan by an inch. Put a strainer on the deep cooking pan. Put broccoli florets on the strainer. Steam the broccoli for about six minutes. Put a big frying pan on moderate heat. Put in sesame oil. When the oil is just warm, put in sesame seeds, chili flakes, ginger, garlic, turmeric powder and salt. Sauté for about 2 minutes until aromatic. Put in steamed broccoli and black beans and sauté until meticulously heated. Put in lime juice and stir. Serve hot.

192. Cauliflower Broccoli Mash

Time To Prepare: five minutes Time to Cook: ten minutes Yield: Servings 6

Ingredients:

1 big head cauliflower, cut into chunks 1 small head broccoli, cut into florets 1 teaspoon salt 3 tablespoons extra virgin olive oil Pepper, to taste

Directions:

Take a pot and put in oil then heat it Put in the cauliflower and broccoli Sprinkle with salt and pepper to taste Keep stirring to make vegetable soft Put in water if required When is already cooked, use a food processor or a potato masher to puree the vegetables Serve and enjoy!

193. Citrus Couscous with Herb

Time To Prepare:five minutes Time to Cook: fifteen minutes Yield:Servings 2

Ingredients:

¼ cup of water ¼ orange, chopped ½ teaspoon butter 1 teaspoon Italian seasonings 1/3 cup couscous 1/3 teaspoon salt 4 tablespoons orange juice

Directions:

Pour water and orange juice in the pan. Put in orange, Italian seasoning, and salt. Bring the liquid to boil and take it off the heat. Put in butter and couscous. Stir thoroughly and close the lid. Leave the couscous rest for about ten minutes.

Couscous Salad

Time To Prepare: ten minutes Time to Cook: six minutes Yield: Servings 4

Ingredients:

¼ teaspoon ground black pepper ¾ teaspoon ground coriander ½ teaspoon salt ¼ teaspoon paprika ¼ teaspoon turmeric 1 tablespoon butter 2 oz. chickpeas, canned, drained 1 cup fresh arugula, chopped 2 oz. sun-dried tomatoes, chopped 1 oz. Feta cheese, crumbled 1 tablespoon canola oil 1/3 cup couscous 1/3 cup chicken stock

Directions:

Bring the chicken stock to boil. Put in couscous, ground black pepper, ground coriander, salt, paprika, and turmeric. Put in chickpeas and butter. Mix the mixture well and close the lid. Allow the couscous soak the hot chicken stock for about six minutes. In the meantime, in the mixing container mix together arugula, sun-dried tomatoes, and Feta cheese. Put in cooked couscous mixture and canola oil. Mix up the salad well.

194. Crispy Corn

Time To Prepare: 8 minutes Time to Cook: five minutes Yield: Servings 3

Ingredients:

½ teaspoon ground paprika ½ teaspoon salt ¾ teaspoon chili pepper 1 cup corn kernels 1 tablespoon coconut flour 1 tablespoon water 3 tablespoons canola oil

Directions:

In the mixing container, mix together corn kernels with salt and coconut flour. Put in water and mix up the corn with the help of the spoon. Pour canola oil in the frying pan and heat it. Put in corn kernels mixture and roast it for about four minutes. Stir it occasionally. When the corn kernels are crispy, move them in the plate and dry with the paper towel's help. Put in chili pepper and ground paprika. Mix up well

195. Curry Wheatberry Rice

Time To Prepare: ten minutes Time to Cook: 1 hour fifteen minutes Yield: Servings 5

Ingredients:

¼ cup milk ½ cup of rice 1 cup wheat berries 1 tablespoon curry paste 1 teaspoon salt 4 tablespoons olive oil 6 cups chicken stock

Directions:

Put wheatberries and chicken stock in the pan. Close the lid and cook the mixture for an hour over the moderate heat. Then put in rice, olive oil, and salt. Stir thoroughly. Mix up together milk and curry paste. Put in the curry liquid in the rice-wheatberry mixture and stir thoroughly. Boil the meal for fifteen minutes with the closed lid. When the rice is cooked, all the meal is cooked.

196. Feta Cheese Salad

Time To Prepare: ten minutes Time to Cook: 0 minutes Yield: Servings 2

Ingredients:

1 tbsp. olive oil (extra virgin) 1 tsp balsamic vinegar 2 cucumbers 30 g feta cheese 4 spring onions 4 tomatoes Salt

Directions:

Cube the tomatoes and cucumbers. Thinly slice the onions. Crush the feta cheese. Mix tomatoes, onions, and cucumbers. Put olive oil, vinegar, and a small amount of salt. Put in feta cheese. Enjoy your meal!

197. Goat Cheese Salad

Time To Prepare: fifteen minutes Time to Cook: thirty minutes Yield: Servings 4

Ingredients:

½ cup of walnuts ½ head of escarole (medium), torn 1 bunch of trimmed and torn arugula 1/3 cup extra virgin olive oil 2 bunches of medium beets (~1 ½ lbs.) with trimmed tops 2 tbsp. of red wine vinegar 4 oz. crumbled of goat cheese (aged cheese is preferred) Kosher salt + freshly ground black pepper

Directions:

Place the beets in water in a deep cooking pan and apply salt as seasoning. Now, boil them using high heat for approximately twenty minutes or until they're soft. Peel them off when they're cool using your fingers or use a knife. To taste, whisk the vinegar with salt and pepper in a big container. Then mix in the olive oil for the dressing. Toss the beets with the dressing, so they're uniformly coated and marinate them for approximately fifteen minutes – 2 hours. Set the oven to 350F. Bring the nuts on a baking sheet and toast them for approximately 8 minutes (stirring them once) until they turn golden brown. Let them cool. Mix and toss the escarole and arugula with the beets and put them in four plates. Put in the walnuts and goat cheese as toppings before you serve. Enjoy

198. Green, Red and Yellow Rice

TimeTo Prepare:five minutes Time to Cook:fifteen minutes Yield:Servings 10

Ingredients:

¼ cup garlic, finely chopped 1 cup fresh cilantro, chopped 2 cups brown rice, washed 2 cups frozen corn, thawed 2 cups green onions, chopped 2 cups red bell pepper, chopped 2 tablespoons olive oil Cayenne pepper to taste Pepper to taste Salt to taste

Directions:

Put a big deep cooking pan on moderate heat. Put in 4 cups water and brown rice and cook in accordance with the instructions on the package. Once cooked, cover and save for later. Put a big frying pan on moderate heat. Put in oil. When the oil is heated, put in garlic and sauté for approximately one minute until aromatic. Put in corn, red bell pepper, green onion, salt, pepper and cayenne pepper and sauté for at least two minutes. Put in rice and cilantro. Mix thoroughly and heat meticulously. Serve.

199. Lentil Salad

Time To Prepare: ten minutes Time to Cook: 0 minutes Yield: Servings 2

Ingredients:

½ cup parsley 1 red bell pepper 1 tbsp. lime juice 1 tbsp. olive oil 2 cups lentil 3 spring onions A pinch of salt fifteen basil leaves Turmeric – to your taste

Directions:

Cook the lentils based on the package instructions. Put in a garlic clove while cooking. When cooled, remove the garlic clove and put the lentils into a big container. Chop all the vegetables then put in them to the lentils. Put in lime juice, a small amount of salt, and olive oil. Mix thoroughly.

200. Moroccan Style Couscous

Time To Prepare: ten minutes Time to Cook: ten minutes Yield: Servings 4

Ingredients:

½ teaspoon ground cardamom ½ teaspoon red pepper 1 cup chicken stock 1 cup yellow couscous 1 tablespoon butter 1 teaspoon salt

Directions:

Toss butter in the pan and melt it. Put in couscous and roast it for a minute over the high heat. Then put in ground cardamom, salt, and red pepper. Stir it well. Pour the chicken stock and bring the mixture to boil. Simmer couscous for five minutes with the closed lid.

201. Onion and Orange Healthy Salad

Time To Prepare: ten minutes Time to Cook: 0 minutes Yield: Servings 3

Ingredients:

¼ cup of fresh chives, chopped 1 cup olive oil 1 red onion, thinly cut 1 teaspoon of dried oregano 3 tablespoon of red wine vinegar 6 big orange 6 tablespoon of olive oil Ground black pepper

Directions:

Peel the orange and cut each of them in 4-5 crosswise slices Move the oranges to a shallow dish Sprinkle vinegar, olive oil and drizzle oregano Toss Chill for thirty minutes Position cut onion and black olives on top Garnish with an additional drizzle of chives and a fresh grind of pepper Serve and enjoy!

202. Quinoa Salad

Time To Prepare: ten minutes Time to Cook: 0 minutes Yield: Servings 2

Ingredients:

¼ tsp sea salt ½ cup quinoa (uncooked) 1 carrot 1 tbsp. apple cider vinegar 1 tbsp. flaxseed oil 2 brussels sprouts

Directions:

Wash quinoa meticulously. Dice the carrots and brussels sprouts to minuscule pieces. Cook the quinoa based on the instruction on the packaging. Mix flaxseed oil, sea salt, and apple cider vinegar. Sauté brussels sprouts and carrots on a small amount of olive oil for a few minutes. After both brussels sprouts and carrots, and quinoa are ready, combine them all in a container. Put in the dressing and mix meticulously. Serve warm.

203. Rice with Pistachios

Time To Prepare:ten minutes Time to Cook: twenty minutes Yield:Servings 6

Ingredients:

¼ cup of raw pistachios (or more for decoration) ½ cup of chopped and packed dill leaves ½ teaspoon of turmeric 1 ½ cups of Basmati rice (rinsed in a colander and soaked in water for approximately 30 minutes, or more) 1 teaspoon of vegetable oil 1 thinly cut medium onion 2 dry baby leaves 3 cups of vegetable stock or water 5 pods of slightly crushed green cardamom Ground black pepper (to taste) Salt, to taste

Directions:

In a big deep cooking pan, warm the oil and put in the cardamom. Heat it for approximately 1 minute until it turns smildly brown and put in the onion. Sauté for approximately 1-2 minutes. Mix in the dill leaves, turmeric and pistachios. Then put in the rice and stir-fry for approximately one minute. Combine the vegetable stock, black pepper and salt to taste, stir it well and bring it to its boiling point. Cover the pan using lid and cook on moderate to low heat for approximately fifteen minutes. Take it off from the heat then set aside the rice (covered) for approximately ten minutes. Then fluff it using a fork and put in more pistachios as decorate, if you desire. Enjoy!

204. Roasted Curried Cauliflower

Time To Prepare: five minutes Time to Cook: thirty minutes Yield: Servings 4

Ingredients:

¾ teaspoon salt 1 and ½ tablespoon olive oil 1 big head cauliflower, cut into florets 1 teaspoon cumin seeds 1 teaspoon curry powder 1 teaspoon mustard seeds

Directions:

Preheat the oven to 375 degrees F Grease a baking sheet with cooking spray Take a container and place all ingredients Toss to coat well Position the vegetable on a baking sheet Roast for thirty minutes Serve and enjoy!

205. Roasted Portobellos With Rosemary

Time To Prepare:five minutes Time to Cook: fifteen minutes Yield:Servings 4

Ingredients:

¼ cup extra virgin olive oil 1 clove garlic, minced 1 sprig rosemary, torn 2 tablespoons fresh lemon juice 8 portobello mushroom, trimmed Salt and pepper, to taste

Directions:

Preheat the oven to 450 degrees F Take a container and put in all ingredients Toss to coat Put the mushroom in a baking sheet stem side up Roast in your oven for fifteen minutes Serve and enjoy!

206. Spiced Sweet Potato Bread

Time To Prepare: fifteen minutes Time to Cook: 45-55 minutes Yield: Servings 2

Ingredients:

For dry Ingredients: ¼ teaspoon sea salt 1 cup coconut flour 1 teaspoon ground mace 2 tablespoons ground cinnamon 2 teaspoons baking powder 2 teaspoons baking soda 2 teaspoons ground nutmeg Wet Ingredients: 1 cup almond butter 2 teaspoons organic almond extract 4 big sweet potatoes, peeled, thinly cut 4 tablespoons coconut oil 8 big eggs 8 tablespoons melted grass fed butter, unsalted

Directions:

Grease 2 loaf pans of 9 x 5 inches with coconut oil. Coat the bottom of the pan using parchment paper. Set aside. Put a medium deep cooking pan on moderate heat. Put in sweet potatoes. Pour enough water to immerse the sweet potatoes. Cook until the sweet potatoes are soft. Remove the heat and drain the sweet potatoes. Put in the sweet potatoes back into the pan. Mash with a potato masher until the desired smoothness is achieved. Allow it to cool completely. Put all together the dry ingredients into a container and mix thoroughly. Put in eggs into a big container and whisk well. Put in sweet potatoes, butter, almond extract and almond butter and whisk until well blended. Put in the dry ingredients into the container of wet ingredients and whisk until well blended. Split the batter into the prepared loaf pans. Bake in a preheated oven at 350°F for approximately 45 -55 minutes or a toothpick when inserted in the middle of the loaf comes out clean. Remove from oven and cool to room temperature. Slice using a sharp knife into slices of 1-inch thickness.

207. Spicy Roasted Brussels Sprouts

Time To Prepare: five minutes Time to Cook: thirty minutes Yield: Servings 4

Ingredients:

½ cup kimchi with juice 1 and ¼ pound Brussels sprouts, cut into florets 2 tablespoons olive oil Salt and pepper, to taste

Directions:

Set the oven to 425 F. Toss the Brussels sprouts with pepper, salt, and oil. Bake using your oven for about twenty-five minutes Remove from oven and mix with kimchi Return to the oven Cook for five minutes Serve and enjoy!

208. Stir-Fried Almond And Spinach

Time To Prepare:ten minutes Time to Cook: fifteen minutes Yield:Servings 2

Ingredients:

1 tablespoon coconut oil 3 tablespoons almonds 34 pounds spinach Salt to taste

Directions:

Put oil to a big pot and place it on high heat Put in spinach and allow it to cook, stirring regularly Once the spinach is cooked and soft, sprinkle with salt and stir Put in almonds and enjoy!

209. Tender Farro

Time To Prepare: 8 minutes Time to Cook: forty minutes Yield: Servings 4

Ingredients:

1 cup farro 1 tablespoon almond butter 1 tablespoon dried dill 1 teaspoon salt 3 cups beef broth

Directions:

Put farro in the pan. Put in beef broth, dried dill, and salt. Close the lid and put the mixture to boil. Then boil it for a little more than half an hour over the medium-low heat. When the time is done, open the lid and put in almond butter. Mix up the cooked farro well.

210. Tomato Bulgur

Time To Prepare: seven minutes Time to Cook: twenty minutes Yield: Servings 2

Ingredients:

½ cup bulgur ½ white onion, diced 1 ½ cup chicken stock 1 teaspoon tomato paste 2 tablespoons coconut oil

Directions:

Toss coconut oil in the pan and melt it. Put in diced onion and roast it until light brown. Then put in bulgur and stir thoroughly. Cook bulgur in coconut oil for about three minutes. Then put in tomato paste and mix up bulgur until homogenous. Put in chicken stock. Close the lid and cook bulgur for fifteen minutes over the moderate heat. The cooked bulgur should soak all liquid.

211. Sauces And Dressings

Apple and Tomato Dipping Sauce

Time To Prepare: ten minutes Time to Cook: 0 minutes Yield: Servings 2-4

Ingredients:

¼ cup of cider vinegar ¼ tsp of freshly ground black pepper ½ tsp of sea salt 1 garlic clove, finely chopped 1 large-sized shallot, diced 1 tbsp. natural tomato paste 1 tbsp. of extra-virgin olive oil 1 tbsp. of maple syrup 1/8 tsp of ground cloves 3 moderate-sized apples, roughly chopped 3 moderate-sized tomatoes, roughly chopped

Directions:

Put oil into a huge deep cooking pan and heat it up on moderate heat. Put in shallot and cook until light brown for approximately 2 minutes. Stir in the tomato paste, garlic, salt, pepper, and cloves for approximately half a minute. Then put in in the apples, tomatoes, vinegar, and maple syrup. Bring to its boiling point then decrease the heat to allow it to simmer for approximately 30 minutes. Allow to cool for twenty additional minutes before placing the mixture into your blender. Combine the mixture until the desired smoothness is achieved. Keep in a mason jar or an airtight container; place in your fridge for maximum 5 days. Serve it on a burger or with fries.

212. Bean Potato Spread

Time To Prepare: twenty-five minutes Time to Cook: 0 minutes Yield: Servings 7-8

Ingredients:

¼ cup sesame paste ½ teaspoon cumin, ground 1 cup garbanzo beans, drained and washed 1 tablespoon olive oil 2 tablespoons lime juice 2 tablespoons water 4 cups cooked sweet potatoes, peeled and chopped 5 garlic cloves, minced A pinch of salt

Directions: Throw all the ingredients into a blender and blend to make a smooth mix. Move to a container. Serve with carrot, celery, or veggie sticks.

213. Creamy Avocado Dressing

Time To Prepare: ten minutes Time to Cook: 0 minutes Yield: Servings 2-4

Ingredients:

½ cup of extra-virgin olive oil 1 clove of garlic, chopped 1 tsp of honey or maple syrup 2 small or 1 large-sized avocado, pitted and chopped 2 tsp of lemon or lime juice 3 tbsp. of chopped parsley 3 tbsp. of red wine vinegar Onion powder Some Kosher salt and ground black pepper

Directions:

Combine all ingredients into a blender, apart from the oil. As the ingredients are mixed, progressively put in the oil into the mixture. Blend until the desired smoothness is achieved or becomes liquidy. Use as a vegetable or fruit salad dressing. Put in your fridge for maximum 5 days.

214. Creamy Raspberry Vinaigrette

Time To Prepare: ten minutes Time to Cook: 0 minutes Yield: Servings 2-4

Ingredients:

½ cup of raspberries 1 tbsp. of Dijon mustard 1 tbsp. of Greek yogurt 1/3 cup of extra-virgin olive oil 2 tbsp. of honey or maple syrup 2 tbsp. of raspberry vinegar

Directions:

Put all together the ingredients apart from the oil into a blender, in accordance with the ordered list. Cover and blend for ten seconds, by slowly increasing the speed. After 10 seconds, reduce the speed and progressively put in the oil into the mixture. Keep the speed at a stable pace until all of the oil has been poured in. Blend until blended. Store in a mason jar then place in your fridge for maximum 5 days. Serve with a vegetable or fruit salad.

215. Cucumber and Dill Sauce

Time To Prepare: ten minutes Time to Cook: 0 minutes Yield: Servings 2-4

Ingredients:

¼ cup of lemon juice 1 cucumber, peeled and squeezed to remove surplus liquid 1 cup of freshly chopped dill 1 tsp of sea salt 450g of Greek yogurt

Directions:

In a moderate-sized container, put together the yogurt, cucumber, and dill then stir until well blended. Put in in the lemon juice and salt to taste. Cover and place in your fridge for approximately 1-2 hours before you serve to keep its freshness. Best serve with Mediterranean food, chips, fish, or even bread.

216. Herby Raita

Time To Prepare: ten minutes Time to Cook: 0 minutes Yield: Servings 2-4

Ingredients:

¼ cup of freshly chopped mint ¼ tsp of freshly ground black pepper ½ tsp of sea salt 1 cup of Greek yogurt 1 large-sized cucumber, shredded 1 tsp of lemon juice

Directions:

Combine the cucumber with ¼ tsp of salt in a sieve and leave to drain for fifteen minutes. Shake to release any surplus liquid and move to a kitchen towel. Squeeze out as much liquid as you can using the paper towel. Put the cucumber into a medium container then mix in the rest of the ingredients until well blended. Put in your fridge for minimum 2 hours to keep its freshness. Best consume with spicy foods as it could relief the spiciness.

217. Homemade Lemon Vinaigrette

Time To Prepare: ten minutes Time to Cook: 0 minutes Yield: Servings 2-4

Ingredients:

¼ tsp of sea salt ½ tsp of Dijon mustard, without preservatives ½ tsp of lemon zest 1 tsp of honey or maple syrup 2 tbsp. of freshly squeezed lemon juice 3 tbsp. of extra-virgin olive oil Freshly ground black pepper

Directions:

Whisk all together the ingredients apart from olive oil and black pepper in a small container. Then progressively put in 3 tbsp. of olive oil while continuously whisking until well blended. Put in some ground black pepper to taste. Put mason jar and place in your fridge for maximum 3 days. Serve with a garden salads

218. Honey Bean Dip

Time To Prepare: five minutes Time to Cook: 0 minutes Yield: Servings 3-4

Ingredients:

¼ teaspoon ground cumin ¼ teaspoon salt 1 (14-ounce) can each of kidney beans and black beans 1 tablespoon apple cider vinegar 1 teaspoon lime juice 2 cherry tomatoes 2 garlic cloves 2 tablespoons filtered water 2 teaspoons raw honey Freshly ground black pepper to taste Pinch cayenne pepper to taste

Directions:

In a blender or food processor, put together the beans, garlic, tomatoes, water, vinegar, honey, lime juice, cumin, salt, cayenne pepper, and black pepper. Blend until it becomes smooth. Put in the mix in a container. Cover and place in your fridge to chill. You can place in your fridge for maximum 5 days.

219. Strawberry Poppy Seed Dressing

Time To Prepare: ten minutes Time to Cook: 0 minutes Yield: Servings 2-4

Ingredients:

¼ cup of raspberry vinegar ¼ tsp of ground ginger ¼ tsp of sea salt ½ tsp of onion powder ½ tsp of poppy seeds 1/3 cup of extra-virgin olive oil 1/3 cup of honey 2 tbsp. of freshly squeezed orange juice

Directions:

Put all ingredients, apart from the poppy seeds and oil into a blender. Blend until the desired smoothness is achieved and creamy. Next, progressively put the oil into the mixture until blended. Put in in the poppy seeds and stir thoroughly. Put in a mason jar then place in your fridge before you serve. Keep for maximum 3 days. Serve with your garden salads

220. Tomato and Mushroom Sauce

Time To Prepare: ten minutes Time to Cook: 0 minutes Yield: Servings 2-4

Ingredients:

½ cup of water 1 moderate-sized leek, chopped 2 moderate-sized carrots, chopped 2 stalks of celery, chopped 2 tsp of dried oregano 4 cloves of garlic, crushed 450g of button mushrooms, diced 5 tbsp. of coconut milk 680g of unsalted tomato puree Black pepper, seasoning Some sea salt, seasoning

Directions:

In a big frying pan, place a few tablespoons of water and heat on moderate heat. Once it sizzles, put in in the mushrooms and Sautee for approximately five minutes, stir once in a while. Next, put in in the leek, carrots, and celery. Stir thoroughly and cook for approximately five minutes or until the vegetables are soft. Put in more water if required. Mix in the tomato puree with ½ cup of water and dried oregano. Bring to its boiling point and then decrease the heat to allow it to simmer for approximately fifteen minutes. Remove from heat and mix in the garlic, coconut milk, and salt and pepper to taste. Put in an airtight container, then store for maximum four days in your fridge or freeze for maximum 1 month. Serve with a pasta.

221. Almonds and Blueberries Yogurt Snack

Time To Prepare: ten minutes Time to Cook: 0 minutes Yield: Servings 2

Ingredients:

1 ½ cups nonfat Greek yogurt 1 cup blueberries 20 almonds, chopped

Directions:

Take 2 bowls and put in ¾ cup yogurt into each container. Split the blueberries among the bowls and stir. Drizzle half the almonds in each container before you serve

222. Ants on a Log

Time To Prepare: five minutes Time to Cook: 0 minutes Yield: Servings 2

Ingredients:

3 tablespoons of almond butter 3 tablespoons of raisins 6 celery sticks

Directions:

Spread half a tablespoon of almond butter on each celery stick. Top with half a tablespoon of raisins on each celery stick. Split the celery sticks between two plates, and enjoy!

223. Apple Sauce Treat

Time To Prepare: ten minutes Time to Cook: 0 minutes Yield: Servings 1

Ingredients:

½ teaspoon cinnamon 1 ½ teaspoons toasted slivered almonds 1/4 cup low Fat cottage cheese 1/4 cup unsweetened applesauce

Directions:

Combine the cottage cheese and applesauce in a container, stirring well. Drizzle with cinnamon and mix thoroughly. Drizzle the top with almonds, pick up your spoon, and enjoy

224. Avocado Hummus

Time To Prepare: fifteen minutes Time to Cook: 0 minutes Yield: Servings 4

Ingredients: .

25 cup Sunflower seeds .25 cup Tahini .25 tsp. Pepper .5 cup Cilantro .5 cup Coconut oil .5 Lemon juice .5 tsp. Salt 1 clove pressed garlic 3 Avocados 5 tsp. Cumin

Directions:

Halve the avocados, take off the pits, then spoon out the flesh. Put all together ingredients in a blender and stir until super smooth. Put in water, lemon juice, or oil if you need to loosen the mixture bit.

225. Baked Veggie Turmeric Nuggets

Time To Prepare: ten minutes Time to Cook: twenty-five minutes Yield: Servings 24

Ingredients:

¼ tsp. Black pepper powder ¼ tsp. Sea salt ½ cup Almond meal ½ tsp. Turmeric powder 1 big Whole egg 1 cup Chopped carrots 1 tsp. Minced garlic 2 cups Broccoli florets 2 cups Cauliflower florets

Directions:

Preheat your oven to 400°F. Get a parchment-lined baking sheet ready. Pour cauliflower, turmeric, broccoli, carrots, black pepper, garlic, and sea salt in the blender and blitz until it's smooth. Pour in the egg and almond meal and stir until it's blended. Pour the paste into a mixing container. Scoop out a small amount onto your hand and make a circular disc. Put this disc on the baking sheet and repeat the pulse until the mixing container is empty. Slide into the oven then bake for minimum fifteen minutes on one before flipping and baking for about ten minutes on the other side. Serve with a side of Paleo ranch sauce.

226. Berry Energy bites

Time To Prepare: ten minutes Time to Cook: 0 minutes Yield: Servings 6

Ingredients:

¼ cup of dried blueberries ½ - 1 cup of almond milk ½ cup of coconut flour 1 tablespoon of coconut sugar 1 teaspoon of cinnamon

Directions:

In a huge mixing container, put together the coconut flour, cinnamon, coconut sugar, and blueberries, and mix thoroughly. Put in the almond milk slowly until a firm dough is formed. Form into bite-sized balls and place in your fridge for thirty minutes so they can harden up. Store leftovers in your fridge

227. Boiled Okra and Squash

Time To Prepare: five minutes Time to Cook: five minutes Yield: Servings 1

Ingredients:

½ cup of okra, cut in 1" cubes ½ cup of squash, cut in 1" cubes 1 clove garlic, minced 2/3 cup Vegetable stock or fish stock, plain water may be used as well Salt to taste

Directions:

Boil the liquid in high heat. Put in the okra and squash. Bring to its boiling point. Put in the garlic. Reduced the heat and simmer for minimum five minutes or until the squash is soft. Put in salt to taste and serve hot.

228. Bruschetta

Time To Prepare: 60 minutes Time to Cook: 0 minutes Yield: Servings 4

Ingredients:

¼ cup of extra virgin olive oil ¼ teaspoon of ground black pepper 1 red onion, diced 1 teaspoon of sea salt 2 cloves of garlic, minced 2 tablespoons of balsamic vinegar 4 medium tomatoes, diced

Directions:

Put all together the ingredients into a big container, and stir slowly. Place in your fridge for an hour before you serve on gluten-free toast (toast is not included in nutritional information)

229. Buttered Banana Chickpea Cookies

Time To Prepare:ten minutes Time to Cook: twelve minutes Yield:Servings 8

Ingredients:

¼-tsp cinnamon ¼-tsp salt ⅓-cup chocolate chips ⅓-cup coconut sugar ½-cup creamy peanut butter 1-pc small banana, very ripe 1-tsp baking powder 2-Tbsps ground flaxseed 2-tsp vanilla extract fifteen-oz. chickpeas, washed and drained

Directions:

Preheat the oven to 350F. Grease a baking pan with cooking spray. Mix in all the ingredients apart from the chocolate chips in your blender. Combine the batter for two minutes, or until turning into a smooth consistency. Mix in the chocolate chips. Ladle the batter to make cookies. Put the cookies in the pan, and bake for about twelve minutes

230. Carrot Sticks with Avocado Dip

Time To Prepare: ten minutes Time to Cook: 0 minutes Yield: Servings 6

Ingredients:

½ cup cilantro, firmly packed ½ onion 1 big avocado, pitted 1 tablespoon of chili-garlic sauce or chili sauce 2 tablespoon olive oil 6 ounces shelled edamame Juice of one lemon Salt and pepper

Directions:

Put the edamame, cilantro, onion, and chili sauce in a blender or food processor. Pulse it to cut and mix the ingredients. Put in the avocado and the lemon juice. Slowly put in the olive oil as you blend. Move to a jar. Scoop 2 spoons and serve with carrot sticks

231. Grams Cashew Cheese

Time To Prepare: 2 hours Time to Cook: 0 minutes Yield: Servings 6

Ingredients:

¼ cup of fresh basil 1 cup of raw cashews 1 tablespoon of nutritional yeast Juice of ½ lemon Salt and pepper to taste

Directions:

In a 1 cup of water, soak the cashew for minimum 2 hours. Drain. Put the cashews, lemon juice, nutritional yeast, and fresh basil into a food processor and pulse until the desired smoothness is achieved. Put in 1 tablespoon of water at a time to make it creamy, but not runny. Flavor it with pepper and salt, then spread it on gluten-free bread or toast. Store in an airtight jar in your fridge.

232. Cereal Chia Chips

Time To Prepare: ten minutes Time to Cook: thirty minutes Yield: Servings 10

Ingredients:

¼-cup rolled oats, gluten-free ½-cup maple syrup ½-cup white quinoa, uncooked ¾-cup pecans, chopped 2-Tbsps chia seeds 2-Tbsps coconut oil 2-Tbsps coconut sugar A pinch of sea salt (not necessary)

Directions:

Preheat the oven to 325°F. Coat a baking pan using parchment paper. Mix in the first six ingredients in a mixing container. Mix thoroughly until meticulously blended. Set aside. Pour the oil and syrup in a small deep cooking pan placed on moderate to low heat. Heat the mixture for about three minutes, stirring once in a while. Fold in the dry ingredients; stir thoroughly to coat completely. Pour the mixture in the baking pan, and spread to a uniform layer using a spoon. Place the pan in your oven. Bake for fifteen minutes. Turn the pan around to cook uniformly. Bake for 8-ten minutes until the mixture turns golden brown. Allow cooling completely before breaking the chips into bite-size pieces

233. Chia Cashew Cream

Time To Prepare: 2 hours and five minutes Time to Cook: 0 minutes Yield: Servings 1

Ingredients:

¼-cup quinoa, cooked ¼-tsp vanilla powder ¾-cup cashew milk 2-Tbsps chia seeds 2-Tbsps hemp hearts 2-Tbsps maple syrup or a dash of liquid stevia A pinch of cinnamon

Directions:

Mix all the ingredients in a jar. Mix thoroughly until meticulously blended. Cover the jar and place in your fridge for about two hours. To serve, top with your desired toppings

234. Coconut Porridge

Time To Prepare: twenty minutes Time to Cook: ten minutes Yield: Servings 2

Ingredients:

1 tbsp. coconut oil 1 tsp cinnamon 1 vanilla bean 2 cups oats 2 tbsp. maple syrup 2 tsp ginger 2 tsp turmeric 330ml vaporized coconut milk 750 ml of water Coconut milk Fresh, shredded coconut (for serving)

Directions:

Mix 750 ml water and turmeric in a container. Allow it to sit for about ten minutes. Combine all ingredients apart from coconut milk and shredded coconut in a deep cooking pan. Heat it on medium heat while stirring continuously, and cook for eight minutes. Allow it to cool for about ten minutes. Split into serving bowls. Put in coconut milk and shredded coconut on top. Put in some extra cinnamon to your taste. Eat warm.

235. Cucumber Rolls Hors D'oeuvres

Time To Prepare: twenty minutes Time to Cook: 0 minutes Yield: Servings 8-10

Ingredients:

¼ cup fresh dill, finely chopped ½ cup capers ½ cup fresh parsley + extra to decorate, finely chopped 1 teaspoon Himalayan pink salt 2 big organic English cucumbers or 4 normal cucumbers 5-6 ripe avocadoes, peeled, pitted, mashed For the avocado spread: Freshly cracked pepper to taste

Directions:

Peel the cucumbers and cut thin slices along the length on a mandolin slicer. Put the cucumber slices on your countertop. To make the avocado spread: Put in all the ingredients of avocado spread into a container and stir until well blended. Spread the avocado mixture uniformly and thinly on the cucumber slices. Begin rolling from one of the shorter ends to the other end and place on a serving platter with its seam side facing down. Repeat the above step with the rest of the cucumber slices. Serve instantly as the cucumbers tend to get soggy after a while.

236. Delectable Cookies

Time To Prepare: twenty minutes Time to Cook: fifteen-twenty minutes Yield: Servings 6

Ingredients:

1 cup of almonds ¼ cup of arrowroot flour 1 tbsp. of coconut flour 1 tsp. ground turmeric Salt, to taste Freshly ground black pepper, to taste 1 organic egg ¼ cup of olive oil 3 tbsp. of raw honey 1 tsp. of organic vanilla extract 1 1/3 cups of almond flour

Directions:

Use a food processor to put the almonds and pulse till chopped roughly Move the chopped almonds in a big container. Place the flours and spices and mix thoroughly. In another container, put the rest of the ingredients then beat till well blended. Put the flour mixture into the egg mixture and mix till well blended. Position a plastic wrap over the cutting board. Put the dough over the cutting board. Use your hands to pat into approximately 1-inch thick circle. Gently chop the circle in 6 wedges. Set the scones onto a cookie sheet in a single layer. Bake for approximately fifteen-20 minutes.

237. Easy Guacamole

Time To Prepare: ten minutes Time to Cook: 0 minutes Yield: Servings 3

Ingredients:

½ Teaspoon Sea Salt 1 Teaspoon Garlic Powder 4 Avocados, Halved & Pitted

Directions:

Scoop your avocado flesh out, placing it in a container. Put in in your salt and garlic powder mashing until it's creamy. You can place in your fridge it, and it'll keep for two days.

238. Energetic Oat Bars

Time To Prepare: ten minutes Time to Cook: twenty-five minutes Yield: Servings 6

Ingredients:

½ cup of gluten-free rolled oats ¾ cup fresh blueberries 1 peeled and mashed banana 1 tbsp. of chopped walnuts 1 tbsp. of fresh pomegranate juice 1 tbsp. of sunflower seeds 2 tbsp. of flax seeds 2 tbsp. of pitted and chopped finely dates 2 tbsp. of raisins

Directions:

Set the oven to 350F. Lightly, oil an 8-inch baking dish. In a huge mixing container, put all ingredients and mix till well blended. Put the mixture into the readied baking dish uniformly. Bake for approximately twenty-five minutes. Remove from the oven then cool. Using a knife, split the bars into the size your desired pieces then serve.

239. Flavorsome Almonds

Time To Prepare: ten minutesTime to Cook: fifteen minutes Yield:Servings 8

Ingredients:

¼ tsp. of cayenne pepper ¼ tsp. of ground cumin ½ tsp. of chili powder ½ tsp. of ground cinnamon 1 tbsp. of filtered water 1 tsp. of extra-virgin olive oil 2 cups of whole almonds 3 tbsp. of raw honey Salt, to taste

Directions:

Preheat your oven to 350 degrees F. Position the almonds onto a big rimmed baking sheet in a single layer. Roast for approximately ten minutes. In the meantime, in a microwave-safe container, put in honey and microwave on Hugh for approximately half a minute. Remove from microwave and mix in oil and water. In a small container, combine all spices. Take away the almonds from the oven, put in it into the container of honey mixture, and stir until blended well. Move the almond mixture onto the baking sheet in a single layer. Drizzle with spice mixture uniformly. Roast for approximately 3-4 minutes. Take off from oven and keep aside to cool to room temperature and serve. You can preserve these roasted almonds in an airtight jar.

240. Ginger Flour Banana Ginger Bars

Time To Prepare:ten minutes Time to Cook:forty minutes Yield: Servings 4-6

Ingredients:

1 ½ tbsp. Grated ginger 1 cup Coconut flour 1 tsp. Baking soda 1 tsp. Ground cardamom 1/3 cup Honey or maple syrup 1/3 cup melted butter 2 big Ripe bananas 2 tsp. Apple cider vinegar 2 tsp. Cinnamon 6 medium While eggs

Directions:

Preheat your oven to 350°F. Coat a glass baking dish using parchment paper. If you do not have any paper, just grease the pan. Put all the ingredients apart from the baking soda and apple cider vinegar through a food processor and pulse until it's all mixed up. Now put in the last two ingredients and blitz once before pouring the mix into the glass dish. Bake up to a toothpick inserted into the center comes out clean. This usually takes forty minutes.

241. Hummus Deviled Eggs

Time To Prepare: ten minutes Time to Cook: 0 minutes Yield: Servings 6

Ingredients:

½ cup hummus 6 hard-boiled eggs Paprika

Directions:

Cut the hardboiled eggs in half along the length and remove the yolk. Fill the egg whites with hummus and drizzle with paprika before you serve.

242. Kale Chips

Time To Prepare: ten minutes Time to Cook: 2 hours Yield: Servings 8

Ingredients:

½ teaspoon sea salt 1 cup cashews, soaked and softened in water about 2 hours 1 cup grated sweet potato 2 bunches of curly kale with stems removed, washed and torn into bite-sized pieces 2 tablespoons honey 2 tablespoons nutritional yeast (found at health food stores) 2 tablespoons water The juice of 1 lemon

Directions:

Place the kale in a huge container and save for later. In a blender or food processor, process the sweet potato, softened cashews yeast, lemon juice, honey, salt, and water until the desired smoothness is achieved. Place the mixture on the kale and toss with your hands to coat the leaves. Spread the kale leaves out on a big cookie sheet in a single cover without touching. Set the oven to its lowest setting. Prop the oven door slightly ajar and dehydrate the chips for approximately 2 hours flipping the cookie sheet and watching to ensure the chips do not burn. When crunchy, take it out of the oven and allow to cool. Store in an airtight container

243. Low Cholesterol-Low Calorie Blueberry Muffin

Time To Prepare: ten minutes Time to Cook: twenty-five minutes Yield: Servings 12

Ingredients:

½ cup skim milk or non-fat milk ½ cup white sugar 1 and ½ cup of flour, all-purpose 1 cup blueberries, fresh 1 egg white 1 tablespoon coconut oil 2 tablespoons melted margarine 2 teaspoons baking powder Pinch of salt

Directions:

Set the oven to 205C. Grease a 12-cup muffin pan using oil. In a small container, put the blueberries. Put in ¼ cup of the flour and mix it together. Set aside. In another container, whisk the egg white and the coconut oil. Put in the melted margarine. In a different container, mix all together the dry ingredients and sift. Sift again over the egg white mixture. Mix to moisten the flour. The flour should look lumpy, so do not overmix. Fold in the blueberries. Separate the blueberries, so that each scoop will have blueberries. Scoop the mixture into the muffin pans. Fill only up to two-thirds of the pan. Bake for about twenty-five minutes or until the muffin turns golden brown.

244. Mini Pepper Nachos

Time To Prepare: five minutes Time to Cook: ten minutes Yield: Servings 8

Ingredients: .

25 tsp. Red pepper flakes .5 cup Tomato, chopped .5 tsp. Oregano 1 tbsp. Chili powder 1 tsp. Cumin, ground 1 tsp. Garlic powder 1 tsp. Paprika 16 oz. Ground beef 16 oz. Mini peppers, seeded, halved 5 tsp. Pepper 5 tsp. Salt cup Cheddar cheese, shredded

Directions:

Mix seasonings together in a container. On moderate heat, brown the meat, be sure all the clumps are broken up. Stir in the spices and continue to sauté until the seasoning has gone through all of the meat. Heat the oven to 400F. Put the peppers in a single line. They can touch. Coat with the beef mix. Drizzle with cheese. Bake for minimum ten minutes or until cheese has melted. Pull out of the oven and top with the toppings.

245. Olive and Tomato Balls

Time To Prepare: ten minutes Time to Cook: thirty-five minutes Yield: Servings 5

Ingredients: .

25 cup Coconut oil .25 tsp. Salt .5 cup Cream cheese 2 cloves Garlic, crushed 2 tbsp. Basil, chopped 2 tbsp. Oregano, chopped 2 tbsp. Thyme, chopped 4 Kalamata olives, pitted 4 pcs. Sun-dried tomatoes, drained 5 tbsp. Parmesan cheese, grated Black pepper (as you wish)

Directions:

Cut the coconut oil, put in it to a small mixing container with the cream cheese, and allow them to tenderize for approximately 30 minutes. Mash together and mix thoroughly to blend. Put in in the Kalamata olives and sun-dried tomatoes and mix thoroughly before you put in in the herbs and seasonings. Mix meticulously before placing the mixing container in your fridge to allow the results to solidify. Once it has solidified, make the mixture into a total of 5 balls using an ice cream scoop. Roll each of the finished balls into the parmesan cheese before plating. Stored the extra's in your refrigerator in an air-tight container for maximum 7 days.

246. Paleo Ginger Spiced Mixed Nuts

Time To Prepare: five minutes Time to Cook: forty minutes Yield: Servings 8

Ingredients:

½ tsp. Fine sea salt ½ tsp. Vietnamese cinnamon 1 tsp. Grated fresh ginger 2 cups Mix nuts; Cashew, goji berries, raw almonds, pumpkin seeds, etc. 2 Large Egg, Coconut oil spray Egg whites

Directions:

Prepare the oven by preheating to 250°F. Whisk egg whites in a container until it gets fluffy. Pour in sea salt, grated ginger, and Vietnamese cinnamon. Whisk until it's one big mix. Pour in the mixed nuts and stir to combine. Coat the parchment-lined baking sheet with coconut oil spray and spread the nut mixture all across the baking sheet. Allow it to bake for approximately twenty minutes, rotate the sheet then bake for another twenty minutes. Take off the baking sheet from the oven and leave to cool. Once it's fully cool and hard, break them into bits with clean hands. Serve or store

247. Peanut Butter and Honey Oat Bars

Time To Prepare: ten minutes Time to Cook: twenty-five minutes Yield: Servings 18

Ingredients:

¼ cup honey ¼ cup honey roasted peanuts, chopped ¼ teaspoon cinnamon powder ¼ teaspoon vanilla extract 1 cup oats 2 teaspoons coconut oil 3 tablespoons peanut butter

Directions: Coat a small baking pan using a parchment paper such that the parchment paper is hanging over the sides of the baking pan. Put in honey, oil, and peanut butter into a microwave-safe container. Microwave on High for around 20 -half a minute or until the peanut butter melts completely. If it takes longer than half a minute, stir and cook in increments of 10 seconds, stirring every time. Remove from the microwave and put in the remaining ingredients. Mix thoroughly and pour into the readied baking pan. Spread the mixture and press using a spatula. Bake in a preheated oven 300° F for approximately twenty minutes or until the top is light brown. Take out of the oven and press once once more. Cool for a while and slice. Cool thoroughly before you serve. Move leftover bars into an airtight container. Place in your fridge until use.

248. Roasted Beets

Time To Prepare: ten minutes Time to Cook: 35-45 minutes Yield: Servings 6

Ingredients:

1 tablespoon of coconut oil, melted 1 teaspoon of salt 2 and a ½ pounds of beets, peeled and diced

Directions: Preheat your oven to 400°F. Spread the beets onto a baking sheet and sprinkle with melted coconut oil. Put in salt and mix thoroughly. Roast the beets in your oven for 35-45 minutes, until the beets are tender.

249. Grams Salmon & Avocado Toast

Time To Prepare: ten minutes Time to Cook: five minutes Yield: Servings 1

Ingredients:

¼ tsp red pepper ½ avocado 1 tsp lemon juice 2 slices of gluten-free bread oz. pink salmon (wild) salt and pepper - to taste

Directions:

Cut the avocado. Toast the bread to your taste. Combine the salmon and lemon juice. When the toast is ready, lay avocado slices onto it. Cover with salmon. Put in some red pepper, salt, and pepper to your taste. Feel free to put the other ingredients you prefer (tomatoes, onions) Enjoy your salmon snack!

250. Grams Soft Flourless Cookies

Time To Prepare: ten minutes Time to Cook: twenty-five minutes Yield: Servings 4

Ingredients:

¼ teaspoon of organic vanilla extract ¾ cup of shredded unsweetened coconut 1 peeled big banana Pinch of ground cinnamon

Directions:

Set the oven to 350F. Coat a cookie sheet with a big greased parchment paper. In a big food processor, put all ingredients and pulse till well blended. Ladle the mixture onto the prepared cookie sheet. Use your hands to flatten the cookies slightly. Bake for minimum twenty-five minutes or till golden brown.

251. Grams Spicy Bean Dip

Time To Prepare: ten minutes Time to Cook: 0 minutes Yield: Servings 3

Ingredients:

¼ Teaspoon Ground Cumin ¼ Teaspoon Sea Salt 1 Tablespoon Apple Cider Vinegar 1 Teaspoon Lime Juice, Fresh 14 Ounce Can Black Beans, Drained & Rinsed 14 Ounce Can Kidney Beans, Drained & Rinsed 2 Cherry Tomatoes 2 Cloves Garlic 2 Tablespoons Water 2 Teaspoon Honey, Raw Black Pepper to Taste Pinch Cayenne Pepper

Directions:

Mix all of your ingredients in a food processor, and blend until it's smooth. Cover, and place in your fridge before you serve.

252. Sweet Potato Muffins

Time To Prepare: fifteen minutes Time to Cook: 20-twenty-five minutes Yield: Servings 12

Ingredients:

¼ Cup Almond Butter ¼ Teaspoon Sea Salt ½ Teaspoon Baking Soda 1 ½ Cups Rolled Oats 1 Cup Almond Milk 1 Cup Sweet Potato, Cooked & Pureed 1 Egg 1 Teaspoon Baking Powder 1 Teaspoon Ground Cinnamon 1 Teaspoon Vanilla Extract, Pure 1/3 Cup Coconut Sugar 2 Tablespoons Olive Oil

Directions:

Begin by heating the oven to 375. Coat your muffin tin with liners, and get out a food processor. Pulse your oats until it forms a course flour. Move it to a small container before setting it to the side. Put in all of your ingredients apart from for the oat flour, blending until the desired smoothness is achieved. Slowly put in in your oat flour, pulsing until it's well blended. Cut between your cupcake liners, and bake for about twenty minutes. Let them cool for minimum five minutes before you serve.

253. Tangy Turmeric Flavored Florets

Time To Prepare: ten minutes Time to Cook: 55 minutes Yield: Servings 1

Ingredients:

1-head cauliflower, chopped into florets 1-Tbsp olive oil 1-Tbsp turmeric A dash of salt A pinch of cumin

Directions:

Set the oven to 400°F. Combine all ingredients in a baking pan. Mix thoroughly until meticulously blended. Cover the pan using foil. Roast for forty minutes. Take away the foil cover and roast additionally for fifteen minutes.

254. Tofu Pudding

Time To Prepare: ten minutes Time to Cook: 0 minutes Yield: Servings 4

Ingredients:

1 cup strawberries 1 teaspoon honey 1 teaspoon pumpkin pie spice 1 teaspoon vanilla 12 ounces silken tofu, softened and well-drained 2 scoops of Protein powder 3/4 cup blueberries 4 almonds Fresh mint leaves

Directions:

Combine the tofu and Protein powder in a blender until thoroughly combined. Put in the blueberries, strawberries, honey, pumpkin pie spice, and vanilla. Blend until the desired smoothness is achieved. Cover and put on the refrigerator to chill for minimum 2 hours. Ladle into four dessert bowls and top with an almond and a mint leaf before you serve.

255. Turmeric Coconut Flour Muffins

Time To Prepare: five minutes Time to Cook: twenty-five minutes Yield: Servings 8

Ingredients:

½ cup Unsweetened coconut milk ½ tsp. Baking soda ½ tsp. Ginger powder ¾ cup & 2 tbsp. Coconut flour 1 tsp. Vanilla extract 1/3 cup Maple syrup 2 tsp. Turmeric 6 big Whole eggs Pepper and salt

Directions:

Preheat your oven to 350°F. Coat 8 muffin tins with 8 muffin liners. Whisk eggs, maple syrup, milk, and vanilla extract in a mixing container until the egg begins to make bubbles. In a different container, combine the coconut flour, turmeric powder, pepper, baking soda, ginger powder, and salt. Place the dry mixture into the wet mixture then stir until it's all mixed and thick. Ladle out the batter into prepared muffin tins. Leave to bake for about twenty-five minutes or until it looked golden. Allow the muffins cool for a couple of minutes before transferring them to a rack.

256. Spinach & Berries Smoothie

Yield: 1 serving Preparation Time: 10 minutes

Ingredients:

1 cup mixed frozen berries (blueberries, strawberries, cranberries) • 2 cups fresh spinach • 1 cup celery stalk, chopped • 2-inch pieces fresh ginger, peeled and chopped • 3 tablespoons hemp Protein powder • ½ cup filtered water

Directions:

In an increased speed blender, add all ingredients and pulse till smooth. 2. Transfer right into a glass and serve immediately.

257. Nutty Berries & Spinach Smoothie

Yield: 3 servings Preparation Time: 10 min

Ingredients:

¾ cup frozen blackberries • ¾ cup frozen blueberries • 1 frozen banana, peeled and sliced • 1 cup fresh baby spinach • ¼ cup raw walnuts • 1 teaspoon bee pollen • 1½ cups unswee10ed almond milk

Directions:

1. In an increased speed blender, add all ingredients and pulse till smooth. 2. Transfer into 2 glasses and serve immediately.

258. Veggies & Turmeric Smoothie

Yield: 2 servings Preparation Time: 10 minutes

Ingredients:

1 small avocado, peeled, pitted and chopped • ½ of green bell pepper, seeded and chopped • 1-inch fresh turmeric piece, peeled and grated • 1 cup fresh baby spinach, chopped • 1 cup fresh arugula, chopped • 1-inch fresh ginger piece, peeled and chopped • ¾ cups fresh parsley • Pinch of cayenne • Pinch of salt • 1 cup fresh coconut water

Directions:

1. In a top speed blender, add all ingredients and pulse till smooth. 2. Transfer into 2 glasses and serve immediately.

259. Pineapple & Green Tea Smoothie

Yield: 1 servings Preparation Time: 10 min

Ingredients:

1 cup pineapple, chopped • 1 small little bit of ginger, peeled and chopped • ½ teaspoon ground turmeric • 1 teaspoon natural immune support • 1 teaspoon chia seeds • 1 cup cold teas • ½ cup Ice, crushed

Directions: 1. In an increased speed blender, add all ingredients and pulse till smooth. 2. Transfer in a glass and serve immediately.

260. Spiced Peach Smoothie

Yield: 2 servings Preparation Time: 10 minutes

Ingredients:

½ of frozen banana, peeled and chopped • 1 cup frozen peaches, pitted and chopped • ½ teaspoon ground ginger • ½ teaspoon chia seeds • 1 teaspoon ground turmeric • 1 teaspoon ground cinnamon • 1 teaspoon raw honey • 10-ounce unswee10ed almond milk

Directions: 1. In a higher speed blender, add all ingredients and pulse till smooth. 2. Transfer right into a glass and serve immediately.

261. Pineapple, Avocado & Spinach Smoothie

Yield: 2 servings Preparation Time: 10 minutes

Ingredients:

¼ of pineapple, peeled and chopped • 3 cups spinach, chopped • ¼ of avocado, peeled, pitted and chopped • ¼ cup fresh cilantro, chopped • ½-inch fresh ginger piece, peeled and chopped • 1 tablespoon chia seeds • 1 tablespoon ground turmeric • Fresh cracked black pepper, to taste

Directions: 1. In a high speed blender, add all ingredients and pulse till smooth. 2. Transfer right into a glass and serve immediately.

262. Strawberry & Beet Smoothie

Yield: 2 servings Preparation Time: 10 minutes

Ingredients:

2 cups frozen strawberries, pitted and chopped • 2/3 cup roasted and frozen beet, chopped • 1 teaspoon fresh ginger, peeled and grated • 1 teaspoon fresh turmeric, peeled and grated • ½ cup fresh orange juice • 1 cup almond milk

Directions:

1. In a top speed blender, add all ingredients and pulse till smooth. 2. Transfer into 2 glasses and serve immediately.

263. Pineapple & Coconut Smoothie

Yield: 1 serving Preparation Time: 10 minutes

Ingredients:

• 1 cup fresh pineapple, diced • 1 tablespoon coconut, shredded • ½ lime, peeled and seeded • 1 tablespoon chia seeds • 1 teaspoon ground turmeric • Pinch of freshly ground black pepper • ½ cup coconut water

Directions:

1. In a high speed blender, add all ingredients and pulse till smooth. 2. Transfer in a glass and serve immediately.

264. Pineapple & Mango Smoothie

Yield: 1 serving Preparation Time: 10 min

Ingredients:

2¼ cups mixed mango and pineapple, peeled and chopped • 1 tablespoon chia seeds • 1 teaspoon ground turmeric • ½ teaspoon ground ginger • ½ teaspoon ground cinnamon • Pinch of vanilla powder • 1 cup coconut milk • 1 teaspoon coconut oil

Directions:

1. In a higher speed blender, add all ingredients and pulse till smooth. 2. Transfer into a glass and serve immediately.

265. Berries, Watermelon & Avocado

Yield: 1 serving Preparation Time: 10 minutes

Ingredients:

1½ cups mixed frozen berries • 1 cup watermelon, peeled, seeded and chopped • ¼ avocado, peeled, pitted and chopped • 1 inch fresh ginger piece, peeled and chopped • 2 teaspoons chia seeds • ¾ cup fresh coconut water

Directions:

1. In a high speed blender, add all ingredients and pulse till smooth. 2. Transfer into a glass and serve immediately.

266. Apple, Strawberry & Beet Smoothie

Yield: 4 servings Preparation Time: 10 min

Ingredients:

2 cups frozen strawberries, hulled and sliced • 1 beet, peeled and chopped • 1 cup apple, peeled, cored and sliced • 3 Medjool dates, pitted and chopped • ¼ cup extra virgin coconut oil • ½ cup unswee10ed almond milk

Directions:

1. In an increased speed blender, add all ingredients and pulse till smooth. 2. Transfer into a glass and serve immediately.

267. Spiced Banana Smoothie

Yield: 1 serving Preparation Time: 10 min

Ingredients:

2 bananas, peeled and sliced • 2 teaspoons ground ginger • ½ teaspoon ground turmeric • ½ teaspoon organic organic vanilla flavor • 1 tablespoon honey • 1 cup coconut milk • 6-8 ice cubes, crushed

Directions:

1. In a high speed blender, add all ingredients and pulse till smooth. 2. Transfer right into a glass and serve immediately.

268. Papaya & Pineapple Smoothie

Yield: 1 serving Preparation Time: 10 minutes

Ingredients:

1½ cups pineapple, peeled and chopped • ½ of papaya, peeled and chopped • 2 dates, pitted • 1½ cups coconut water

Directions:

1. In a higher speed blender, add all ingredients and pulse till smooth. 2. Transfer in a glass and serve immediately.

269. Cherry & Pineapple Smoothie

Yield: 1 serving Preparation Time: 10 min

Ingredients:

¼ of pineapple, peeled and chopped • 12 fresh cherries, pitted • ¼ of beetroot, peeled and chopped • 1 tablespoon chia seeds • 1 cup coconut water • ½ cup ice, crushed

Directions:

1. In a high speed blender, add all ingredients and pulse till smooth. 2. Transfer in to a glass and serve immediately.

270. Pineapple, Mango & Coconut Smoothie

Yield: 2 servings Preparation Time: 10 min

Ingredients:

1 cup pineapple, chopped • ½ cup mango, peeled, pitted and chopped • Flesh and water of your coconut • 1 tablespoon Goji berries • ½ teaspoon fresh turmeric, chopped • 1 teaspoon chia seeds • 1 cup brewed teas

Directions:

1. In a higher speed blender, add all ingredients and pulse till smooth. 2. Transfer into 2 glasses and serve immediately.

271. Tangy Ginger & Radish Smoothie

Yield: 2 servings Preparation Time: 10 minutes

Ingredients:

1 orange, peeled, seeded and sliced • 1 radish, trimmed and chopped • 1 tablespoon fresh ginger, peeled and chopped • 5-10 fresh mint leaves • 1 tablespoon ground chia seeds • 1 teaspoon organic honey • 1 cup spring water • ½ cup fresh orange juice • 1 tablespoon freshly squeezed lemon juice • Ice, as required

Directions:

In a higher speed blender, add all ingredients and pulse till smooth. 2. Transfer into 2 glasses and serve immediately.

1.

272. Strawberry & Kale Smoothie

Yield: 1 serving Preparation Time: 10 min

Ingredients:

½ fresh strawberries, hulled and sliced • 1 cup fresh kale, trimmed and chopped • 1 celery stalk, chopped • ½ of lime, peeled • 1 cup coconut water

Directions:

1. In a higher speed blender, add all ingredients and pulse till smooth. 2. Transfer in a glass and serve immediately.

273. Almond Butter Smoothies

Time To Prepare: five minutes Time to Cook: 0 minutes Yield: Servings 1

Ingredients:

1 banana, if possible frozen for a creamier shake 1 cup of hemp milk 1 scoop of hemp protein 1 Tablespoon natural almond butter few ice cubes

Directions:

Blend all ingredients together and enjoy!

274. Baby Kale Pineapple Smoothie

Time To Prepare: five minutes Time to Cook: 0 minutes Yield: Servings 1

Ingredients:

1 cup almond milk 1 cup Kale 1 tablespoon hemp protein powder 1/2 cup frozen pineapple

Directions:

Put the almond milk, pineapple, and greens in the blender and blend until the desired smoothness is achieved.

275. Beet Smoothie

Time To Prepare: ten minutes Time to Cook: 0 minutes Yield: Servings 2

Ingredients:

1 tbsp. almond butter 1/2 banana, peeled and frozen 1/2 cup cherries, pitted 10 oz. almond milk, unsweetened 2 beets, peeled and quartered

Directions:

In your blender, combine the milk with the beets, banana, cherries, and butter. Pulse thoroughly, pour into glasses, before you serve. Enjoy!

276. Blackberry & Ginger Milkshake

Time To Prepare: five minutes Time to Cook: 0 minutes Yield: Servings 2

Ingredients:

1 thumb-sized piece of ginger, grated 2 cups of almond milk 2 cups of blackberries, washed 2 cups of chopped peaches

Directions:

Combine all ingredients to a blender or juicer and blend until the desired smoothness is achieved. Serve with a scattering of fresh blackberries and enjoy!

277. Blended Coconut Milk and Banana Breakfast Smoothie

Time To Prepare: ten minutes Time to Cook: 0 minutes Yield: Servings 4

Ingredients:

2 cups almond milk 2 cups coconut milk 4 ripe moderate-sized bananas 4 tbsp. flax seeds 4 tsp. cinnamon

Directions:

Peel the banana and cut it into ½-inch pieces. Put all the ingredients in the blender and blend into a smoothie. Put in a dash of cinnamon at the top of the smoothie before you serve.

278. Blueberry Lime Juice

Time To Prepare: five minutes Time to Cook: five minutes Yield: Servings 4

Ingredients:

1 cup fresh blueberries Water to cover contents Zest and juice of 1 lime

Directions:

Put ingredients in a mesh steamer basket for instant pot. Put in pot. Pour in water to immerse contents. Secure the lid. Cook on HIGH pressure five minutes. When done, depressurize swiftly. Remove steamer basket. Discard cooked produce. Let flavored water cool. Chill completely before you serve.

279. Blueberry Pomegranate Smoothie

Time To Prepare: five minutes Time to Cook: 0 minutes Yield: Servings 2

Ingredients:

¼ cup of canned coconut milk 1 cup of pomegranate juice, unsweetened 1 tbsp. of hemp seeds 2 cup of frozen blueberries 6 to 8 ice cubes

Directions:

Mix the smoothie ingredients in your high-speed blender. Pulse the ingredients a few times to cut them up. Combine the mixture on the highest speed setting for thirty to 60 seconds. Pour into glasses and serve.

280. Broccoli Smoothie

Time To Prepare: five minutes Time to Cook: 0 minutes Yield: Servings 4

Ingredients:

1 ½ cups strawberries 1 ½ cups water 1 cup broccoli florets 1 cup chopped spinach 2 bananas, cut, frozen 2 cups frozen mango chunks 2 cups pineapple juice

Directions: Combine all ingredients into a blender and blend until the desired smoothness is achieved. Pour into 4 tall glasses before you serve.

281. Cherry Smoothie

Time To Prepare: five minutes Time to Cook: 0 minutes Yield: Servings 4-6

Ingredients:

1 ½ cups vanilla Greek yogurt 2 bananas, cut 3 cups cherry juice 3 cups pitted, froze dark sweet cherries Fresh cherries, pitted Mint sprigs To decorate: Optional

Directions:

Combine all ingredients into a blender and blend until the desired smoothness is achieved. Pour into 4 tall glasses. Decorate using optional ingredients if using before you serve.

282. Chocolate Latte with Reishi

Time To Prepare: five minutes Time to Cook: ten minutes Yield: Servings 2

Ingredients:

1 teaspoon Reishi powder 2 tablespoons coconut butter 4 cups almond milk, unsweetened 4 teaspoons raw cacao powder A pinch ground cinnamon A pinch sea salt Sweetener of your choice

Directions:

Put in almond milk into a deep cooking pan. Put the deep cooking pan using low heat. When the milk is warm and just starts to bubble, remove the heat. Move into a blender. Put in the remaining ingredients and blend for 30 – 40 seconds or until the desired smoothness is achieved. Pour into mugs before you serve.

283. Cucumber Kiwi Green Smoothie

Time To Prepare: five minutes Time to Cook: 0 minutes Yield: Servings 2

Ingredients:

¼ cup of canned coconut milk 1 cup of coconut water 1 cup of seedless cucumber, chopped 2 ripe kiwi fruit 2 tbsps. of fresh chopped cilantro 6 to 8 ice cubes ice cubes

Directions:

Mix the smoothie ingredients in your high-speed blender. Pulse the ingredients a few times to cut them up. Combine the mixture on the highest speed setting for thirty to 60 seconds. Pour into glasses and serve.

284. Dreamy Yummy Orange Cream Smoothie

Time To Prepare: five minutes Time to Cook: 0 minutes Yield: Servings 2

Ingredients:

¼ cup of fresh orange juice ½ cup of canned full-fat coconut milk 1 cup of almond milk 1 navel orange, peel removed 6 to 8 ice cubes

Directions:

Mix the smoothie ingredients in your high-speed blender. Pulse the ingredients a few times to cut them up. Combine the mixture on the highest speed setting for thirty to 60 seconds. Pour into glasses and serve.

285. Flu Fighting Tonic

Time To Prepare: five minutes Time to Cook: ten minutes Yield: Servings 2

Ingredients:

½ teaspoon turmeric powder 2 tablespoons clear honey if possible manuka Boiling water, as required Juice of 2 lemons Lemon slices to decorate

Directions:

Split the lemon juice into 2 mugs. Put in ¼ teaspoon turmeric powder into each mug. Put in a tablespoon of honey into each mug. Pour boiling water to fill up the mugs. Stir. Decorate using a slice of lemon before you serve.

286. Fresh Tropical Juice

Time To Prepare: five minutes Time to Cook: 0 minutes Yield: Servings 2

Ingredients:

1 whole pineapple, peeled and slice into chunks. 1 cup of water 1/2 can of low-fat coconut milk

Directions: Put in all ingredients to a juicer and blend until the desired smoothness is achieved. Serve over ice

287. Ginger, Carrot, and Turmeric Smoothie

Time To Prepare: five minutes Time to Cook: 0 minutes Yield: Servings 2

Ingredients:

½ cup Mango, fresh or frozen chunks 1 big Carrot, peeled and chopped 1 cup Coconut water 1 Orange, peeled and separated 1 tbsp. Hemp seeds, raw, shelled 1 tsp. Ginger, ground 1 tsp. Turmeric, ground 1/8 tsp. Cayenne pepper

Directions:

Puree all of the ingredients with one-half cup of ice until the desired smoothness is achieved and drink instantly.

288. Green Vanilla Smoothie

Time To Prepare: ten minutes Time to Cook: 0 minutes Yield: Servings 1

Ingredients:

1 1/2 cups fresh spinach leaves 1 banana, cut in chunks 1 cup grapes 1 tub (6 oz.) vanilla yogurt 1/2 apple, cored and chopped

Directions:

Put in everything to a blender jug. Cover the jug firmly. Blend until the desired smoothness is achieved. Serve and enjoy!

289. Hot Apple Cider

Time To Prepare: five minutes Time to Cook: fifteen minutes Yield: Servings 4

Ingredients:

½ cup fresh cranberries ½ cup honey ½ star of anise ½ tsp whole cloves 1 lemon, peeled, cut into segments 1 orange, peeled, cut into segments 2 cinnamon sticks 7 medium apples, cored, quarter Water to cover ingredients

Directions:

Put in apples, lemon, orange, and cranberries to the instant pot. Put in cinnamon stick, star anise, and cloves. Pour in water to immerse ingredients. Secure the lid. Cook on HIGH pressure fifteen minutes. Depressurize naturally. Mash fruit using a masher to release juices. Strain the liquid. Chill completely before you serve

290. Instant Horchata

Time To Prepare: five minutes Time to Cook: five minutes Yield: Servings 4

Ingredients:

1 cinnamon stick, broken into little chunks 32 ounces rice milk 6 tbsp. honey

Directions:

Put in listed ingredients to the instant pot. Secure the lid. Cook on HIGH pressure five minutes. When done, depressurize naturally over ten minutes. Cool thoroughly. Chill before you serve.

291. Kale Smoothie

Time To Prepare: ten minutes Time to Cook: 0 minutes Yield: Servings 2

Ingredients:

10 kale leaves 2 pears, chopped 5 bananas, peeled and slice into chunks 5 cups almond milk 5 tbsp. almond butter

Directions:

In your blender, combine the kale with the bananas, pears, almond butter, and almond milk. Pulse thoroughly, split into glasses, before you serve. Enjoy!

292. Lemon Ginger Iced Tea

Time To Prepare: five minutes Time to Cook: ten minutes Yield: Servings 2-3

Ingredients:

¼ teaspoon turmeric 1 tablespoon fresh lemon juice or to taste (not necessary) 1 tablespoon maple syrup 2 – 3 lemon slices 2 inches fresh ginger, peeled, thinly cut or to taste 3-4 cups water A pinch ground cinnamon

Directions:

Pour water into a deep cooking pan. Put in ginger, turmeric, lemon slices, and cinnamon. Put the deep cooking pan on moderate heat. Cover and simmer for eight - ten minutes. Strain and pour into a jar. Place the maple syrup, and lemon juice, then stir. Chill for eight – 10 hours. Stir thoroughly. Pour into glasses before you serve.

293. Mango Tomato Smoothie

Time To Prepare: five minutes Time to Cook: 0 minutes Yield: Servings 4

Ingredients:

1 cup almond milk 2 cups chopped cilantro 2 cups pineapple chunks 2 mangoes, peeled, pitted 4 Campari tomatoes, chopped 6 cups fresh baby spinach

Directions:

Combine all ingredients into a blender and blend until the desired smoothness is achieved. Pour into 4 tall glasses before you serve.

294. Parsley Ginger Green Juice

Time To Prepare: five minutes Time to Cook: 0 minutes Yield: Servings 2

Ingredients:

2 cucumbers, chopped 2 green apples, cored 2 lemons, peeled, halved 4 cups chopped parsley 4 cups chopped spinach 4 inches fresh ginger, peeled, cut 6 stalks celery, chopped

Directions:

Juice together all the ingredients in a juicer. Pour into 2 glasses before you serve.

295. Peach Maple Smoothie

Time To Prepare: ten minutes Time to Cook: 0 minutes Yield: Servings 1

Ingredients:

1 cup fat-free yogurt 1 cup ice 2 tbsp. maple syrup 4 big peaches, peeled and chopped

Directions:

Put in everything to a blender jug. Cover the jug firmly. Blend until the desired smoothness is achieved. Serve and enjoy!

296. Pineapple & Ginger Juice

Time To Prepare: five minutes Time to Cook: 0 minutes Yield: Servings 2

Ingredients:

2 apples, cored, chopped 2 cucumbers, chopped 2 cups chopped pineapple 2 cups spinach 2 inches ginger, peeled, cut 2 lemons, peeled, halved 8 celery stalks, chopped

Directions:

Juice together all the ingredients in a juicer. Pour into 2 glasses before you serve.

297. Pineapple- Ginger Smoothie

Time To Prepare: five minutes Time to Cook: 0 minutes Yield: Servings 1

Ingredients:

½ inch thick ginger, cut 1 cup coconut milk 1 cup pineapple slice

Directions:

Put all ingredients in a blender. Pulse until the desired smoothness is achieved. Chill before you serve.

298. Pink California Smoothie

Time To Prepare: ten minutes Time to Cook: 0 minutes Yield: Servings 1

Ingredients:

1 container (8 oz.) lemon yogurt 1/3 cup orange juice 7 big strawberries

Directions:

Put in everything to a blender jug. Cover the jug firmly. Blend until the desired smoothness is achieved. Serve and enjoy!

299. Grams Purple Fruit Smoothie

Time To Prepare: ten minutes Time to Cook: 0 minutes Yield: Servings 1

Ingredients:

2 frozen bananas, cut in chunks 1 cup orange juice 1 tbsp. honey, optional 1 tsp. vanilla extract, optional 1/2 cup frozen blueberries

Directions:

Put in everything to a blender jug. Cover the jug firmly. Blend until the desired smoothness is achieved. Serve and enjoy!

300. Raspberry Smoothie

Time To Prepare: ten minutes Time to Cook: 0 minutes Yield: Servings 2

Ingredients:

1 avocado, pitted and peeled 1/2 cup raspberries 3/4 cup raspberry juice 3/4 cup orange juice

Directions:

In your blender, combine the avocado with the raspberry juice, orange juice, and raspberries. Pulse thoroughly, split into 2 glasses, before you serve. Enjoy!

301. Strawberry Oatmeal Smoothie

Time To Prepare: ten minutes Time to Cook: 0 minutes Yield: Servings 1

Ingredients:

1 cup soy milk 1 banana, broken into chunks 14 frozen strawberries 1/2 cup rolled oats 1/2 tsp. vanilla extract 1 1/2 tsp. honey

Directions:

Put in everything to a blender jug. Cover the jug firmly. Blend until the desired smoothness is achieved. Serve and enjoy

302. Sweet Cranberry Juice

Time To Prepare: five minutes Time to Cook: 8 minutes Yield: Servings 4

Ingredients:

½ cup honey 1 cinnamon stick 1 gallon filtered water 4 cups fresh cranberries Juice of 1 lemon

Directions:

Put in cranberries, ½ of water, cinnamon cling to the instant pot. Secure the lid. Cook on HIGH pressure 8 minutes. Depressurize naturally. Once cool, strain liquid. Put in remaining water. Mix in honey and lemon. Cool thoroughly. Chill before you serve.

303. Tropical Mango Coconut Smoothie

Time To Prepare: five minutes Time to Cook: 0 minutes Yield: Servings 2

Ingredients:

½ cup of canned coconut milk ½ cup of fresh orange juice 1 ½ cups of frozen mango 1 ½ tsp of honey 1 medium frozen banana 1 tbsp. of fresh lemon juice

Directions:

Mix the smoothie ingredients in your high-speed blender. Pulse the ingredients a few times to cut them up. Combine the mixture on the highest speed setting for thirty to 60 seconds. Pour into glasses and serve.

304. Turmeric and Ginger Tonic

Time To Prepare: five minutes Time to Cook: ten minutes Yield: Servings 4

Ingredients:

1/8 teaspoon cayenne pepper 2 tablespoons grated, fresh ginger 2 tablespoons grated, fresh turmeric 6 cups water Juice of 2 lemons Maple syrup or honey to taste The rind of 2 lemons, peeled

Directions: Put in water, ginger, turmeric, cayenne pepper, and lemon rind into a deep cooking pan. Put the deep cooking pan on moderate to high heat. (Do not boil) Once the mixture is hot, remove from heat. Strain into 4 mugs. Put in honey and lemon juice and stir. Serve warm.

305. Turmeric Hot Chocolate

Time To Prepare: five minutes Time to Cook: ten minutes Yield: Servings 2

Ingredients:

1/8 tsp. cayenne pepper, optional 1/8 tsp. pepper 2 cups milk 2 tsp. ground turmeric 3 tbsp. cacao or cocoa powder 4 tsp. coconut oil 4 tsp. honey

Directions: Put in milk, turmeric, cocoa, and coconut oil into a deep cooking pan. Put the deep cooking pan on moderate heat. Coconut oil and pepper are added because it helps to absorb the turmeric. Whisk regularly until well blended. When it starts to boil, remove from heat. Put in honey, cayenne pepper, and pepper and whisk well. Split into 2 cups before you serve.

306. Vanilla Avocado Smoothie

Time To Prepare: ten minutes Time to Cook: 0 minutes Yield: Servings 1

Ingredients:

1 cup almond milk 1 ripe avocado, halved and pitted 1/2 cup vanilla yogurt 3 tbsp. honey 8 ice cubes

Directions:

Put in everything to a blender jug. Cover the jug firmly. Blend until the desired smoothness is achieved. Serve and enjoy!

307. Vanilla Turmeric Orange Juice

Time To Prepare: five minutes Time to Cook: 0 minutes Yield: Servings 2

Ingredients:

½ teaspoon turmeric powder 1 teaspoon ground cinnamon 2 cups unsweetened almond milk 2 teaspoons vanilla extract 6 oranges, peeled, separated into segments, deseeded Pepper to taste

Directions:

Juice the oranges. Put in the remaining ingredients. Pour into 2 glasses before you serve.

308. Wassail

Time To Prepare: five minutes Time to Cook: ten minutes Yield: Servings 4

Ingredients:

½ tsp nutmeg 1 inch peeled ginger 10 cloves 2 vanilla beans, split or 2 Tbsp pure vanilla extract 4 cups orange juice 5 cinnamon sticks 8 cups apple cider Zest and juice of 2 lemons

Directions:

Pour cider and orange juice in the instant pot. Put cinnamon sticks, nutmeg piece, cloves, lemon zest, vanilla beans in the steamer basket. If you didn't use vanilla beans, pour in vanilla extract. Put in lemon juice. Secure the lid. Cook on HIGH pressure ten minutes. When done, depressurize naturally. Discard contents of the steamer basket. Serve hot from the pot.

309. Wonderful Watermelon Drink

Time To Prepare: five minutes Time to Cook: 0 minutes Yield: Servings 2

Ingredients:

1 cup of coconut water 1 cup of watermelon chunks 1/2 cup of tart cherries 2 cups of frozen mixed berries 2 tbsp. of chia seeds

Directions:

Combine all ingredients in a blender or juicer then blend until pureed. Serve instantly and enjoy!

310. Sides Beet Hummus

Time To Prepare: five minutes Time to Cook: 0 minutes Yield: Servings 2

Ingredients:

¼ tsp of chili flakes ½ cup of olive oil ½ tsp of oregano ½ tsp of salt 1 ½ tsp of cumin 1 ¾ cup of chickpeas 1 clove of garlic 1 nub of fresh ginger 1 skinless roasted beet 1 tsp of curry 1 tsp of maple syrup 2 tbsp. of sunflower seeds Juice of one lemon

Directions: Blend all together the ingredients in a food processor until they're smooth and decorate them with sunflower seeds. Enjoy!

311. Caramelized Pears and Onions

Time To Prepare: five minutes Time to Cook: thirty-five minutes Yield: Servings 4

Ingredients:

1 tablespoon olive oil 2 firm red pears, cored and quartered 2 red onion, cut into wedges Salt and pepper, to taste

Directions:

Preheat the oven to 425 degrees F Put the pears and onion on a baking tray Sprinkle with olive oil Sprinkle with salt and pepper Bake using your oven for a little more than half an hour Serve and enjoy!

312. Cilantro And Avocado Platter

Time To Prepare: ten minutes Time to Cook: 0 minutes Yield: Servings 6

Ingredients:

¼ cup of fresh cilantro, chopped ½ a lime, juiced 1 big ripe tomato, chopped 1 green bell pepper, chopped 1 sweet onion, chopped 2 avocados, peeled, pitted and diced Salt and pepper as required

Directions:

Take a moderate-sized container and put in onion, bell pepper, tomato, avocados, lime and cilantro Mix thoroughly and give it a toss Sprinkle with salt and pepper in accordance with your taste Serve and enjoy!

313. Cool Garbanzo and Spinach Beans

Time To Prepare: 5-ten minutes Time to Cook: 0 minute Yield: Servings 4

Ingredients:

½ onion, diced ½ teaspoon cumin 1 tablespoon olive oil 10 ounces spinach, chopped 12 ounces garbanzo beans

Directions:

Take a frying pan and put in olive oil Put it on moderate to low heat Put in onions, garbanzo and cook for five minutes Mix in cumin, garbanzo beans, spinach and flavor with sunflower seeds Use a spoon to smash gently Cook meticulously Serve and enjoy

314. Creamy Polenta

Time To Prepare: 8 minutes Time to Cook: forty-five minutes Yield: Servings 4

Ingredients:

½ cup cream 1 ½ cup water 1 cup polenta 1/3 cup Parmesan, grated 2 cups chicken stock

Directions:

Put polenta in the pot. Put in water, chicken stock, cream, and Parmesan. Mix up polenta well. Then preheat oven to 355F. Cook polenta in your oven for about forty-five minutes. Mix up the cooked meal with the help of the spoon cautiously before you serve

315. Cucumber Yogurt Salad with Mint

Time To Prepare: ten minutes Time to Cook: 0 minutes Yield: Servings 2

Ingredients:

¼ cup organic coconut milk ¼ cup organic mint leaves ¼ teaspoon pink Himalayan sea salt ½ cup chopped organic red onion 1 tablespoon extra virgin olive oil 1 tablespoon plain organic goat yogurt 1 teaspoon organic dill weed 2 chopped organic cucumbers 3 tablespoons fresh organic lime juice

Directions:

Cut the red onion, dill, cucumbers, and mint and mix them in a big container. Blend them until they're smooth. Top the dressing onto the cucumber salad and mix meticulously. Chill for minimum 1 hour and serve. Enjoy!

316. Farro Salad with Arugula

Time To Prepare: ten minutes Time to Cook: thirty-five minutes Yield: Servings 2

Ingredients:

½ cup farro ½ teaspoon ground black pepper ½ teaspoon Italian seasoning ½ teaspoon olive oil 1 ½ cup chicken stock 1 cucumber, chopped 1 tablespoon lemon juice 1 teaspoon salt 2 cups arugula, chopped

Directions:

Mix up together farro, salt, and chicken stock and move mixture in the pan. Close the lid and boil it for a little more than half an hour. In the meantime, place all rest of the ingredients in the salad container. Chill the farro to the room temperature and put in it in the salad container too. Mix up the salad well.

317. Fresh Strawberry Salsa

Time To Prepare: ten minutes Time to Cook: 0 minutes Yield: Servings 6-8

Ingredients:

¼ cup fresh lime juice ½ cup fresh cilantro ½ cup red onion, finely chopped ½ teaspoon lime zest, grated 1-2 jalapeños, deseeded, finely chopped 2 kiwi fruit, peeled, chopped 2 pounds fresh ripe strawberries, hulled, chopped 2 teaspoons pure raw honey

Directions:

Put in lime juice, lime zest and honey into a big container and whisk well. Put in remaining ingredients then mix thoroughly. Cover and set aside for a while for the flavors to set in and serve

318. Green Beans

Time To Prepare: five minutes Time to Cook: ten minutes Yield: Servings 5

Ingredients:

½ teaspoon kosher salt ½ teaspoon of red pepper flakes 1½ lbs. green beans, trimmed 2 garlic cloves, minced 2 tablespoons of extra-virgin olive oil 2 tablespoons of water

Directions:

Heat oil in a frying pan on medium temperature. Include the pepper flake. Stir to coat in the olive oil. Include the green beans. Cook for seven minutes. Stir frequently. The beans must be brown in some areas. Put in the salt and garlic. Cook for a minute, while stirring. Pour water and cover instantly. Cook covered for 1 more minute

319. Hot Pink Coconut Slaw

Time To Prepare: five minutes Time to Cook: 0 minutes Yield: Servings 3

Ingredients:

¼ cup fresh cilantro, chopped ¼ teaspoon salt ½ cup big coconut flakes, unsweetened or shredded coconut, unsweetened ½ cup radish, thinly cut or shredded carrots ½ small jalapeño, deseeded, discard membranes, chopped ½ tablespoon honey or maple syrup 1 cup red onion, thinly cut 1 tablespoon olive oil 2 cups purple cabbage, thinly cut 2 tablespoons apple cider vinegar 2 tablespoons lime juice

Directions:

Combine all ingredients into a container and toss thoroughly. Cover and set aside for about forty minutes. Toss thoroughly before you serve.

320. Mascarpone Couscous

Time To Prepare: fifteen minutes Time to Cook: 7.5 hours Yield: Servings 4

Ingredients:

½ cup mascarpone 1 cup couscous 1 teaspoon ground paprika 1 teaspoon salt 3 ½ cup chicken stock

Directions:

Put chicken stock and mascarpone in the pan and bring the liquid to boil. Put in salt and ground paprika. Stir gently and simmer for a minute. Take off the liquid from the heat and put in couscous. Stir thoroughly and close the lid. Leave couscous for about ten minutes. Mix the cooked side dish well before you serve.

321. Mushroom Millet

Time To Prepare:ten minutes Time to Cook: fifteen minutes Yield:Servings 3

Ingredients:

¼ cup mushrooms, cut ½ cup millet ¾ cup onion, diced 1 cup of water 1 tablespoon olive oil 1 teaspoon butter 1 teaspoon salt 3 tablespoons milk

Directions:

Pour olive oil in the frying pan then put the onion. Put in mushrooms and roast the vegetables for about ten minutes over the moderate heat. Stir them occasionally. In the meantime, pour water in the pan. Put in millet and salt. Cook the millet with the closed lid for fifteen minutes over the moderate heat. Then put in the cooked mushroom mixture in the millet. Put in milk and butter. Mix up the millet well.

322. Parmesan Roasted Broccoli

Time To Prepare:ten minutes Time to Cook: twenty minutes Yield:Servings 6

Ingredients:

½ teaspoon of Italian seasoning 1 tablespoon of lemon juice 1 tablespoon parsley, chopped 3 tablespoons of olive oil 3 tablespoons of vegan parmesan, grated 4 cups of broccoli florets Pepper and salt to taste

Directions:

Preheat the oven to 450 degrees F. Apply cooking spray on your pan. Keep the broccoli florets in a freezer bag. Now put in the Italian seasoning, olive oil, pepper, and salt. Seal your bag. Shake it. Coat well. Pour your broccoli on the pan. It must be in a single layer. Bake for about twenty minutes. Stir midway through. Take out from the oven. Drizzle parsley and parmesan. Sprinkle some lemon juice. You can decorate with lemon wedges if you wish.

323. Red Cabbage with Cheese

Time To Prepare:five minutes Time to Cook: twelve minutes Yield:Servings 4

Ingredients:

¼ cup & 1 tbsp. of extra virgin olive oil ¼ tsp of freshly ground pepper ¼ tsp of salt 1 cup of walnuts 1 Tbsp. of crumbled blue cheese 1 tbsp. of Dijon mustard 1 tsp of butter 2 thinly cut scallions 3 tbsp. of pure maple syrup 3 tbsp. of red wine vinegar 8 cups of red cabbage, thinly cut

Directions: For the vinaigrette: Combine the blue cheese, ¼ cup of olive oil, mustard, vinegar, salt, and pepper in a food processor or blender until the mixture has a creamy consistency. For the salad: Put a parchment paper near the stove. Heat 1 tbsp. Of oil on moderate heat in a moderate-sized frying pan and mix in the walnuts, cooking them for approximately 2 minutes. Now mix salt and pepper, sprinkle maple syrup and cook for approximately three to five minutes while stirring the mixture up to the nuts are uniformly coated. Move to the paper and pour the rest of the syrup over them using a spoon. Separate the nuts and cool down for approximately five minutes. In a big container, put in the cabbage and scallions and toss them with the vinaigrette. Put in the walnuts and blue cheese as toppings.

324. Roasted Carrots

Time To Prepare: ten minutes Time to Cook: forty minutes Yield: Servings 4

Ingredients:

¼ teaspoon ground pepper ½ teaspoon rosemary, chopped ½ teaspoon salt 1 onion, peeled & cut 1 teaspoon thyme, chopped 2 tablespoons of extra-virgin olive oil 8 carrots, peeled & cut

Directions:

Preheat the oven to 425 degrees F. Combine the onions and carrots by tossing in a container with rosemary, thyme, pepper, and salt. Spread on your baking sheet. Roast for forty minutes. The onions and carrots must be browning and soft

325. Roasted Parsnips

Time To Prepare: five minutes Time to Cook: thirty minutes Yield: Servings 4

Ingredients:

1 tablespoon of extra-virgin olive oil 1 teaspoon of kosher salt 1½ teaspoon of Italian seasoning 2 lbs. parsnips Chopped parsley for decoration

Directions:

Preheat the oven to 400 degrees F. Peel the parsnips. Cut them into one-inch chunks. Now toss with the seasoning, salt, and oil in a container. Spread this on your baking sheet. It must be in a single layer. Roast for half an hour Stir every ten minutes. Move to a plate. Decorate using parsley.

326. Shoepeg Corn Salad

Time To Prepare: ten minutes Time to Cook: 0 minute Yield: Servings 4

Ingredients:

¼ cup Greek yogurt ½ cup cherry tomatoes halved 1 cup shoepeg corn, drained 1 jalapeno pepper, chopped 1 tablespoon chives, chopped 1 tablespoon lemon juice 3 tablespoons fresh cilantro, chopped

Directions:

In the salad container, mix up together shoepeg corn, cherry tomatoes, jalapeno pepper, chives, and fresh cilantro. Put in lemon juice and Greek yogurt. Mix yo the salad well. Put in your fridge and store it for maximum 1 day.

327. Spicy Barley

Time To Prepare: seven minutes Time to Cook: 42 minutes Yield: Servings 5

Ingredients:

½ teaspoon cayenne pepper ½ teaspoon chili pepper ½ teaspoon ground black pepper 1 cup barley 1 teaspoon butter 1 teaspoon olive oil 1 teaspoon salt 3 cups chicken stock

Directions:

Put barley and olive oil in the pan. Roast barley on high heat for a minute. Stir it well. Then put in salt, chili pepper, ground black pepper, cayenne pepper, and butter. Put in chicken stock. Close the lid and cook barley for forty minutes over the medium-low heat.

328. Spicy Wasabi Mayonnaise

Time To Prepare: fifteen minutes Time to Cook: 0 minute Yield: Servings 4

Ingredients:

½ tablespoon wasabi paste 1 cup mayonnaise

Directions:

Take a container and mix wasabi paste and mayonnaise Mix thoroughly Allow it to chill, use as required Serve and enjoy

329. Stir-Fried Farros

Time To Prepare: five minutes Time to Cook: thirty-five minutes Yield: Servings 2

Ingredients:

½ cup farro ½ teaspoon ground coriander ½ teaspoon paprika ½ teaspoon turmeric 1 ½ cup water 1 carrot, grated 1 tablespoon butter 1 teaspoon chili flakes 1 teaspoon salt 1 yellow onion, cut

Directions:

Put farro in the pan. Put in water and salt. Close the lid and boil it for half an hour In the meantime, toss the butter in the frying pan. Heat it and put in cut onion and grated carrot. Fry the vegetables for about ten minutes over the moderate heat. Stir them with the help of spatula occasionally. When the farro is cooked, put in it in the roasted vegetables and mix up well. Cook stir-fried farro for five minutes over the moderate to high heat.

330. Thyme with Honey-Roasted Carrots

Time To Prepare: five minutes Time to Cook: thirty minutes Yield: Servings 4

Ingredients:

½ teaspoon of sea salt ½ teaspoon thyme, dried 1 tablespoon of honey 1/5 lb. carrots, with the tops 2 tablespoons of olive oil

Directions:

Preheat the oven to 425 degrees F. Place parchment paper on your baking sheet. Toss your carrots with honey, oil, thyme, and salt. Coat well. Keep in a single layer. Bake in the oven for half an hour Allow to cool before you serve

331. Wheatberry Salad

Time To Prepare: ten minutes Time to Cook: 50 minutes Yield: Servings 2

Ingredients:

¼ cup fresh parsley, chopped ¼ cup of wheat berries 1 cup of water 1 tablespoon canola oil 1 tablespoon chives, chopped 1 teaspoon chili flakes 1 teaspoon salt 2 oz. pomegranate seeds 2 tablespoons walnuts, chopped

Directions: Put wheat berries and water in the pan. Put in salt and simmer the ingredients for about fifty minutes over the moderate heat. In the meantime, mix up together walnuts, chives, parsley, pomegranate seeds, and chili flakes. When the wheatberry is cooked, move it in the walnut mixture. Put in canola oil and mix up the salad well.

332. Balsamic Vinaigrette

Time To Prepare: ten minutes Time to Cook: 0 minutes Yield: Servings 2-4

Ingredients:

¼ tsp of freshly ground black pepper ½ cup of extra-virgin olive oil ½ cup of rice vinegar 1 clove of freshly minced garlic 1 tbsp. of honey or maple syrup 1 tsp of sea or kosher salt 2 tsp of Dijon mustard

Directions: Put all ingredients in a mason jar and cover firmly. Shake thoroughly until all ingredients are blended. Keep in your fridge for minimum 30 minutes before you serve to keep its freshness. Serve with a salad or as your meat marinate.

333. Cashew Ginger Dip

Time To Prepare: five minutes Time to Cook: 0 minutes Yield: Servings 1

Ingredients:

¼ cup filtered water ¼ teaspoon salt ½ teaspoon ground ginger 1 cup cashews, soaked in water for about twenty minutes and drained 1 tablespoon extra-virgin olive oil 1 teaspoon lemon juice 2 garlic cloves 2 teaspoons coconut aminos Pinch cayenne pepper

Directions: I

n a blender or food processor, put together the cashews, garlic, water, olive oil, aminos, lemon juice, ginger, salt, and cayenne pepper. Put in the mix in a container. Cover and place in your fridge until chilled. You can use store it for 4-5 days in your fridge

334. Creamy Homemade Greek Dressing

Time To Prepare: ten minutes Time to Cook: 0 minutes Yield: Servings 2-4

Ingredients:

¼ cup non-dairy milk (e.g., almond, rice milk) ½ cup of high-quality mayonnaise, without preservatives ½ tsp dried basil ½ tsp dried oregano ½ tsp parsley ½ tsp thyme 1/3 cup of extra-virgin olive oil 1/4 cup of white wine vinegar 2 cloves of garlic, minced 2 tbsp. of lemon or lime juice 2 tsp of honey A few tablespoons of water Some Kosher salt and pepper

Directions:

Put all together ingredients in a mason jar and shake, cover firmly, and shake thoroughly. Place in your fridge for a few hours before you serve or serve instantly on your favorite vegetable or fruit salad. Shake well before use. Put in your fridge for maximum 5 days. You may put in a few tablespoons of water to tune the consistency as per your preference.

335. Creamy Siamese Dressing

Time To Prepare: ten minutes Time to Cook: 0 minutes Yield: Servings 2-4

Ingredients:

¼ cup of non-dairy milk (e.g., almond, rice, soymilk) ¼ cup of unsweetened peanut sauce 1 cup of mayonnaise 1 tbsp. of honey or maple syrup 1 tbsps. freshly chopped cilantro 2 tbsp. of unsalted peanuts 2 tbsp. rice vinegar

Directions:

Put all ingredients apart from the cilantro and peanuts into a blender and blend until the desired smoothness is achieved and creamy. Next, put in in the cilantro and peanuts and pulse the blender a few times until completely crushed and well blended. Put in a mason jar and bring it in your fridge. Serve with a garden salad, pasta or as a dipping sauce.

336. Dairy-Free Creamy Turmeric Dressing

Time To Prepare: ten minutes Time to Cook: 0 minutes Yield: Servings 2-4

Ingredients:

½ cup of extra-virgin olive oil ½ cup of tahini 1 tbsp. of turmeric powder 2 tbsp. of lemon juice 2 tsp of honey Some sea salt and pepper

Directions:

In a container, whisk all ingredients until well blended. Store in a mason jar and place in your fridge for maximum 5 days.

337. Homemade Ginger Dressing

Time To Prepare: ten minutes Time to Cook: 0 minutes Yield: Servings 2-4

Ingredients:

¼ cup of chopped celery ¼ cup of honey or maple syrup ¼ cup of water ½ cup of chopped carrots ½ tsp of white pepper 1 cup of chopped onion 1 cup of extra-virgin olive oil 1 tsp of freshly minced garlic 1 tsp of kosher salt 2 ½ tbsp. of unsalted, gluten-free soy sauce 2 tbsp. of ketchup 2/3 cup of rice vinegar 6 tbsp. of freshly grated ginger

Directions:

Put the onion, ginger, celery, carrots, and garlic into a blender. Blend until the mixture are fine but still lumpy from the small vegetable chunks. Put in in the vinegar, water, ketchup, soy sauce, honey or maple syrup, lemon juice, salt, and pepper. Pulse until the ingredients are well blended. Slowly put in the oil while blending, until everything is thoroughly combined. The mixture must be runny but still grainy. Serve with a winter salad.

338. Homemade Ranch

Time To Prepare: ten minutes Time to Cook: 0 minutes Yield: Servings 2-4

Ingredients:

¼ cup of Greek yogurt ¼ tsp Kosher salt ½ cup of natural mayonnaise, without preservatives ½ tsp of dried dill ½ tsp of dried parsley ½ tsp of garlic powder ½ tsp of onion powder ¾ cup of non-dairy milk 1/8 tsp Freshly ground black pepper 2 tsp of dried chives

Directions:

Combine all ingredients apart from the milk into a medium container. Mix together until well blended. Put in in the milk and mix thoroughly. Pour in a mason jar or an airtight container. Serve instantly or place in your fridge for maximum 2 hours to keep the freshness. Put in your refrigerator for maximum 5 days. Serve with a garden or fruit salad.

339. Soy with Honey and Ginger Glaze

Time To Prepare: ten minutes Time to Cook: 0 minutes Yield: Servings 2-4

Ingredients:

¼ cup of honey 1 tbsp. of rice vinegar 1 tsp of freshly grated ginger 2 tbsp. gluten-free soy sauce

Directions:

Put all together the ingredients into a small container and whisk well. Serve with a vegetables, chickens, or seafood. Keep the glaze in a mason jar, firmly covered, and place in your fridge for maximum four days.

340. Tahini Dip

Time To Prepare: ten minutes Time to Cook: 0 minutes Yield: Servings 2-4

Ingredients:

¼ cup of tahini ½ tsp of maple syrup 1 small grated or thoroughly minced clove of garlic (this is optional) 1 tbsp. of apple cider vinegar 1 tbsp. of freshly squeezed lemon juice 1 tbsp. of tamari 1 tsp of finely grated ginger, or ½ tsp of ground ginger 1 tsp of turmeric 1/3 cup of water

Directions:

Blend or whisk all ingredients together. Place the dressing in an airtight container then place in your fridge for approximately 5 days. Enjoy!

341. Snacks Almond and Honey Homemade Bar

Time To Prepare: fifteen minutes + thirty minutes refrigerator time Time to Cook: fifteen minutes Yield: Servings 8

Ingredients:

¼ cup almond butter ¼ cup honey ¼ cup sugar (or another sweetener to your taste in adjusted amount) ¼ cup sunflower seeds ½ teaspoon vanilla extract 1 cup oats 1 cup whole-grain puffed cereal (unsweetened) 1 tbsp. flaxseeds 1 tbsp. sesame seeds 1/3 cup apricots (dried and chopped) 1/3 cup currants 1/3 cup raisins (chopped) 1/8 tsp salt A ¼ cup of almonds

Directions:

Preheat your oven to 350 degrees Fahrenheit. Place a baking paper to an 8-inch pan or coat it with cooking spray/oil. Combine the almonds, oats, and seeds and spread the mixture on a rimmed baking sheet. Bake the mixture until you notice that the oats are mildly toasted (for approximately ten minutes). Move the mixture to a container. Put in cereal, raisins, currants, and apricots to the container. Toss thoroughly to blend. Mix honey, almond butter, vanilla, salt, and sugar in a deep cooking pan. Heat on moderate heat. Stir regularly for 2-5 minutes until you see light bubbles. Once you notice the bubbles, pour the mixture over the dry mixture with apricots and oats you prepared previously. Mix thoroughly using a spatula. There mustn't be any dry spots. Move the new mixture to the previously prepared pan. Push it to the pan to make a firm and flat layer. Place in your refrigerator for half an hourChop the layer into eight equal bars or squares, to your taste. Consume instantly or place in your refrigerator up to seven days

342. Anti-Inflammatory Key Lime Pie

Time To Prepare: twenty minutes + thirty-five minutes refrigerator time Time to Cook: 0 Yield: Servings 8

Ingredients:

½ cup honey ½ cup Medjool dates, chopped and pitted 1 cup unsweetened shredded coconut 1 cup walnuts 1 teaspoon lime zest 1/4 teaspoon sea salt 3 firm avocados 3 tablespoons lime juice Lime slices Pinch of sea salt

Directions:

Use a food processor to put all together the walnuts, coconut, and the salt, then pulse until crudely ground. Place the dates and pulse until the mixture resembles bread crumbs, trying to stick together. Push the mixture into the edges and bottom of a non-stick greased 9-inch pie pan. Use your fingers or the back of a spoon to press the crust into a uniform layer. Bring the crust into the freezer for minimum fifteen minutes while preparing the filling. Use the food processor again and mix the avocado, honey, lime juice, lime zest, and salt. Process until the desired smoothness is achieved. Pour the filling into the now-chilled piecrust and place it in your fridge for about twenty minutes. Decorate using fresh lime slices and serve cold. Store any left overs in your fridge

343. Apple Crisp

Time To Prepare: fifteen minutes Time to Cook: twenty-five minutes Yield: Servings 6-8

Ingredients:

Topping: 1 ½ cups old-fashioned rolled oats 1 teaspoon salt ½ cup stevia 2 teaspoons ground cinnamon 1 cup nuts, crudely chopped 3 tablespoon melted coconut oil. 1/3 cup almond meal 2/3 cup shredded, unsweetened coconut 1/4 teaspoon ground nutmeg Apple filling: ½ cup stevia 1 tablespoon ground cinnamon 1 teaspoon vanilla 1/4 cup arrowroot flour 1/4 teaspoon salt 10 tart apples 2 tablespoons fresh-squeezed lemon juice 3 tablespoons melted coconut oil The zest of 1 orange

Directions:

Set the oven to 350 F then grease a 9 by a 13-inch baking pan with coconut oil. Put together the topping ingredients in a container, then mix and save for later. Combine the filling ingredients (except for the apples) in a second big container. Leave the skins on the apples, if you wish. Core them and slice super slim (1/8 inch thick). Toss the apples in the filling ingredients to coat uniformly. Put the apple mixture in a baking pan and spread the topping over it all, pushing down tightly. Put in your oven with a pan underneath to catch any drips. Bake for about twenty-five minutes or until the topping is brown and juices are bubbling. Apples must be tender. Cool slightly on a rack then serve

344. Avocado and Egg Sandwich

Time To Prepare: ten minutes Time to Cook: 0 minutes Yield: Servings 2

Ingredients:

½ lime juice 1 avocado (ripe) 1 egg, organic 1 scallion 2 radishes 2 slices of who wheat, seed bread A pinch of salt (sea or Himalayan) Black pepper – to your taste Mixed seeds – to your choice

Directions:

Peel the avocado. Boil the egg (soft boiled). Chop the radishes to thin slices. Dice the scallion (finely). Mix avocado, salt, and lime juice in a container. Mash the mixture meticulously. Spread the mixture onto the bread. Put in some radish. Put tender boiled eggs on top. Put in some scallion, seeds, and pepper.

345. Avocado with Tomatoes and Cucumber

Time To Prepare: ten minutes Time to Cook: 0 minutes Yield: Servings 2

Ingredients:

¼ cup cilantro ¼ cup olives – to your choice ½ red onion 1 cucumber 1 lemon 1 Tbsp. turmeric 1/8 cup parsley 2 avocados 4 Roma tomatoes Salt and pepper – to your taste

Directions:

Dice the tomatoes, cucumber, avocado, and olives. Cut the cilantro, parsley, and onion. Put in the above ingredients into a container. Squeeze the lemon juice then put in to the vegetables. Put in olive oil, turmeric, salt, and pepper. Toss thoroughly. Consume instantly after putting in lemon juice and olive oil. If you prefer to consume the salad later, put in the dressing instantly before consuming it.

346. Berry Delight

Time To Prepare: fifteen minutes Time to Cook: 0 minutes Yield: Servings 6

Ingredients:

¼ cup of raw honey 1 cup of fresh organic blackberries 1 cup of fresh organic blueberries 1 cup of fresh organic raspberries 1 tablespoon of cinnamon

Directions:

Mix all the berries together in a big container, put in in the honey, and slowly stir. Drizzle with the cinnamon.

347. Blueberry & Chia Flax Seed Pudding

Time To Prepare:ten minutes Time to Cook:fifteen minutes Yield: Servings 4

Ingredients:

¼ cup of blueberries 2 cups of almond milk 3 tablespoons of chia seeds 3 tablespoons of ground flaxseed

Directions:

Warm a pan on moderate heat then put all together of the ingredients apart from the blueberries. Stir all the ingredients until the pudding is thick, this will take around three minutes. Place the pudding into a container then top with blueberries.

348. Brownies Avocado

Time To Prepare: ten minutes Time to Cook: twenty-five minutes Yield: Servings 6-8

Ingredients:

½ cup almond meal 1 ½ teaspoon instant coffee (with or without caffeine, as you wish) 2 teaspoons ground cinnamon ½ teaspoon salt 2 cups nuts or seeds, chopped 1 avocado 1 apple, cored and chopped, with the skin on 1 cup cooked and diced sweet potato 4 tablespoons ground chia seeds 1 teaspoon vanilla ½ cup almond butter ½ cup coconut butter, softened 1/4 cup coconut oil 2 1/4 cup stevia 3/4 cup cocoa powder

Directions:

Set the oven to 350F then line a 9 by 13-inch pan with parchment. Allow it to overlap the sides to make handles for lifting the brownies out when done. In a container, mix the almond meal, cocoa, coffee, cinnamon, salt, and nuts. Whisk and save for later. Bring the remaining ingredients in a food processor and mix until the desired smoothness is achieved. Put in the ingredients in the container and pulse. This combination must be lumpy. Pour into pan and bake for minimum twenty-five minutes. Allow to cool and chill in your fridge for a couple of hours before cutting. The baked product will be a little gooey, so refrigerating it makes the brownies easier to cut. The chilled results will be fairly crumbly.

349. Brussels Sprout Chips

Time To Prepare: ten minutes Time to Cook: ten minutes Yield: Servings 4

Ingredients:

2 cups Brussels sprout leaves 2 tablespoons ghee Kosher salt Lemon zest

Directions:

Set the oven to 350F, then cover two cookie sheets using parchment paper. Place the leaves in a huge container and pour melted ghee over the top, and put in salt. Bake for minimum 8 to ten minutes or until the leaves are crunchy. If they are tender at all, put them back in your oven. While still hot, drizzle the lemon zest over the leaves. Serve warm

350. Candied Dates

Time To Prepare: five minutes Time to Cook: 0 minutes Yield: Servings 2

Ingredients:

2 tablespoons of dark cocoa nibs 2 tablespoons of peanut butter 4 pitted Medjool dates

Directions:

Cut the pitted dates in half, and spread half a tablespoon of peanut butter on each date. Top each date with half a tablespoon of dark cocoa nibs. Split the candied dates between two plates, and enjoy!

351. Cashew "Humus"

Time To Prepare: ten minutes Time to Cook: 0 minutes Yield: Servings 1

Ingredients:

¼ Cup Water ¼ Teaspoon Sea Salt, Fine ½ Teaspoon Ground Ginger 1 Cup Cashews, Raw & Soaked in Water for fifteen Minutes & Drained 1 Tablespoon Olive Oil 1 Teaspoon Lemon juice, Fresh 2 Cloves Garlic 2 Teaspoon Coconut Aminos Pinch Cayenne Pepper

Directions:

Blend all ingredients together, and ensure to scrape the sides. Continue to combine until the desired smoothness is achieved, and then place in your fridge it before you serve

352. Cauliflower Snacks

Time To Prepare: ten minutes Time to Cook: 60 minutes Yield: Servings 4

Ingredients:

1 head of cauliflower 1 teaspoon salt 4 tablespoons extra virgin olive oil

Directions:

Set the oven to 425F, then prepare two cookie sheets by lining them using parchment paper. Trim off the cauliflower florets and discard the core. Chop the florets into golf-ball-sized pieces. Put the cauliflower in a container, and pour olive oil over them and drizzle with salt. Mix to coat. Spread in a single layer, not touching. Roast approximately 1 hour flipping the cauliflower three to four times until a golden-brown color is achieved. Serve warm

353. Chewy Blackberry Leather

Time To Prepare: fifteen minutes Time to Cook: 5-6 hours Yield: Servings 8

Ingredients:

¼ cup of raw honey 1 tbsp. of fresh mint leaves 1 tsp. of ground cinnamon 1/8 tsp. of fresh lemon juice 2 cups of fresh blackberries

Directions:

Set the oven to 170F. Coat baking sheet using parchment paper. Use a food processor to put all ingredients and pulse till smooth. Take the mixture onto the readied baking sheet and, using the backside of a spoon, smooth the top. Bake for approximately 5-6 hours. Chop the leather into equal-sized strips. Now, roll each rectangle to make fruit rolls

354. Coco Cherry Bake-less Bars

Time To Prepare: ten minutes Time to Cook: 0 minutes Yield: Servings 6

Ingredients:

¼-cup pure maple syrup ⅓-cup coconut, unsweetened and shredded ⅓-cup dried cherries or cranberries ⅓-cup ground flaxseed ½-cup almond butter 1-cup old-fashioned oats 1-Tbsp almond milk 1-Tbsp vanilla extract 3-scoops vanilla plant-based Protein powder

Directions:

Coat a loaf pan using parchment paper. Mix in the first four ingredients in your blender. Blend until the mixture becomes powdery. Move the mixture to a mixing container. Put in in all the rest of the ingredients. Mix thoroughly until meticulously blended. Put the mixture in the pan, and press down onto a consistently flat surface. Freeze for thirty minutes before cutting into six bars.

355. Cottage Cheese with Apple Sauce

Time To Prepare: five minutes Time to Cook: 0 minutes Yield: Servings 2

Ingredients:

½ teaspoon cinnamon powder 5-6 tablespoons cottage cheese two to three tablespoons applesauce or more if required

Directions:

Split the cottage cheese into 2 bowls. Spread applesauce over the cottage cheese. Drizzle ¼ teaspoon cinnamon powder on each before you serve.

356. Cucumber Yogurt

Time To Prepare: five minutes Time to Cook: 0 minutes Yield: Servings 1

Ingredients:

1 cup cucumbers, skin removed and chopped in chunks 1 teaspoon fresh dill, chopped fine 1/4 cup fat-free Greek yogurt 2 tablespoons chopped cashews 2 teaspoons fresh-squeezed lemon juice

Directions:

Peel and cut the cucumbers, then put them in a container. Put in the cashews, yogurt, lemon juice, and dill. Mix thoroughly, grab a spoon, and enjoy.

357. Dried Dates & Turmeric Truffles

Time To Prepare: fifteen minutes Time to Cook: 0 minutes Yield: Servings 4

Ingredients:

¼-tsp black pepper ⅓-cup walnuts ½-cup rolled oats ¾-cup dates, pitted 1-Tbsp turmeric powder + more for rolling

Directions:

Mix in all the ingredients, excluding the dates in a food processor. Blend until meticulously blended. Put in the dates progressively until forming into the dough. Shape and roll balls from the mixture. Roll each ball with the additional turmeric powder until coating fully. Store the truffles in an airtight jar until ready to serve.

358. Grams Easy Peasy Ginger Date

Time To Prepare: twenty minutes Time to Cook: ten minutes Yield: Servings 8

Ingredients:

¼ cup Almond milk ¾ cup Dates 1 or 1 ½ cup Almonds or almond flour 1 tsp. Ground ginger

Directions:

Preheat your oven to 350°F. If you're using fresh almonds, put it through a blender to turn it to almond flour. Blitz for a couple of minutes or so until it looks and feels smooth. Do not blitz for too long, or you might end up making nut butter. Now that you have your almond powder put it in a container and set it aside. Pour the dates and almond milk into your blender and pulse for five minutes. If it doesn't resemble a paste, pulse for another two minutes. Pour in the ground ginger and almond flour. Pulse for three to four minutes to combine. Place the mixture to a baking dish and bake for approximately twenty minutes. Take out of the oven and leave to cool before cutting into bits. Serve or store.

359. Energy Dates Balls

Time To Prepare: ten minutes Time to Cook: twenty-five minutes Yield: Servings 7

Ingredients:

¼ cup of fresh lemon juice ½ cup of shredded sweetened coconut 1 cup of pitted and chopped dates 1 cup of toasted almonds

Directions:

Coat a big baking sheet using a parchment paper. Keep aside. Use a food processor to add almonds and pulse till chopped crudely. Put in dates and lemon juice and pulse till a tender dough forms. Make equal sized balls from the mixture. In a shallow, dish place shredded coconut. Roll the balls in shredded coconut uniformly. Place the balls onto the baking sheet in a single layer. Place in your fridge to set completely before you serve.

360. Flourless & Flaky Muffin Munchies

Time To Prepare: twenty-five minutes Time to Cook: twenty minutes Yield: Servings 4

Ingredients:

⅛-tsp baking soda ¼-cup peanut butter or allergy-friendly substitution ¼-cup pure maple syrup or honey ¼-tsp salt ½-cup quick oats or quinoa flakes, loosely packed ¾-tsp baking powder 1-cup white beans, cooked 1-pc medium mashed banana, very ripe 2-tsp pure vanilla extract A handful of mini chocolate chips, crushed walnuts, shredded coconut, pinch cinnamon, etc. (not necessary)

Directions:

Preheat your oven to 350 F. Coat 8-muffin cups with glassine. Mix all the ingredients in your blender. Blend to a smooth consistency. Pour the mixture into the muffin cups at ⅔ full. Place the cups in your oven, and bake for about twenty minutes. Allow the muffins to sit and cool for about twenty minutes.

361. Ginger Turmeric | Protein: Bars

Time To Prepare: ten minutes + 20 cooling time Time to Cook: twenty-five minutes Yield: Servings 7

Ingredients:

½ cup coconut 1 cup cashews 1 scoop turmeric Protein bone broth 1 Tbsp. ginger 1/3 cup sunflower butter 2 Tbsp. maple syrup

Directions:

Put in coconut pieces and cashews to a blender or food processor. Use the pulse option to obtain a coarse mixture. Put in butter, broth, maple syrup, and ginger and pulse the mixture to make a coarse, yet even and fairly sticky mass. Evenly put the mixture to a baking pan (8x8 inches) with your hands or a spoon. Push tightly to the baking pan. Bring it in a fridge and allow it to cool for about twenty minutes. Chop the mixture into even squares. You can consume instantly or store in a glass container in the refrigerator (up to 7 days

362. Hummus with Celery

Time To Prepare: fifteen minutes Time to Cook: 0 minutes Yield: Servings 4

Ingredients:

3 cloves of garlic, crushed 2 tablespoons extra virgin olive oil ½ teaspoon salt ½ teaspoon cumin 1 (fifteen–ounce) can chickpeas two to three tablespoons water Dash of paprika 6 stalks celery, cut into two-inch pieces 3 tablespoons salsa 1/4 cup lemon juice 1/4 cup tahini

Directions:

Using a food processor mix the lemon juice and tahini for approximately one minute, until it is smooth. Scrape the sides down and process for 30 more seconds. Put in the garlic, olive oil, salt, and cumin. Blend for approximately one minute. Drain the chickpeas, put the half of them on the food processor, and blend for one more minute. Scrape down the sides, put in the other half of the chickpeas, and pulse until smooth, approximately 2 minutes. If it like a little too thick, put in water, 1 tablespoon at a time until you reach the desired consistency. Fill the celery sticks with hummus and drizzle paprika on top. Serve with salsa for dipping.

363. Lemony Ginger Cookies

Time To Prepare: fifteen minutes + thirty minutes chill time Time to Cook: 10-twelve minutes Yield: Servings 25

Ingredients:

½ cup arrowroot flour ½ teaspoon baking soda 1 ½ cup coconut butter, softened 1 ½ cups stevia 1 teaspoon nutritional yeast 2 teaspoons vanilla 3 inches of ginger root, peeled and diced 3/4 teaspoon salt Zest of 1 lemon

Directions:

Set the oven to 350F, then line two or three cookie sheets using parchment paper. Combine the arrowroot flour, stevia, salt, soda, and yeast in a container. In another container, put the rest of the ingredients and mix thoroughly. Put in the dry ingredients progressively until well blended. If the dough is too soft, put an additional one to 2 tablespoons of arrowroot powder. The dough will stiffen when chilled, so be careful. Cover the dough in parchment and push it flat. Chill for half an hour Take a chunk of the chilled dough and flatten it between two pieces of parchment until it is 1/8 inch thick. Sprinkle with a little arrowroot powder and slice into shapes. Put on baking sheets approximately 1 inch apart and bake ten to twelve minutes. Cool on cookie sheets for fifteen minutes before removing.

364. Mandarin Cottage Cheese

Time To Prepare: five minutes Time to Cook: 0 minutes Yield: Servings 1

Ingredients:

½ cup canned mandarin oranges ½ cup low-fat cottage cheese 1 ½ tablespoons slivered almonds

Directions:

Put the cottage cheese in a container. Drain the mandarin oranges, put them atop the cottage cheese, and drizzle with almonds

365. Mushroom Chips

Time To Prepare: ten minutes Time to Cook: 45-60 minutes Yield: Servings 2-4

Ingredients:

16 ounces of king oyster mushrooms 2 tablespoons ghee Kosher salt and ground pepper to taste

Directions:

Set the oven to 300F, then line two cookie sheets using parchment paper. Cut every mushroom in half along the length, then cut with a mandolin into 1/8 inch slices or strips. Put them on cookie sheets with some room in between. Melt the ghee and brush it over the mushrooms, then flavor with the salt and pepper. Bake for minimum 45 minutes to an hour, until they are completely crunchy. Store in airtight containers.

366. Oven Crisp Sweet Potato

Time To Prepare:ten minutes Time to Cook: twenty minutes Yield:Servings 2

Ingredients:

1 moderate-sized sweet potato, raw 1 teaspoon coconut oil 1 teaspoon sugar

Directions:

Preheat your oven to 160C. Using a mandolin slicer or a peeler, slice the sweet potato into thin chips or strips. Rinse and pat dry. Sprinkle the coconut oil over the potatoes. Toss until all chips are coated. Position in an oven baking sheet. Bake for about ten minutes. Check the crispiness. If it is not that crunchy enough, bake for an extra five or 10 minutes or until the chips attain the crispiness desired. Take out the crunchy sweet potatoes. Drizzle with sugar before you serve.

367. Party-Time Chicken Nuggets

Time To Prepare: ten minutes Time to Cook: twenty-five minutes Yield: Servings 6

Ingredients:

½ cup tapioca flour ½ tsp. of garlic powder ½ tsp. of onion powder ½ tsp. of paprika 1½ cups of blanched almond flour 2 (6-ounce) grass-fed skinless, boneless chicken breasts 2 big organic eggs Freshly ground black pepper, to taste Salt, to taste

Directions:

Set the oven to 400F then grease a big baking sheet. With a rolling pin, roll the chicken breasts to a uniform thickness. Cut each breast into bite-sized pieces. In a shallow dish, crack the eggs and beat thoroughly. In another shallow dish, combine flours and spices. Immerse the chicken nuggets in beaten eggs. Then roll in flour mixture completely. Position the nuggets onto the readied baking sheet in a single layer. Bake for approximately 10-twelve minutes, turning once after five minutes

368. Protein-Packed Croquettes

Time To Prepare: ten minutes Time to Cook: five minutes Yield: Servings 12

Ingredients:

¼ cup of chopped fresh cilantro leaves ¼ cup plus 1 tbsp. of olive oil, divided ¼ tsp. of ground turmeric ½ cup of thawed frozen peas ½ tsp. of paprika 1 cup of cooked quinoa 2 big peeled and mashed boiled potatoes 2 minced garlic cloves 2 tsp. of ground cumin Freshly ground black pepper, to taste Salt, to taste

Directions:

In a frying pan, heat 1 tbsp. of oil on moderate heat. Put in peas and garlic and sauté for approximately one minute. Move the peas mixture into a big container. Put rest of the ingredients then mix till well blended. Make equal sized oblong shaped patties from the mixture. In a huge frying pan, warm remaining oil on moderate to high heat. Put in croquettes in batches and fry for approximately 4 minutes per side

369. Roasted Garlic Chickpeas

Time To Prepare: five minutes Time to Cook: twenty minutes Yield: Servings 2

Ingredients:

1 Teaspoon Garlic Powder 1 Teaspoon Sea Salt 2 Tablespoons Olive Oil 4 Cups Cooked Chickpeas, Rinsed, Drained & Dried Black Pepper to Taste

Directions:

Begin by heating the oven to 400. Spread your chickpeas on a baking sheet, coating them with your olive oil. Bake of 20 minutes, ensuring to stir them at the ten-minute mark. Put your hot chickpeas in a container, seasoning before securing them in an airtight container. They'll keep at room temperature for maximum two days

370. Salt & Vinegar Kale Crisps

Time To Prepare: five minutes Time to Cook: 20-twenty-five minutes Yield: Servings 2

Ingredients:

1 Teaspoon Sea Salt, Fine 2 Tablespoon Apple Cider Vinegar 2 Tablespoons Olive Oil 4 Cups Kale, Torn into 2 Inch Pieces

Directions:

Begin by heating the oven to 350. Get out a container, and mix all of your ingredients. Put your kale on a baking sheet, baking for twenty to twenty-five minutes. Toss midway through this time. Put at room temperature in an airtight container. They'll keep for two days.

371. Spiced Nuts

Time To Prepare: ten minutes Time to Cook: 10-fifteen minutes Yield: Servings 2

Ingredients:

¼ Cup Pumpkin Puree ¼ Cup Sunflower Seeds ¼ Teaspoon Garlic Powder ¼ Teaspoon Red Pepper Flakes ½ Cup Walnuts ½ Teaspoon Ground Cumin 1 Cup Almonds 1 Teaspoon Ground Turmeric

Directions:

Begin by heating the oven to 350. Mix all ingredients together, and then get out a baking sheet. Spread your nuts over your baking sheet, cooking for ten to fifteen minutes. Allow it to cool well before you store it.

372. Grams Spicy Roasted chickpeas

Time To Prepare: ten minutes Time to Cook: forty minutes Yield: Servings 6

Ingredients:

¼ teaspoon of cayenne pepper 1 teaspoon of paprika 1 teaspoon of turmeric 2 (fifteen ounce) cans of chickpeas, drained and washed 2 teaspoons of coconut oil, melted

Directions:

Set the oven to 425°F. Coat a baking sheet using a paper towels, then put the chickpeas on them and use more paper towels to take off the surplus water in the chickpeas. Remove all of the paper towels. Place the oil and spices to the chickpeas and mix thoroughly. Roast your chickpeas for forty minutes, stirring every ten minutes. Once the chickpeas are done, take it off from the oven and let fully cool.

373. Grams Sweet Sunup Seeds

Time To Prepare: five minutes Time to Cook: 60 minutes Yield: Servings 8

Ingredients:

¼-cup pure maple syrup ¼-cup sunflower oil ¼-sesame seeds ⅓-cup honey ½-cup flaxseed 1-cup dried cranberries 1-cup raw pumpkin seeds 1-tsp vanilla extract 3-tsp cinnamon 4-cups rolled oats

Directions:

Preheat your oven to 350°F. Prepare two units of baking sheets by lining them using parchment paper. In a large-sized mixing container, mix the rolled oats, pumpkin seeds, flaxseed, sesame seeds, and cinnamon. Mix gently until meticulously blended. Pour all the liquid ingredients into the mixture and stir until mixed well. On the baking sheets, spread the mixture uniformly. Place the sheets in your oven. Cook for minimum an hour. While baking, stir the mixture every quarter of an hour to achieve uniform color on its surfaces. Take away the sheets from the oven. Allow cooling completely. Put in the cup of dried cranberries, and mix thoroughly. Store the granola in an airtight container to maintain its freshness and crunchiness.

374. Toasted Pumpkin Seeds

Time To Prepare: five minutes Time to Cook: thirty minutes Yield: Servings 2-4

Ingredients:

½ teaspoon extra virgin olive oil 1 teaspoon salt 1 to 2 cups pumpkin seeds Sea salt Water

Directions:

Put seeds in a deep cooking pan and cover with water. Put in salt. Bring it to its boiling point and boil for about ten minutes. Simmer uncovered for ten more minutes. This makes the seeds very crunchy when baked. Drain the seeds and pat dry using a paper towel. Coat a baking sheet using parchment paper and spread out the seeds in a single layer. Sprinkle with salt, then bake in an oven at 325F for minimum ten minutes, stirring midway through. Cool, then store in an airtight container

375. Turmeric Chickpea Cakes

Time To Prepare: twenty minutes Time to Cook: thirty minutes Yield: Servings 8

Ingredients:

½ cup fresh parsley, minced 1 teaspoon cayenne pepper, to taste (not necessary) 1 teaspoon salt or to taste 2 cans (15oz.) chickpeas, washed, drained 2 small onions, minced 2 teaspoons turmeric powder 4 cloves garlic, minced 4 tablespoons cornstarch 8-10 tablespoons chickpea flour Avocado dipping sauce to serve Freshly ground pepper to taste Grapeseed oil to fry

Directions:

Put a frying pan on moderate heat. Put in a little oil. When the oil is heated, put onion and garlic and sauté until translucent. Remove the heat and cool to room temperature. Put in chickpeas into the food processor container and pulse until very finely chopped. Put in the onion mixture, salt, pepper, cayenne pepper, and turmeric powder and pulse again until well blended. Move into a container. Put in parsley and mix thoroughly. Make small balls of the mixture (of approximately 1 inch diameter) and mould into patties. Put chickpea flour on a plate. Put a nonstick pan on moderate heat. Put in a little oil and swirl the pan so that the oil spreads. Immerse the patties in the chickpea flour and place a few on the pan. Cook in batches. Cook until the underside is golden brown. Flip then cook the other side till it's golden brown. Repeat steps 6-8 to fry the rest of the patties. Serve with avocado dipping sauce

376. Turmeric Gummies

Time To Prepare: five minutes Time to Cook: 4 hours and ten minutes Yield: Servings 4

Ingredients:

¼ tsp. Ground pepper 1 tsp. Ground turmeric 3 ½ cups Water 6 tbsp. Maple syrup 8 tbsp. Unflavored gelatin powder

Directions:

Combine the ground turmeric, maple syrup, and water in a pot set on moderate heat. Stir continuously for five minutes before removing from heat and pouring in the gelatin powder. Stir using a wooden spoon to dissolve the gelatin. Put back the pan on the heat and stir for another two minutes. Remove the heat and take the mixture to a deep container that you will seal using plastic wrapimmediately after. Place in your fridge the mixture for approximately 4 hours. It must be firm now, cut it into little squares, and serve or store.

377. Pineapple & Carrot Smoothie

Yield: 2 servings Preparation Time: 10 minutes

Ingredients:

1 cup frozen pineapple • 1 large ripe banana, peeled and sliced • ½ tablespoon fresh ginger, peeled and chopped • ¼ teaspoon ground turmeric • 1 cup unswee10ed almond milk • ½ cup fresh carrot juice • 1 tablespoon freshly squeezed lemon juice

Directions:

1. In a high speed blender, add all ingredients and pulse till smooth. 2. Transfer into 2 glasses and serve immediately.

378. Cherry & Kale Smoothie

Yield: 1 serving Preparation Time: 10 minutes

Ingredients:

2 ripe bananas, peeled and sliced • 1 cup fresh cherries, pitted • 1 cup fresh kale, trimmed • 1 teaspoon fresh ginger, peeled and chopped • 1 tablespoon chia seeds, soaked for quarter-hour • ½ teaspoon ground turmeric • ¼ teaspoon ground cinnamon • 1 cup coconut water

Directions:

1. In a top speed blender, add all ingredients and pulse till smooth. 2. Transfer in a glass and serve immediately.

379. Banana & Ginger Smoothie

Yield: 1 serving Preparation Time: 10 min

Ingredients:

1-inch fresh ginger piece, peeled and chopped • 1 frozen banana, peeled and sliced • ½ teaspoon ground cinnamon • 1 cup coconut milk

Directions:

1. In a higher speed blender, add all ingredients and pulse till smooth. 2. Transfer in to a glass and serve immediately.

380. Pineapple, Kale & Ginger Smoothie

Yield: 1 serving Preparation Time: 10 min

Ingredients:

1 cup frozen pineapple, chopped • 1 tablespoon fresh ginger, peeled and chopped • 1 cup fresh kale, trimmed and chopped • ½ cup fresh mixed berries • ¼-½ teaspoon ground turmeric, to taste • 2 teaspoons ground flax seeds • 1 cup unswee10ed coconut milk • ½ cup ice, crushed

Directions:

1. In a higher speed blender, add all ingredients and pulse till smooth. 2. Transfer into 1 glass and serve immediately.

381. Fruit & Veggie Smoothie

Yield: 2 servings Preparation Time: fifteen minutes

Ingredients:

¾ cups pineapple, chopped • ½ cup cucumber, peeled and chopped • ½ of pear, peeled, cored and chopped • 1 small avocado, peeled, pitted and chopped • ½ tablespoon fresh dill • 1 cup fresh spinach, chopped • 1 celery stalk, chopped • ¼ teaspoon ground turmeric • 1 piece fresh ginger, peeled • 1 tablespoon fresh lime juice • 2 cups water

Directions:

1. In a top speed blender, add all ingredients and pulse till smooth. 2. Transfer into 2 glasses and serve immediately.

382. Tangy Mango & Spinach Smoothie

Yield: 2 servings Preparation Time: 10 minutes

Ingredients:

2 cups frozen mango, peeled, pitted and chopped • 3 cups fresh spinach, chopped • 1 teaspoon ground turmeric • 16-ounce fresh coconut water • 1 tablespoon fresh lemon juice • 1 tablespoon lime juice

Directions:

1. In a high speed blender, add all ingredients and pulse till smooth. 2. Transfer into 2 glasses and serve immediately.

383. Kale & Avocado Smoothie

Yield: 2 servings Preparation Time: 10 min

Ingredients:

3 stalks fresh kale, trimmed and chopped • 1-2 celery stalks, chopped • ½ of avocado, peeled, pitted and chopped • ½-1 ginger herb, chopped • ½-1 turmeric root, chopped • 2 cups coconut milk

Directions: 1. In a higher speed blender, add all ingredients and pulse till smooth. 2. Transfer into 2 glasses and serve immediately.

384. Pineapple & Orange Smoothie

Yield: 1 serving Preparation Time: 10 minutes

Ingredients: •

1 fresh orange, peeled and chopped • 1½ cups fresh pineapple, chopped • 1 small thumb of ginger, peeled and chopped/grated • 1 frozen banana, peeled and sliced • 1 teaspoon ground turmeric • 1 tablespoon chia seeds • 1 cup unswee10ed almond milk

Directions:

1. In a higher speed blender, add all ingredients and pulse till smooth. 2. Transfer in a glass and serve immediately.

385. Pineapple & watermelon Smoothie

Yield: 2 servings Preparation Time: 10 min

Ingredients:

1 cup frozen pineapple, chopped • 1 fresh orange, peeled and sliced (white pith and seeds removed) • 2 cups frozen watermelon, peeled, pitted and chopped • 1 teaspoon fresh ginger, peeled and chopped • ½ teaspoon ground turmeric • ½ cup coconut milk • 1 teaspoon organic honey • 1½ cups coconut water

Directions:

1. In a higher speed blender, add all ingredients and pulse till smooth. 2. Transfer into 2 glasses and serve immediately.

386. Cherry & Blueberry Smoothie

Ingredients:

2 cups escarole • ½ cup frozen blueberries • ½ cup frozen cherries • ¼ teaspoon ground cinnamon • ¼ teaspoon ground turmeric • 1 scoop of chocolate Protein powder • 1 cup filtered water • 5 ice cubes, crushed

Directions:

1. In an increased speed blender, add all ingredients and pulse till smooth. 2. Transfer in a glass and serve immediately.

387. Pear, Peach & Papaya Smoothie

Yield: 3 servings Preparation Time: 10 min

Ingredients:

½ cup pear, peeled, cored and chopped • ¾ cup peaches, pitted and chopped • ¾ cup papaya, peeled and chopped • 1 teaspoon fresh ginger, peeled and chopped • 2 fresh mint leaves • ½ cup coconut water • 1 cup ice, crushed

Directions:

1. In an increased speed blender, add all ingredients and pulse till smooth. 2. Transfer into 3 glasses and serve immediately.

388. Cherry & Beet Smoothie

Yield: 1 serving Preparation Time: 10 minutes

Ingredients:

¾ cup frozen pineapple, chopped • 1 cup frozen berries • ¼ cup frozen red beets, peeled and chopped • ¼ small avocado, peeled, pitted and chopped • 1 tablespoon chia seeds • 1 teaspoon fresh ginger, peeled and chopped • ½ teaspoon fresh turmeric, grated • 2 teaspoon raw honey • 1 cup unswee10ed almond milk

Directions:

1. In a high speed blender, add all ingredients and pulse till smooth. 2. Transfer in a glass and serve immediately.

389. Pineapple & Almond Smoothie

Yield: 3 servings Preparation Time: 10 minutes

Ingredients:

1 cup fresh pineapple, peeled and chopped • ¼ cup blanched almonds • ½ cup fresh pineapple juice • ½ teaspoon pure maple syrup • ½ cup fresh pineapple juice • ¼ cup rice milk • ½ cup ice cubes, crushed

Directions:

1. In a top speed blender, add all ingredients and pulse till smooth. 2. Transfer in to a glass and serve immediately.

390. Watermelon, Berries & Avocado Smoothie

Yield: 1 serving Preparation Time: 10 minutes

Ingredients:

1½ cups mixed frozen berries • 1 cup watermelon, peeled, seeded and chopped • ¼ of avocado, peeled, pitted and chopped • 1-inch fresh ginger piece, peeled and chopped • 2 teaspoons chia seeds • ¾ cup fresh coconut water

Directions:

1. In a top speed blender, add all ingredients and pulse till smooth. 2. Transfer right into a glass and serve immediately.

391. Nutty Banana & Ginger Smoothie

Yield: 4 servings Preparation Time: 10 min

Ingredients:

1 frozen banana, peeled and sliced • ¼-inch fresh turmeric root, grates • ½-inch fresh ginger root, peeled and chopped • 1 cup pecans, chopped • 1 cup walnuts, chopped • 1 tablespoon flax seeds • 1 tablespoon chia seeds • 1 tablespoon fresh maca powder • ½ teaspoon ground cinnamon • 1½ cups unswee1oed almond milk

Directions:

1. In a high speed blender, add all ingredients and pulse till smooth. 2. Transfer into 4 glasses and serve immediately.

392. Tangy Avocado & Ginger Smoothie

Yield: 1 serving Preparation Time: 10 min

Ingredients:

½ cup frozen berries • 2 tablespoons unswee1oed coconut, shredded • 1/3 cup low- Fat cottage cheese • 1 packet stevia • 8-ounce coconut water • ½ cup ice, crushed

Directions:

1. In a top speed blender, add all ingredients and pulse till smooth. 2. Transfer in a glass and serve immediately.

393. Sweet Potato & Orange Smoothie

Yield: 2 servings Preparation Time: 10 min

Ingredients:

1 medium banana, peeled and sliced • 1 cup sweet potato puree • 1 teaspoon fresh ginger, chopped • ½ tablespoon flax seeds meal • 1 tablespoon almond butter • ¼ teaspoon ground turmeric • ¼ teaspoon ground cinnamon • ¾ cup unswee1oed almond milk • ¼ cup fresh orange juice • Ice, as required

Directions: 1. In an increased speed blender, add all ingredients and pulse till smooth. 2. Transfer into 2 glasses and serve immediately.

394. Blueberry & Cucumber Smoothie

Yield: 1 serving Preparation Time: 10 min

Ingredients:

½ cup cucumber, peeled and chopped • ½ of small banana, peeled and sliced • 1 cup frozen blueberries • 1 tablespoon chia seeds • 1 cup water

Directions:

1. In a top speed blender, add all ingredients and pulse till smooth. 2. Transfer in to a glass and serve immediately.

MEAT

395. Beef with Mushroom & Broccoli

Yield: 4 servings Preparation Time: quarter-hour Cooking Time: 12 minutes

Ingredients:

For Beef Marinade: • 1 garlic clove, minced • 1 (2-inch) piece fresh ginger, minced • Salt and freshly ground black pepper, to taste • 3 tablespoons white wine vinegar • ¾ cup beef broth • 1 pound flank steak, trimmed and sliced into thin strips For Vegetables: • 2 tablespoons coconut oil, divided • 2 minced garlic cloves • 3 cups broccoli rabe, chopped • 4-ounce shiitake mushrooms, halved • 8-ounce cremini mushrooms, sliced

Directions:

1. For marinade in a substantial bowl, mix together all ingredients except beef. 2. Add beef and coat with marinade generously. 3. Refrigerate to marinate for around quarter-hour. 4. In a substantial skillet, heat oil on medium-high heat. 5. Remove beef from bowl, reserving the marinade. 6. Add beef and garlic and cook for about 3-4 minutes or till browned. 7. With a slotted spoon, transfer the beef in a bowl. 8. In exactly the same skillet, add reserved marinade, broccoli and mushrooms and cook for approximately 3-4 minutes. 9. Stir in beef and cook for about 3-4 minutes.

396. Beef with Zucchini Noodles

Yield: 4 servings Preparation Time: 15 minutes Cooking Time: 9 minutes

Ingredients:

1 teaspoon fresh ginger, grated • 2 medium garlic cloves, minced • ¼ cup coconut aminos • 2 tablespoons fresh lime juice • 1½ pound NY strip steak, trimmed and sliced thinly • 2 medium zucchinis, spiralized with Blade C • Salt, to taste • 3 tablespoons essential olive oil • 2 medium scallions, sliced • 1 teaspoon red pepper flakes, crushed • 2 tablespoons fresh cilantro, chopped

Directions:

1. In a big bowl, mix together ginger, garlic, coconut aminos and lime juice. 2. Add beef and coat with marinade generously. 3. Refrigerate to marinate approximately 10 minutes. 4. Place zucchini noodles over a large paper towel and sprinkle with salt. 5. Keep aside for around 10 minutes. 6. In a big skillet, heat oil on medium-high heat. 7. Add scallion and red pepper flakes and sauté for about 1 minute. 8. Add beef with marinade and stir fry for around 3-4 minutes or till browned. 9. Add zucchini and cook for approximately 3-4 minutes. 10. Serve hot with all the topping of cilantro.

397. Spiced Ground Beef

Yield: 5 servings Preparation Time: 10 min Cooking Time: 22 minutes

Ingredients:

2 tablespoons coconut oil • 2 whole cloves • 2 whole cardamoms • 1 (2-inch) piece cinnamon stick • 2 bay leaves • 1 teaspoon cumin seeds • 2 onions, chopped • Salt, to taste • ½ tablespoon garlic paste • ½ tablespoon fresh ginger paste • 1 pound lean ground beef • 1½ teaspoons fennel seeds powder • 1 teaspoon ground cumin • 1½ teaspoons red chili powder • 1/8 teaspoon ground turmeric • Freshly ground black pepper, to taste • 1 cup coconut milk • ¼ cup water • ¼ cup fresh cilantro, chopped

Directions: 1. In a sizable pan, heat oil on medium heat. 2. Add cloves, cardamoms, cinnamon stick, bay leaves and cumin seeds and sauté for about 20-a few seconds. 3. Add onion and 2 pinches of salt and sauté for about 3-4 minutes. 4. Add garlic-ginger paste and sauté for about 2 minutes. 5. Add beef and cook for about 4-5 minutes, entering pieces using the spoon. 6. Cover and cook approximately 5 minutes. 7. Stir in spices and cook, stirring for approximately 2-2½ minutes. 8. Stir in coconut milk and water and cook for about 7-8 minutes. 9. Season with salt and take away from heat. 10. Serve hot using the garnishing of cilantro.

398. Ground Beef with Veggies

Yield: 2-4 servings Preparation Time: quarter-hour Cooking Time: twenty or so minutes

Ingredients

1-2 tablespoons coconut oil • 1 red onion, sliced • 2 red jalapeño peppers, seeded and sliced • 2 minced garlic cloves • 1 pound lean ground beef • 1 small head broccoli, chopped • ½ of head cauliflower, chopped • 3 carrots, peeled and sliced • 3 celery ribs, sliced • Chopped fresh thyme, to taste • Dried sage, to taste • Ground turmeric, to taste • Salt and freshly ground black pepper, to taste

Directions:

1. In a large skillet, melt coconut oil on medium heat. 2. Add onion, jalapeño peppers and garlic and sauté for about 5 minutes. 3. Add beef and cook for around 4-5 minutes, entering pieces using the spoon. 4. Add remaining ingredients and cook, stirring occasionally for about 8-10 min. 5. Serve hot.

399. Ground Beef with Greens & Tomatoes

Yield: 4 servings Preparation Time: fifteen minutes Cooking Time: 15 minutes

Ingredients:

1 tbsp organic olive oil • ½ of white onion, chopped • 2 garlic cloves, chopped finely • 1 jalapeño pepper, chopped finely • 1 pound lean ground beef • 1 teaspoon ground coriander • 1 teaspoon ground cumin • ½ teaspoon ground turmeric • ½ teaspoon ground ginger • ½ teaspoon ground cinnamon • ½ teaspoon ground fennel seeds • Salt and freshly ground black pepper, to taste • 8 fresh cherry tomatoes, quartered • 8 collard greens leaves, stemmed and chopped • 1 teaspoon fresh lemon juice

Directions:

1. In a big skillet, heat oil on medium heat. 2. Add onion and sauté for approximately 4 minutes. 3. Add garlic and jalapeño pepper and sauté for approximately 1 minute. 4. Add beef and spices and cook approximately 6 minutes breaking into pieces while using spoon. 5. Stir in tomatoes and greens and cook, stirring gently for about 4 minutes. 6. Stir in lemon juice and take away from heat.

400. Ground Beef & Veggies Curry

Yield: 6-8 servings Preparation Time: 15 minutes Cooking Time: 36 minutes

Ingredients:

2-3 tablespoons coconut oil • 1 cup onion, chopped • 1 garlic cloves, minced • 1 pound lean ground beef • 1½ tablespoons curry powder • 1/8 teaspoon ground ginger • 1/8 teaspoon ground cinnamon • 1/8 teaspoon ground turmeric • Salt, to taste • 2½-3 cups tomatoes, chopped finely • 2½-3 cups fresh peas, shelled • 2 sweet potatoes, peeled and chopped

Directions:

In a sizable pan, melt coconut oil on medium heat. 2. Add onion and garlic and sauté for around 4-5 minutes. 3. Add beef and cook for about 4-5 minutes. 4. Add curry powder and spices and cook for about 1 minute. 5. Stir in tomatoes, peas and sweet potato and bring to your gentle simmer. 6. Simmer, covered approximately 25 minutes.

401. Curried Beef Meatballs

Yield: 6 servings Preparation Time: twenty minutes Cooking Time: 22 minutes

Ingredients:

For Meatballs: • 1 pound lean ground beef • 2 organic eggs, bea10 • 3 tablespoons red onion, minced • ¼ cup fresh basil leaves, chopped • 1 (1-inch) fresh ginger piece, chopped finely • 4 garlic cloves, chopped finely • 3 Thai bird's eye chilies, minced • 1 teaspoon coconut sugar • 1 tablespoon red curry paste • Salt, to taste • 1 tablespoon fish sauce • 2 tablespoons coconut oil For Curry: • 1 red onion, chopped • Salt, to taste • 4 garlic cloves, minced • 1 (1-inch) fresh ginger piece, minced • 2 Thai bird's eye chilies, minced • 2 tablespoons red curry paste • 1 (14-ounce) coconut milk • Salt and freshly ground black pepper, to taste • Lime wedges, for serving

Directions:

1. For meatballs in a large bowl, add all ingredients except oil and mix till well combined. 2. Make small balls from mixture. 3. In a large skillet, melt coconut oil on medium heat. 4. Add meatballs and cook for about 3-5 minutes or till golden brown all sides. 5. Transfer the meatballs right into a bowl. 6. In the same skillet, add onion as well as a pinch of salt and sauté for around 5 minutes. 7. Add garlic, ginger and chilies and sauté for about 1 minute. 8. Add curry paste and sauté for around 1 minute. 9. Add coconut milk and meatballs and convey to some gentle simmer. 10. Reduce the warmth to low and simmer, covered for around 10 minutes. 11. Serve using the topping of lime wedges.

402. Honey Glazed Beef

Yield: 2-3 servings Preparation Time: quarter-hour Cooking Time: 12 minutes

Ingredients:

2 tablespoons arrowroot flour • Salt and freshly ground black pepper, to taste • 1 pound flank steak, cut into ¼-inch thick slices • ½ cup plus 1 tablespoon coconut oil, divided • 2 minced garlic cloves • 1 teaspoon ground ginger • Pinch of red pepper flakes, crushed • 1/3 cup organic honey • ½ cup beef broth • ½ cup coconut aminos • 3 scallions, chopped

Directions:

1. In a bowl, mix together arrowroot flour, salt and black pepper. 2. Coat beef slices in arrowroot flour mixture evenly after which get rid of excess mixture. 3. Keep aside for about 10-15 minutes. 4. For sauce in a pan, melt 1 tablespoon of coconut oil on medium heat. 5. Add garlic, ginger powder and red pepper flakes and sauté for about 1 minute. 6. Add honey, broth and coconut aminos and stir to mix well. 7. Increase the heat to high and cook, stirring continuously for around 3 minutes. 8. Remove from heat and keep aside. 9. In a large skillet, melt remaining coconut oil on medium heat. 10. Add beef and stir fry approximately 2-3 minutes. 11. Transfer the beef onto a paper towel lined plate to drain. 12. Remove the oil from skillet and return the beef into skillet. 13. Stir fry for around 1 minute. 14. Stir in honey sauce and cook approximately 3 minutes. 15. Stir in scallion and cook approximately 1 minute more. 16. Serve hot.

403. Grilled Skirt Steak Coconut

Yield: 4 servings Preparation Time: quarter-hour Cooking Time: 8-9 minutes

Ingredients:

2 teaspoons fresh ginger herb, grated finely • 2 teaspoons fresh lime zest, grated finely • ¼ cup coconut sugar • 2 teaspoons fish sauce • 2 tablespoons fresh lime juice • ½ cup coconut milk • 1 pound beef skirt steak, trimmed and cut into 4-inch slices lengthwise • Salt, to taste

Directions:

1. In a sizable sealable bag, mix together all ingredients except steak and salt. 2. Add steak and coat with marinade generously. 3. Seal the bag and refrigerate to marinate for about 4-12 hours. 4. Preheat the grill to high heat. Grease the grill grate. 5. Remove steak from refrigerator and discard the marinade. 6. With a paper towel, dry the steak and sprinkle with salt evenly. 7. Cook the steak for approximately 3½ minutes. 8. Flip the medial side and cook for around 2½-5 minutes or till desired doneness. 9. Remove from grill pan and keep side for approximately 5 minutes before slicing. 10. With a clear, crisp knife cut into desired slices and serve.

404. Lamb with Prunes

Yield: 4-6 servings Preparation Time: fifteen minutes Cooking Time: a couple of hours 40 minutes

Ingredients:

3 tablespoons coconut oil • 2 onions, chopped finely • 1 (1-inch) piece fresh ginger, minced • 3 garlic cloves, minced • ½ teaspoon ground turmeric • 2 ½ pound lamb shoulder, trimmed and cubed into 3-inch size • Salt and freshly ground black pepper, to taste • ½ teaspoon saffron threads, crumbled • 1 cinnamon stick • 3 cups water • 1 cup runes, pitted and halved

Directions:

1. In a big pan, melt coconut oil on medium heat. 2. Add onions, ginger, garlic cloves and turmeric and sauté for about 3-5 minutes. 3. Sprinkle the lamb with salt and black pepper evenly. 4. In the pan, add lamb and saffron threads and cook for approximately 4-5 minutes. 5. Add cinnamon stick and water and produce to some boil on high heat. 6. Reduce the temperature to low and simmer, covered for around 1½-120 minutes or till desired doneness of lamb. 7. Stir in prunes and simmer for approximately 20-a half-hour. 8. Remove cinnamon stick and serve hot.

405. Baked Lamb with Spinach

Yield: 6 servings Preparation Time: quarter-hour Cooking Time: couple of hours 55 minutes

Ingredients:

2 tablespoons coconut oil • 2 pound lamb necks, trimmed and cut into 2-inch pieces crosswise • Salt, to taste • 2 medium onions, chopped • 3 tablespoons fresh ginger, minced • 4 garlic cloves, minced • 2 tablespoons ground coriander • 1 tablespoon ground cumin • 1 teaspoon ground turmeric • ¼ cup coconut milk • ½ cup tomatoes, chopped • 2 cups boiling water • 30-ounce frozen spinach, thawed and squeezed • 1½ tablespoons garam masala • 1 tablespoon fresh lemon juice • Freshly ground black pepper, to taste

Directions:

1. Preheat the oven to 300 degrees F. 2. In a substantial Dutch oven, melt coconut oil on medium-high heat. 3. Add lamb necks and sprinkle with salt. 4. Stir fry approximately 4-5 minutes or till browned completely. 5. Transfer the lamb right into a plate and lower the heat to medium. 6. In exactly the same pan, add onion and sauté for about 10 minutes. 7. Add ginger, garlic and spices and sauté for around 1 minute. 8. Add coconut milk and tomatoes and cook approximately 3-4 minutes. 9. With an immersion blender, blend the mix till smooth. 10. Add lamb, boiling water and salt and convey to some boil. 11. Cover the pan and transfer into the oven. 12. Bake approximately 2½ hours. 13. Now, take away the pan from oven and place on medium heat. 14. Stir in spinach and garam masala and cook for about 3-5 minutes. 15. Stir in fresh lemon juice, salt and black pepper and take off from heat. 16. Serve hot.

406. Ground Lamb with Peas

Yield: 4 servings Preparation Time: 15 minutes Cooking Time: 55 minutes

Ingredients:

1 tablespoon coconut oil • 3 dried red chilies • 1 (2-inch) cinnamon stick • 3 green cardamom pods • ½ teaspoon cumin seeds • 1 medium red onion, chopped • 1 (¾-inch) piece fresh ginger, minced • 4 garlic cloves, minced • 1½ teaspoons ground coriander • ½ teaspoon garam masala • ½ teaspoon ground cumin • ½ teaspoon ground turmeric • ¼ teaspoon ground nutmeg • 2 bay leaves • 1 pound lean ground lamb • ½ cup Roma tomatoes, chopped • 1-1½ cups water • 1 cup fresh green peas, shelled • 2 tablespoons plain Greek yogurt, whipped • ¼ cup fresh cilantro, chopped • Salt and freshly ground black pepper, to taste

Directions:

1. In a Dutch oven, melt coconut oil medium-high heat. 2. Add red chilies, cinnamon stick, cardamom pods and cumin seeds and sauté for around thirty seconds. 3. Add onion and sauté for about 3-4 minutes. 4. Add ginger, garlic cloves and spices and sauté for around thirty seconds. 5. Add lamb and cook approximately 5 minutes. 6. Add tomatoes and cook approximately 10 min. 7. Stir in water and green peas and cook, covered approximately 25-thirty minutes. 8. Stir in yogurt, cilantro, salt and black pepper and cook for around 4-5 minutes. 9. Serve hot.

407. Broiled Lamb Shoulder

Yield: 10 servings Preparation Time: 10 minutes Cooking Time: 8-10 minutes

Ingredients:

2 tablespoons fresh ginger, minced • 2 tablespoons garlic, minced • ¼ cup fresh lemongrass stalk, minced • ¼ cup fresh orange juice • ¼ cup coconut aminos • Freshly ground black pepper, to taste • 2 pound lamb shoulder, trimmed

Directions:

1. In a bowl, mix together all ingredients except lamb shoulder. 2. In a baking dish, squeeze lamb shoulder and coat the lamb with half in the marinade mixture generously. 3. Reserve remaining mixture. 4. Refrigerate to marinate for overnight. 5. Preheat the broiler of oven. Place a rack inside a broiler pan and arrange about 4-5-inches from heating unit. 6. Remove lamb shoulder from refrigerator and remove excess marinade. 7. Broil approximately 4-5 minutes from both sides. 8. Serve with all the reserved marinade like a sauce.

408. Roasted Lamb Chops

Yield: 4 servings Preparation Time: 15 minutes Cooking Time: half an hour

Ingredients:

For Lamb Marinade: • 4 garlic cloves, chopped • 1 (2-inch) piece fresh ginger, chopped • 2 green chilies, seeded and chopped • 1 teaspoon fresh lime zest • 2 teaspoons garam masala • 1 teaspoon ground coriander • 1 teaspoon ground cumin • ½ teaspoon ground cinnamon • 1 teaspoon coconut oil, melted • 2 tablespoons fresh lime juice • 6-7 tablespoons plain Greek yogurt • 1 (8-bone) rack of lamb, trimmed • 2 onions, sliced For Relish: • ½ of garlic herb, chopped • 1 (1-inch) piece fresh ginger, chopped • ¼ cup fresh cilantro, chopped • ¼ cup fresh mint, chopped • 1 green chili, seeded and chopped • 1 teaspoon fresh lime zest • 1 teaspoon organic honey • 2 tablespoons fresh apple juice • 2 tablespoons fresh lime juice

Directions:

1. For chops in a very mixer, add all ingredients except yogurt, chops and onions and pulse till smooth. 2. Transfer the mixture in a large bowl with yogurt and stir to combine well. 3. Add chops and coat with mixture generously. 4. Refrigerate to marinate for approximately twenty four hours. 5. Preheat the oven to 375 degrees F. Linea roasting pan with a foil paper. 6. Place the onion wedges in the bottom of prepared roasting pan. 7. Arrange rack of lamb over onion wedges. 8. Roast approximately half an hour. 9. Meanwhile for relish in the blender, add all ingredients and pulse till smooth. 10. Serve chops and onions alongside relish.

409. Lamb Burgers with Avocado Dip

Yield: 4-6 servings Preparation Time: 20 minutes Cooking Time: 10 minutes

Ingredients:

For Burgers: • 1 (2-inch) piece fresh ginger, grated • 1 pound lean ground lamb • 1 medium onion, grated • 2 minced garlic cloves • 1 bunch fresh mint leaves, chopped finely • 2 teaspoons ground coriander • 2 teaspoons ground cumin • ½ teaspoon ground allspice • ½ teaspoon ground cinnamon • Salt and freshly ground black pepper, to taste • 1 tbsp essential olive oil For Dip: • 3 small cucumbers, peeled and grated • 1 avocado, peeled, pitted and chopped • ½ of garlic oil, crushed • 2 tablespoons fresh lemon juice • 2 tablespoons olive oil • 2 tablespoons fresh dill, chopped finely • 2 tablespoons chives, chopped finely • Salt and freshly ground black pepper, to taste

Directions:

Preheat the broiler of oven. Lightly, grease a broiler pan. 2. For burgers in a big bowl, squeeze the juice of ginger. 3. Add remaining ingredients and mix till well combined. 4. Make equal sized burgers from your mixture. 5. Arrange the burgers in broiler pan and broil approximately 5 minutes per side. 6. Meanwhile for dip squeeze the cucumbers juice in a bowl. 7. In a blender, add avocado, garlic, lemon juice and oil and pulse till smooth. 8. Transfer the avocado mixture in a bowl. 9. Add remaining ingredients and stir to mix. 10. Serve the burgers with avocado dip.

410. Baked Meatballs & Scallions

Yield: 4-6 servings Preparation Time: 20 min Cooking Time: 35 minutes

Ingredients:

For Meatballs: • 1 lemongrass stalk, outer skin peeled and chopped • 1 (1½-inch) piece fresh ginger, sliced • 3 garlic cloves, chopped • 1 cup fresh cilantro leaves, chopped roughly • ½ cup fresh basil leaves, chopped roughly • 2 tablespoons plus 1 teaspoon fish sauce • 2 tablespoons water • 2 tablespoons fresh lime juice • ½ pound lean ground pork • 1 pound lean ground lamb • 1 carrot, peeled and grated • 1 organic egg, bea10 For Scallions: • 16 stalks scallions, trimmed • 2 tablespoons coconut oil, melted • Salt, to taste • ½ cup water

Directions:

1. Preheat the oven to 375 degrees F. Grease a baking dish. 2. In a blender, add lemongrass, ginger, garlic, fresh herbs, fish sauce, water and lime juice and pulse till chopped finely. 3. Transfer the amalgamation in a bowl with remaining ingredients and mix till well combined. 4. Make about 1-inch balls from mixture. 5. Arrange the balls into prepared baking dish in a single layer. 6. In another rimmed baking dish, arrange scallion stalks in a very single layer. 7. Drizzle with coconut oil and sprinkle with salt. 8. Pour water in the baking dish 1nd with a foil paper cover it tightly. 9. Bake the scallion for around a half-hour. 10. Bake the meatballs for approximately 30-35 minutes. Pork with Bell Pepper This stir fry not simply tastes wonderful but additionally is packed with nutritious benefits.

411. Pork with Pineapple

Yield: 4 servings Preparation Time: 15 minutes Cooking Time: 14 minutes

Ingredients:

2 tablespoons coconut oil • 1½ pound pork 10derloin, trimmed and cut into bite-sized pieces • 1 onion, chopped • 2 minced garlic cloves • 1 (1-inch) piece fresh ginger, minced • 20-ounce pineapple, cut into chunks • 1 large red bell pepper, seeded and chopped • ¼ cup fresh pineapple juice • ¼ cup coconut aminos • Salt and freshly ground black pepper, to taste

Directions:

1. In a substantial skillet, melt coconut oil on high heat. 2. Add pork and stir fry approximately 4-5 minutes. 3. Transfer the pork right into a bowl. 4. In exactly the same skillet, heat remaining oil on medium heat. 5. Add onion, garlic and ginger and sauté for around 2 minutes. 6. Stir in pineapple and bell pepper and stir fry for around 3 minutes. 7. Stir in pork, pineapple juice and coconut aminos and cook for around 3-4 minutes. 8. Serve hot.

412. Pork Chili

Yield: 8 servings Preparation Time: quarter-hour Cooking Time: 60 minutes

Ingredients:

2 tablespoons extra-virgin organic olive oil • 2 pound ground pork • 1 medium red bell pepper, seeded and chopped • 1 medium onion, chopped • 5 garlic cloves, chopped finely • 1 (2-inch) part of hot pepper, minced • 1 tablespoon ground cumin • 1 teaspoon ground turmeric • 3 tablespoon chili powder • ½ teaspoon chipotle chili powder • Salt and freshly ground black pepper, to taste • 1 cup chicken broth • 1 (28-ounce) can fire-roasted crushed tomatoes • 2 medium bokchoy heads, sliced • 1 avocado, peeled, pitted and chopped

Directions:

In a sizable pan, heat oil on medium heat. 2. Add pork and stir fry for about 5 minutes. 3. Add bell pepper, onion, garlic, hot pepper and spices and stir fry for approximately 5 minutes. 4. Add broth and tomatoes and convey with a boil. 5. Stir in bokchoy and cook, covered for approximately twenty minutes. 6. Uncover and cook approximately 20-half an hour. 7. Serve hot while using topping of avocado.

413. Glazed Pork chops with Peach

Yield: 2 servings Preparation Time: quarter-hour Cooking Time: 16 minutes

Ingredients:

2 boneless pork chops • Salt and freshly ground black pepper, to taste • 1 ripe yellow peach, peeled, pitted, chopped and divided • 1 tbsp organic olive oil • 2 tablespoons shallot, minced • 2 tablespoons garlic, minced • 2 tablespoons fresh ginger, minced • 1 tablespoon organic honey • 1 tablespoon balsamic vinegar • 1 tablespoon coconut aminos • ¼ teaspoon red pepper flakes, crushed • ¼ cup water

Directions:

1. Sprinkle the pork chops with salt and black pepper generously. 2. In a blender, add 1 / 2 of peach and pulse till a puree forms. 3. Reserve remaining peach. 4. In a skillet, heat oil on medium heat. 5. Add shallots and sauté approximately 1-2 minutes. 6. Add garlic and ginger and sauté approximately 1 minute. 7. Add remaining ingredients and lower heat to medium-low. 8. Bring to your boil and simmer for approximately 4-5 minutes or till a sticky glaze forms. 9. Remove from heat and reserve 1/3 with the glaze and keep aside. 10. Coat the chops with remaining glaze. 11. Heat a nonstick skillet on medium-high heat. 12. Add chops and sear for around 4 minutes from both sides. 13. Transfer the chops in a plate and coat with all the remaining glaze evenly. 14. Top with reserved chopped peach and serve.

414. Baked Pork & Mushroom Meatballs

Yield: 6 servings Preparation Time: 15 minutes Cooking Time: fifteen minutes

Ingredients:

1 pound lean ground pork • 1 organic egg white, bea10 • 4 fresh shiitake mushrooms, stemmed and minced • 1 tablespoon fresh parsley, minced • 1 tablespoon fresh basil leaves, minced • 1 tablespoon fresh mint leaves, minced • 2 teaspoons fresh lemon zest, grated finely • 1½ teaspoons fresh ginger, grated finely • Salt and freshly ground black pepper, to taste

Directions:

1. Preheat the oven to 425 degrees F. Arrange the rack inside center of oven. 2. Line a baking sheet with a parchment paper. 3. In a sizable bowl, add all ingredients and mix till well combined. 4. Make small equal-sized balls from mixture. 5. Arrange the balls onto prepared baking sheet in a single layer. 6. Bake for approximately 12-quarter-hour or till done completely.

415. Beef with Carrot & Broccoli

Yield: 4 servings Preparation Time: fifteen minutes Cooking Time: 14 minutes

Ingredients:

2 tablespoons coconut oil, divided • 2 medium garlic cloves, minced • 1 pound beef sirloin steak, trimmed and sliced into thin strips • Salt, to taste • ¼ cup chicken broth • 2 teaspoons fresh ginger, grated • 1 tablespoon ground flax seeds • ½ teaspoon red pepper flakes, crushed • ¼ teaspoon freshly ground black pepper • 1 large carrot, peeled and sliced thinly • 2 cups broccoli florets • 1 medium scallion, sliced thinly

Directions:

In a substantial skillet, heat 1 tablespoon of oil on medium-high heat. 2. Add garlic and sauté approximately 1 minute. 3. Add beef and salt and cook for approximately 4-5 minutes or till browned. 4. With a slotted spoon, transfer the beef in a bowl. 5. Remove the liquid from skillet. 6. In a bowl, mix together broth, ginger, flax seeds, red pepper flakes and black pepper. 7. In a similar skillet, heat remaining oil on medium heat. 8. Add carrot, broccoli and ginger mixture and cook for approximately 3-4 minutes or till desired doneness. 9. Stir in beef and scallion and cook for around 3-4 minutes.

416. Citrus Beef with Bok Choy

Yield: 4 servings Preparation Time: fifteen minutes Cooking Time: 11 minutes

Ingredients:

For Marinade: • 2 minced garlic cloves • 1 (1-inch) piece fresh ginger, grated • 1/3 cup fresh orange juice • ½ cup coconut aminos • 2 teaspoons fish sauce • 2 teaspoons Sriracha • 1¼ pound sirloin steak, trimmed and sliced thinly For Veggies: • 2 tablespoons coconut oil, divided • 3-4 wide strips of fresh orange zest • 1 jalapeño pepper, sliced thinly • ½ pound string beans, stemmed and halved crosswise • 1 tablespoon arrowroot powder • ½ pound bokchoy, chopped • 2 teaspoons sesame seeds

Directions:

1. For marinade in a big bowl, mix together garlic, ginger, orange juice, coconut aminos, fish sauce and Sriracha. 2. Add beef and coat with marinade generously. 1. Refrigerate to marinate for around couple of hours. 2. In a substantial skillet, heat oil on medium-high heat. 3. Add orange zest and sauté approximately 2 minutes. 4. Remove beef from bowl, reserving the marinade. 5. In the skillet, add beef and increase the heat to high. 6. Stir fry for about 2-3 minutes or till browned. 7. With a slotted spoon, transfer the beef and orange strips right into a bowl. 8. With a paper towel, wipe out the skillet. 9. In a similar skillet, heat remaining oil on medium-high heat. 10. Add jalapeño pepper and string beans and stir fry for about 3-4 minutes. 11. Meanwhile add arrowroot powder in reserved marinade and stir to mix. 12. In the skillet, add marinade mixture, beef and bokchoy and cook for about 1-2 minutes. 13. Serve hot with garnishing of sesame seeds.

417. Beef with Asparagus & Bell Pepper

Yield: 4-5 servings Preparation Time: fifteen minutes Cooking Time: 13 minutes

Ingredients:

4 garlic cloves, minced • 3 tablespoons coconut aminos • 1/8 teaspoon red pepper flakes, crushed • 1/8 teaspoon ground ginger • Freshly ground black pepper, to taste • 1 bunch asparagus, trimmed and halved • 2 tablespoons olive oil, divided • 1 pound flank steak, trimmed and sliced thinly • 1 red bell pepper, seeded and sliced • 3 tablespoons water • 2 teaspoons arrowroot powder

Directions:

1. In a bowl, mix together garlic, coconut aminos, red pepper flakes, crushed, ground ginger and black pepper. Keep aside. 2. In a pan of boiling water, cook asparagus for about 2 minutes. 3. Drain and rinse under cold water. 4. In a substantial skillet, heat 1 tablespoon of oil on medium-high heat. 5. Add beef and stir fry for around 3-4 minutes. 6. With a slotted spoon, transfer the beef in a bowl. 7. In a similar skillet, heat remaining oil on medium heat. 8. Add asparagus and bell pepper and stir fry for approximately 2-3 minutes. 9. Meanwhile in the bowl, mix together water and arrowroot powder. 10. Stir in beef, garlic mixture and arrowroot mixture and cook for around 3-4 minutes or till desired thickness.

418. Ground Beef with Cabbage

Yield: 6 servings Preparation Time: 10 minutes Cooking Time: quarter-hour

Ingredients:

1 tbsp olive oil • 1 onion, sliced thinly • 2 teaspoons fresh ginger, minced • 4 garlic cloves, minced • 1 pound lean ground beef • 1½ tablespoons fish sauce • 2 tablespoons fresh lime juice • 1 small head purple cabbage, shredded • 2 tablespoons peanut butter • ½ cup fresh cilantro, chopped

Directions:

In a large skillet, heat oil on medium heat. 2. Add onion, ginger and garlic and sauté for about 4-5 minutes. 3. Add beef and cook for approximately 7-8 minutes, getting into pieces using the spoon. 4. Drain off the extra liquid in the skillet. 5. Stir in fish sauce and lime juice and cook for approximately 1 minute. 6. Add cabbage and cook approximately 4-5 minutes or till desired doneness. 7. Stir in peanut butter and cilantro and cook for about 1 minute. 8. Serve hot.

419. Ground Beef with Cashews & Veggies

Yield: 4 servings Preparation Time: 15 minutes Cooking Time: quarter-hour

Ingredients:

1½ pound lean ground beef • 1 tablespoon garlic, minced • 2 tablespoons fresh ginger, minced • ¼ cup coconut aminos • Salt and freshly ground black pepper, to taste • 1 medium onion, sliced • 1 can water chestnuts, drained and sliced • 1 large green bell pepper, seeded and sliced • ½ cup raw cashews, toasted

Directions:

1. Heat a nonstick skillet on medium-high heat. 2. Add beef and cook for about 6-8 minutes breaking into pieces with all the spoon. 3. Add garlic, ginger, coconut aminos, salt and black pepper and cook approximately 2 minutes. 4. Add vegetables and cook approximately 5 minutes or till desired doneness. 5. Stir in cashews and immediately remove from heat. 6. Serve hot.

420. Beef & Veggies Chili

Yield: 6-8 servings Preparation Time: 15 minutes Cooking Time: one hour

Ingredients:

2 pounds lean ground beef • ½ head cauliflower, chopped into large pieces • 1 onion, chopped • 6 garlic cloves, minced • 2 cups pumpkin puree • 1 teaspoon dried oregano, crushed • 1 teaspoon dried thyme, crushed • 1 teaspoon ground cumin • 1 teaspoon ground turmeric • 1-2 teaspoons chili powder • 1 teaspoon paprika • 1 teaspoon cayenne pepper • ¼ teaspoon red pepper flakes, crushed • Salt and freshly ground black pepper, to taste • 1 (26-ounce) can tomatoes, drained • ½ cup water • 1 cup beef broth

Directions:

1. Heat a substantial pan on medium-high heat. 2. Add beef and stir fry for around 5 minutes. 3. Add cauliflower, onion and garlic and stir fry for approximately 5 minutes. 4. Add spices and herbs and stir to mix well. 5. Stir in remaining ingredients and provide to a boil. 6. Reduce heat to low and simmer, covered approximately 30-45 minutes. 7. Serve hot.

421. Spicy & Creamy Ground Beef Curry

Yield: 4 servings Preparation Time: quarter-hour Cooking Time: 32 minutes

Ingredients:

1-2 tablespoons coconut oil • 1 teaspoon black mustard seeds • 2 sprigs curry leaves • 1 Serrano pepper, minced • 1 large red onion, chopped finely • 1 (1-inch) piece fresh ginger, minced • 4 garlic cloves, minced • 1 teaspoon ground coriander • 1 teaspoon ground cumin • ½ teaspoon ground turmeric • ¼ teaspoon red chili powder • Salt, to taste • 1 pound lean ground beef • 1 potato, peeled and chopped • 3 medium carrots, peeled and chopped • ¼ cup water • 1 (14-ounce) can coconut milk • Salt and freshly ground black pepper, to taste • Chopped fresh cilantro, for garnishing

Directions:

In a big pan, melt coconut oil on medium heat. 2. Add mustard seeds and sauté for about thirty seconds. 3. Add curry leaves and Serrano pepper and sauté approximately half a minute. 4. Add onion, ginger and garlic and sauté for about 4-5 minutes. 5. Add spices and cook for about 1 minute. 6. Add beef and cook for about 4-5 minutes. 7. Stir in potato, carrot and water and provide with a gentle simmer. 8. Simmer, covered for around 5 minutes. 9. Stir in coconut milk and simmer for around fifteen minutes. 10. Stir in salt and black pepper and remove from heat. 11. Serve hot while using garnishing of cilantro.

422. Beef Meatballs in Tomato Gravy

Yield: 4 servings Preparation Time: 20 minutes Cooking Time: 37 minutes

Ingredients:

For Meatballs: • 1 pound lean ground beef • 1 organic egg, bea10 • 1 tablespoon fresh ginger, minced • 1 garlic oil, minced • 2 tablespoons fresh cilantro, chopped finely • 2 tablespoons tomato paste • 1/3 cup almond meal • 1 tablespoon ground cumin • Pinch of ground cinnamon • Salt and freshly ground black pepper, to taste • ¼ cup coconut oil For Tomato Gravy: • 2 tablespoons coconut oil • ½ of small onion, chopped • 2 garlic cloves, chopped • 1 teaspoon fresh lemon zest, grated finely • 2 cups tomatoes, chopped finely • Pinch of ground cinnamon • 1 teaspoon red pepper flakes, crushed • ¾ cup chicken broth • Salt and freshly ground black pepper, to taste • ¼ cup fresh parsley, chopped

Directions:

1. For meatballs in a sizable bowl, add all ingredients except oil and mix till well combined. 2. Make about 1-inch sized balls from mixture. 3. In a substantial skillet, melt coconut oil on medium heat. 4. Add meatballs and cook for approximately 3-5 minutes or till golden brown all sides. 5. Transfer the meatballs in to a bowl. 6. For gravy in a big pan, melt coconut oil on medium heat. 7. Add onion and garlic and sauté approximately 4 minutes. 8. Add lemon zest and sauté approximately 1 minute. 9. Add tomatoes, cinnamon, red pepper flakes and broth and simmer approximately 7 minutes. 10. Stir in salt, black pepper and meatballs and reduce the warmth to medium-low. 11. Simmer for approximately twenty minutes. 12. Serve hot with all the garnishing of parsley.

423. Pan Grilled Flank Steak

Yield: 3-4 servings Preparation Time: 10 minutes Cooking Time: 12-16 minutes

Ingredients:

8 medium garlic cloves, crushed • 1 (5-inch) piece fresh ginger, sliced thinly • 1 tablespoon organic honey • ¼ cup organic olive oil • Salt and freshly ground black pepper, to taste • 1½ pound flank steak, trimmed

Directions:

1. In a large sealable bag, mix together all ingredients except steak. 2. Add steak and coat with marinade generously. 3. Seal the bag and refrigerate to marinate for approximately one day. 4. Remove from refrigerator and in room temperature approximately 15 minutes. 5. Lightly, grease a grill pan as well as heat to medium-high heat. 6. Discard the surplus marinade from steak and place in grill pan. 7. Cook for about 6-8 minutes from each party. 8. Remove from grill pan and keep side for around 10 min before slicing. 9. With a clear, crisp knife cut into desired slices and serve.

424. Spicy Lamb Curry

Yield: 6-8 servings Preparation Time: 15 minutes Cooking Time: 2 hours quarter-hour

Ingredients:

For Spice Mixture: • 4 teaspoons ground coriander • 4 teaspoons ground coriander • 4 teaspoons ground cumin • ¾ teaspoon ground ginger • 2 teaspoons ground cinnamon • ½ teaspoon ground cloves • ½ teaspoon ground cardamom • 2 tablespoons sweet paprika • ½ tablespoon cayenne pepper • 2 teaspoons chili powder • 2 teaspoons salt For Curry: • 1 tablespoon coconut oil • 2 pounds boneless lamb, trimmed and cubed into 1-inch size • Salt and freshly ground black pepper, to taste • 2 cups onions, chopped • 1¼ cups water • 1 cup coconut milk

Directions:

For spice mixture in a bowl, mix together all spices. Keep aside. 2. Season the lamb with salt and black pepper. 3. In a large Dutch oven, heat oil on medium-high heat. 4. Add lamb and stir fry for around 5 minutes. 5. Add onion and cook approximately 4-5 minutes. 6. Stir in spice mixture and cook approximately 1 minute. 7. Add water and coconut milk and provide to some boil on high heat. 8. Reduce the heat to low and simmer, covered for approximately 1-120 minutes or till desired doneness of lamb. 9. Uncover and simmer for approximately 3-4 minutes. 10. Serve hot.

425. Lamb with Zucchini & Couscous

Yield: 2 servings Preparation Time: 15 minutes Cooking Time: 8 minutes

Ingredients:

¾ cup couscous • ¾ cup boiling water • ¼ cup fresh cilantro, chopped • 1 tbsp olive oil • 5-ounces lamb leg steak, cubed into ¾-inch size • 1 medium zucchini, sliced thinly • 1 medium red onion, cut into wedges • 1 teaspoon ground cumin • 1 teaspoon ground coriander • ¼ teaspoon red pepper flakes, crushed • Salt, to taste • ¼ cup plain Greek yogurt • 1 garlic herb, minced

Directions:

1. In a bowl, add couscous and boiling water and stir to combine, 2. Cover whilst aside approximately 5 minutes. 3. Add cilantro and with a fork, fluff completely. 4. Meanwhile in a substantial skillet, heat oil on high heat. 5. Add lamb and stir fry for about 2-3 minutes. 6. Add zucchini and onion and stir fry for about 2 minutes. 7. Stir in spices and stir fry for about 1 minute 8. Add couscous and stir fry approximately 2 minutes. 9. In a bowl, mix together yogurt and garlic. 10. Divide lamb mixture in serving plates evenly. 11. Serve using the topping of yogurt.

426. Ground Lamb with Harissa

Yield: 4 servings Preparation Time: 15 minutes Cooking Time: one hour 11 minutes

Ingredients:

1 tablespoon extra-virgin olive oil • 2 red peppers, seeded and chopped finely • 1 yellow onion, chopped finely • 2 garlic cloves, chopped finely • 1 teaspoon ground cumin • ½ teaspoon ground turmeric • ¼ teaspoon ground cinnamon • ¼ teaspoon ground ginger • 1½ pound lean ground lamb • Salt, to taste • 1 (14½-ounce) can diced tomatoes • 2 tablespoons harissa • 1 cup water • Chopped fresh cilantro, for garnishing

Directions:

1. In a sizable pan, heat oil on medium-high heat. 2. Add bell pepper, onion and garlic and sauté for around 5 minutes. 3. Add spices and sauté for around 1 minute. 4. Add lamb and salt and cook approximately 5 minutes, getting into pieces. 5. Stir in tomatoes, harissa and water and provide with a boil. 6. Reduce the warmth to low and simmer, covered for about 1 hour. 7. Serve hot while using garnishing of harissa.

427. Roasted Leg of Lamb

Yield: 8 servings Preparation Time: quarter-hour Cooking Time: 75-100 minutes

Ingredients:

1/3 cup fresh parsley, minced • 4 garlic cloves, minced • 1 teaspoon fresh lemon zest, grated finely • 1 tablespoon ground coriander • 1 tablespoon ground cumin • 1 teaspoon ground cinnamon • 1 teaspoon ground turmeric • 1 tablespoon sweet paprika • ½ teaspoon allspice • 20 saffron threads, crushed • 1/3 cup essential olive oil • 1 (5-pound) leg of lamb, trimmed

Directions:

In a bowl, mix together all ingredients except lamb. 2. Coat the leg of lamb with marinade mixture generously. 3. With a plastic wrap, cover the leg of lamb and refrigerate to marinate for about 4-8 hours. 4. Remove from refrigerator and keep in room temperature for about a half-hour before roasting. 5. Preheat the oven to 350 degrees F. Arrange the rack inside the center of the oven. 6. Lightly, grease a roasting pan make a rack inside roasting pan. 7. Place the lower limb of lamb in the rack in prepared roasting pan. 8. Roast for approximately 75-100 minutes or till desired doneness, rotating once inside the middle way.

428. Pan-Seared Lamb Chops

Yield: 4 servings Preparation Time: 10 minutes Cooking Time: 4-6 minutes

Ingredients:

4 garlic cloves, peeled • Salt, to taste • 1 teaspoon black mustard seeds, crushed finely • 2 teaspoons ground cumin • 1 teaspoon ground ginger • 1 teaspoon ground coriander • ½ teaspoon ground cinnamon • Freshly ground black pepper, to taste • 1 tablespoon coconut oil • 8 medium lamb chops, trimmed

Directions:

1. Place garlic cloves onto a cutting board and sprinkle with a few salt. 2. With a knife, crush the garlic till a paste forms. 3. In a bowl, mix together garlic paste and spices. 4. With a clear, crisp knife, make 3-4 cuts on both side in the chops. 5. Rub the chops with garlic mixture generously. 6. In a large skillet, melt butter on medium heat. 7. Add chops and cook for approximately 2-3 minutes per side or till desired doneness.

429. Grilled Lamb Chops

Yield: 4 servings Preparation Time: 10 min Cooking Time: 6 minutes

Ingredients:

1 tablespoon fresh ginger, grated • 4 garlic cloves, chopped roughly • 1 teaspoon ground cumin • ½ teaspoon red chili powder • Salt and freshly ground black pepper, to taste • 1 tbsp essential olive oil • 1 tablespoon fresh lemon juice • 8 lamb chops, trimmed

Directions:

1. In a bowl, mix together all ingredients except chops. 2. With a hand blender, blend till a smooth mixture forms. 3. Add chops and coat with mixture generously. 4. Refrigerate to marinate for overnight. 5. Preheat the barbecue grill till hot. Grease the grill grate. 6. Grill the chops for approximately 3 minutes per side.

430. Lamb & Pineapple Kebabs

Yield: 4-6 servings Preparation Time: 15 minutes Cooking Time: 10 minutes

Ingredients:

1 large pineapple, cubed into 1½-inch size, divided • 1 (½-inch) piece fresh ginger, chopped • 2 garlic cloves, chopped • Salt, to taste • 16-24-ounce lamb shoulder steak, trimmed and cubed into 1½-inch size • Fresh mint leaves coming from a bunch • Ground cinnamon, to taste

Directions:

In a blender, add about 1½ servings of pineapple, ginger, garlic and salt and pulse till smooth. 2. Transfer the amalgamation right into a large bowl. 3. Add chops and coat with mixture generously. 4. Refrigerate to marinate for about 1-2 hours. 5. Preheat the grill to medium heat. Grease the grill grate. 6. Thread lam, remaining pineapple and mint leaves onto pre-soaked wooden skewers. 7. Grill the kebabs approximately 10 min, turning occasionally.

431. Fresh lime juice

Yield: 4 servings Preparation Time: 15 minutes Cooking Time: 13 minutes

Ingredients:

1 tablespoon fresh ginger, chopped finely • 4 garlic cloves, chopped finely • 1 cup fresh cilantro, chopped and divided • ¼ cup plus 1 tbsp olive oil, divided • 1 pound 10der pork, trimmed, sliced thinly • 2 onions, sliced thinly • 1 green bell pepper, seeded and sliced thinly • 1 tablespoon fresh lime juice

Directions:

In a substantial bowl, mix together ginger, garlic, ½ cup of cilantro and ¼ cup of oil. • Add pork and coat with mixture generously. • Refrigerate to marinate approximately a couple of hours. • Heat a big skillet on medium-high heat. • Add pork mixture and stir fry for approximately 4-5 minutes. • Transfer the pork right into a bowl. • In the same skillet, heat remaining oil on medium heat. • Add onion and sauté for approximately 3 minutes. • Stir in bell pepper and stir fry for about 3 minutes. • Stir in pork, lime juice and remaining cilantro and cook for about 2 minutes. • Serve hot.

432. Spiced Pork One

Yield: 6 servings Preparation Time: fifteen minutes Cooking Time: 60 minutes 52 minutes

Ingredients:

1 (2-inch) piece fresh ginger, chopped • 5-10 garlic cloves, chopped • 1 teaspoon ground cumin • ½ teaspoon ground turmeric 1 tablespoon hot paprika • 1 tablespoon red pepper flakes • Salt, to taste • 2 tablespoons cider vinegar • 2 pounds pork shoulder, trimmed and cubed into 1½-inch size • 2 cups domestic hot water, divided • 1 (1-inch wide) ball tamarind pulp • ¼ cup olive oil • 1 teaspoon black mustard seeds, crushed • 4 green cardamoms • 5 whole cloves • 1 (3-inch) cinnamon stick • 1 cup onion, chopped finely • 1 large red bell pepper, seeded and chopped

Directions:

1. In a food processor, add ginger, garlic, cumin, turmeric, paprika, red pepper flakes, salt and cider vinegar and pulse till smooth. 2. Transfer the amalgamation in to a large bowl. 3. Add pork and coat with mixture generously. 4. Keep aside, covered for around an hour at room temperature. 5. In a bowl, add 1 cup of warm water and tamarind and make aside till water becomes cool. 6. With the hands, crush the tamarind to extract the pulp. 7. Add remaining cup of hot water and mix till well combined. 8. Through a fine sieve, strain the tamarind juice inside a bowl. 9. In a sizable skillet, heat oil on medium-high heat. 10. Add mustard seeds, green cardamoms, cloves and cinnamon stick and sauté for about 4 minutes. 11. Add onion and sauté for approximately 5 minutes. 12. Add pork and stir fry for approximately 6 minutes. 13. Stir in tamarind juice and convey with a boil. 14. Reduce the heat to medium-low and simmer 1½ hours. 15. Stir in bell pepper and cook for about 7 minutes.

433. Ground Pork with Water Chestnuts

Yield: 4 servings Preparation Time: fifteen minutes Cooking Time: 12 minutes

Ingredients:

1 tablespoon plus 1 teaspoon coconut oil • 1 tablespoon fresh ginger, minced • 1 bunch scallion (white and green parts separated), chopped • 1 pound lean ground pork • Salt, to taste • 1 tablespoon 5-spice powder • 1 (18-ounce) can water chestnuts, drained and chopped • 1 tablespoon organic honey • 2 tablespoons fresh lime juice

Directions:

In a big heavy bottomed skillet, heat oil on high heat. 2. Add ginger and scallion whites and sauté for approximately ½-1½ minutes. 3. Add pork and cook for approximately 4-5 minutes. 4. Drain the extra Fat from skillet. 5. Add salt and 5-spice powder and cook for approximately 2-3 minutes. 6. Add scallion greens and remaining ingredients and cook, stirring continuously for about 1-2 minutes.

434. Pork chops in Creamy Sauce

Yield: 4 servings Preparation Time: fifteen minutes Cooking Time: 14 minutes

Ingredients:

2 garlic cloves, chopped • 1 small jalapeño pepper, chopped • ¼ cup fresh cilantro leaves • 1½ teaspoons ground turmeric, divided • 1 tablespoon fish sauce • 2 tablespoons fresh lime juice • 1 (13½-ounce) can coconut milk • 4 (½-inch thick) pork chops • Salt, to taste • 1 tablespoon coconut oil • 1 shallot, chopped finely

Directions:

1. In a blender, add garlic, jalapeño pepper, cilantro, 1 teaspoon of ground turmeric, fish sauce, lime juice and coconut milk and pulse till smooth. 2. Sprinkle the pork with salt and remaining turmeric evenly. 3. In a skillet, melt butter on medium-high heat. 4. Add shallots and sauté approximately 1 minute. 5. Add chops and cook for approximately 2 minutes per side. 6. Transfer the chops inside a bowl. 7. Add coconut mixture and convey to your boil. 8. Reduce heat to medium and simmer, stirring occasionally for approximately 5 minutes. 9. Stir in pork chops and cook for about 3-4 minutes. 10. Serve hot.

Soups and Stews

435. Spring Pea Soup

Time To Prepare: five minutes Time to Cook: fifteen minutes Yield: Servings 6

Ingredients:

½ tsp. Black pepper powder ½ tsp. ground cumin 1 liter Vegetable stock 1 medium Chopped onion 2 tbsp. Coconut oil 2 tsp. Celtic sea salt 700 g. Fresh peas Chopped flat-leaf parsley Chopped mint leaves Fresh lemon juice Grated nutmeg Toasted sunflower seeds

Directions:

Warm the coconut oil in a pan set on moderate heat. Mix in onions and stir fry for approximately five minutes. Put in the stock and raise the heat. Throw in fresh peas and cook for five minutes. If you're using frozen peas, it should take half the time. Pour in the lemon juice, salt, pepper, herbs, and spices. Stirring continuously Remove the heat and allow it to cool before running it through a food processor to whatever consistency you prefer. Serve with sunflower seed sprinkles and mint or parsley leaves. Enjoy!

436. Bacon & Cheese Soup

Time To Prepare: fifteen minutes Time to Cook: forty minutes Yield: Servings 6

Ingredients:

½ cup sour cream, for serving ½ teaspoon cumin ½ teaspoon onion powder ½ teaspoon paprika 1 cup heavy cream 1 cup shredded cheddar cheese 1 pound of lean ground beef 1 tablespoon coconut oil, for cooking 1 teaspoon garlic powder 1 yellow onion, chopped 6 cups beef broth 6 slices uncured bacon

Directions:

Put in the coconut oil to a frying pan and cook the bacon until crunchy. Allow the bacon to cool and cut into little pieces. Set aside. Once cooked, put in the lean ground beef to the same frying pan with the bacon fat and cook until browned. Put in the onions and cook for an extra two to three minutes. Put in all the ingredients minus the bacon, heavy cream, sour cream and cheese to a stockpot and stir. Cook for about twenty-five minutes. Warm the heavy cream, and then put in the warmed cream and cheese and serve with the bacon and a spoonful of sour cream

437. Broccoli Cheddar & Bacon Soup

Time To Prepare: ten minutes Time to Cook: ten minutes Yield: Servings 6

Ingredients:

¼ teaspoon black pepper ½ teaspoon salt ½ white onion, chopped 1 cup broccoli florets finely chopped 1 cup heavy cream 1 cup shredded cheddar cheese 2 cloves garlic, chopped 2 cups chicken broth 3 slices cooked bacon, crumbled for serving

Directions:

Put in all the ingredients minus the heavy cream, cheddar cheese and bacon to a stockpot on moderate heat. Heat to a simmer and cook for 5 minutes. Warm the cream, and then put in the warm cream and cheddar cheese. Whisk until the desired smoothness is achieved. Serve with crumbled bacon.

438. Brown Rice and Shitake Miso Soup with Scallion

Time To Prepare: ten minutes Time to Cook: forty-five minutes Yield: Servings 4

Ingredients:

½ teaspoon salt 1 (1½-inch) piece fresh ginger, peeled and cut 1 cup medium-grain brown rice 1 cup thinly cut shiitake mushroom caps 1 garlic clove, minced 1 tablespoon white miso 2 scallions, thinly cut 2 tablespoons finely chopped fresh cilantro 2 tablespoons sesame oil

Directions:

In a large pot, heat the oil on moderate to high heat. Put in the mushrooms, garlic, and ginger and sauté until the mushrooms start to tenderize, approximately five minutes. Place the rice and stir to uniformly coat with the oil. Put in 2 cups of water and salt and place it to its boiling point. Reduce the heat then cook until the rice is soft, thirty to forty minutes. Use a little of the soup broth to tenderize the miso, then mix it into the pot until well mixed. Stir in the scallions and cilantro, then serve.

439. Butternut Squash Soup with Shrimp

Time To Prepare:ten minutes Time to Cook: twenty minutes Yield:Servings 4

Ingredients:

¼ cup slivered almonds (not necessary) ¼ teaspoon freshly ground black pepper 1 cup unsweetened almond milk 1 garlic clove, cut 1 pound cooked peeled shrimp, thawed if required 1 small red onion, finely chopped 1 teaspoon salt 1 teaspoon turmeric 2 cups peeled butternut squash cut into ¼-inch dice 2 tablespoons finely chopped fresh flat-leaf parsley 2 teaspoons grated or minced lemon zest 3 cups vegetable broth 3 tablespoons unsalted butter

Directions:

In a large pot, melt the butter on high heat. Put in the onion, garlic, turmeric, salt, and pepper and sauté until the vegetables are tender and translucent, five to seven minutes. Put in the broth and squash and bring to its boiling point. Reduce the heat and cook until the squash has tenderized, approximately five minutes. Put in the shrimp and almond milk and cook until thoroughly heated, approximately 2 minutes. Drizzle with the almonds (if using), parsley, and lemon zest before you serve

440. Carrot Broccoli Stew

Time To Prepare: ten minutes Time to Cook: forty-five minutes Yield: Servings 3

Ingredients: 1 cup Broccoli, florets 1 cup Carrots, cut 1 cup Heavy Cream 3 cups Chicken broth Salt and black pepper to taste

Directions:

Put in florets, cream, carrots, salt, and chicken broth; toss thoroughly. Secure the lid and cook on Meat/Stew mode for forty minutes on High. When ready, do a quick pressure release. Move into serving bowls and drizzle black pepper on top

441. Cauliflower And Clam Chowder

Time To Prepare: ten minutes Time to Cook: ten minutes Yield: Servings 6

Ingredients:

½ teaspoon dried thyme 1 small yellow onion 1½ cups heavy whipping cream 3 (6.5-ounce / 184-g) cans chopped clams 3 tablespoons butter 4 cups chopped cauliflower From the cupboard: Salt and freshly ground black pepper, to taste

Directions:

Split the clams and clam juice into two bowls. Thin the clam juice with water to make 2 cups of juice. Place the onion and butter in an instant pot and press the Sauté bottom, then sauté for a couple of minutes or until the onion is translucent. Put in the clam juice and cauliflower into the instant pot. Place the lid on and press the Manual button, and set the temperature to 375°F (190°C), then cook for five minutes. Quick Release the pressure, then open the lid and mix in the heavy cream and clams. Push the Sauté bottom and cook for about three minutes or until the clams are opaque and firm, then drizzle with thyme, salt, and black pepper. Stir to mix thoroughly. Ladle the chowder in a big container and serve warm.

442. Celery Soup

Time To Prepare: ten minutes Time to Cook: twenty minutes Yield: Servings 4

Ingredients:

½ cup brown onion, chopped ½ cup full-fat milk ½ pound with Salsiccia links, casing removed and cut ½ teaspoon dried chili flakes ½ teaspoon ground black pepper 1 carrot, chopped 1 garlic clove, pressed 2 teaspoon coconut oil 3 cups celery, chopped 3 cups roasted vegetable broth Kosher salt, to taste

Directions:

Simply throw all of the above ingredients into your Instant Pot; gently stir until blended. Secure the lid. Choose "Soup/Broth" mode and High pressure; cook for about twenty-five minutes. Once cooking is complete, use a quick pressure release; cautiously remove the lid. Ladle into four soup bowls and serve hot. Enjoy!

443. Cheesy Chicken Soup

Time To Prepare: twenty minutes Time to Cook: 33-40 minutes Yield: Servings 6

Ingredients:

¼ teaspoon black pepper ½ cup shredded cheddar cheese ½ teaspoon cumin ½ teaspoon salt 1 cup whipped cream cheese 1 tablespoon coconut oil, for cooking 1 teaspoon chili powder 1 yellow onion, chopped 2 boneless, skinless chicken breasts 2 cloves garlic, chopped 2 cups chicken broth 2 cups water

Directions:

Heat a big frying pan on moderate heat with a ½ tablespoon of the coconut oil. Brown the chicken breasts until thoroughly cooked. Set aside. Put in the garlic and onion to a big stockpot with the rest of the 1 tablespoon of the coconut oil and sauté until translucent over low to moderate heat. This should take about three to five minutes. Put in this chicken broth and water. Whisk in the cream cheese and keep whisking over low to moderate heat until blended. Put in in the spices and bring to its boiling point. While the water is boiling, chop the chicken into bite-sized pieces and put in to the stockpot. Reduce to a simmer and cook for half an hour. Mix in the cheddar cheese before you serve.

444. Chicken And Cauliflower Curry Stew

Time To Prepare: fifteen minutes Time to Cook: 4 hours Yield: Servings 7

Ingredients:

¼ cup fresh cilantro, chopped ⅓ cup coconut oil 1 green bell pepper, chopped 1 pound (454 g) cauliflower, chopped into little pieces 1.5pounds (680 g) skinless, boneless chicken thighs, cut into bite-sized pieces 14 ounces (397 g) unsweetened coconut milk 2 tablespoons curry powder 2 tablespoons ginger garlic paste Salt and ground black pepper, to taste

Directions:

Warm half of the coconut oil in a nonstick frying pan on moderate heat, then sauté the garlic ginger paste and curry powder for a minutes or until aromatic. Put in the chicken pieces, and drizzle with salt and pepper. sauté for another ten minutes or until the chicken is mildly browned. Remove from the frying pan and set aside in warm. Warm another half of coconut oil in the frying pan, then sauté the cauliflower and bell pepper on moderate to high heat for one to two minutes. Then fold in the coconut milk and reduce the heat to low. Cover with lid and stew for about forty-five minutes. Drizzle with salt and pepper, then put in the sautéed chicken. Move the stew to a big platter and serve with cilantro on top as decorate.

445. Chicken Chili Blanco

Time To Prepare: ten minutes Time to Cook: twenty minutes Yield: Servings 4

Ingredients:

¼ teaspoon cayenne pepper 1 tablespoon ghee 1 teaspoon chili powder 2 (4-ounce) cans diced mild green chiles with their liquid 2 scallions, cut 2 small onions, chopped 2 teaspoons dried oregano 4 cups chicken broth or vegetable broth 4 cups shredded cooked chicken 4 cups white beans, drained and washed well 4 teaspoons ground cumin 6 garlic cloves, minced

Directions:

In a huge soup pot on moderate heat, melt the ghee. Put in the onions and garlic, and sauté for five minutes. Place the chiles, and cook for a couple of minutes, stirring. Mix in the beans, broth, cumin, oregano, chili powder, and cayenne pepper. Heat it until it simmers. Put in the chicken, bring to a simmer, decrease the heat to moderate-low, and cook for about ten minutes. Serve instantly, sprinkled with the scallions.

446. Chickpea Curry Soup

Time To Prepare: ten minutes Time to Cook: twenty-five minutes Yield: Servings 4

Ingredients:

¼ cup extra-virgin olive oil or coconut oil 1 (fifteen-ounce) can chickpeas, drained and washed 1 big apple, cored, peeled, and slice into ¼-inch dice 1 cup full-fat coconut milk 1 medium onion, finely chopped 1 teaspoon salt 2 garlic cloves, cut 2 tablespoons finely chopped fresh cilantro 2 teaspoons curry powder 3 cups peeled butternut squash cut into ½-inch dice 3 cups vegetable broth

Directions:

In a large pot, heat the oil on high heat. Put in the onion and garlic and sauté until the onion starts to brown, six to eight minutes. Place the apple, curry powder, and salt and sauté to toast the curry powder, one to two minutes. Place the squash and broth then bring to its boiling point. Reduce the heat then cook until the squash is soft about ten minutes. Mix in the coconut milk. Use an immersion blender to purée the soup in the pot until the desired smoothness is achieved. Mix in the chickpeas and cilantro, heat through for one to two minutes, before you serve.

447. Coconut Cashew Soup with Butternut Squash

Time To Prepare: ten minutes Time to Cook: twenty minutes Yield: Servings 6

Ingredients:

½ tsp. salt ¾ cup toasted cashews 1 (14-ounce) can full-fat coconut milk 1 cup mung bean sprouts 1 small butternut squash, halved, diced 1 small Napa cabbage, shredded 1 white onion, diced 1½ tbsp. Ginger, peeled and minced 2 carrots, chopped 2 cups green beans, trimmed 2 red chili peppers, seeded and diced 2 tbsp. coconut oil 3 cups vegetable broth 3 garlic cloves, peeled and minced 4 tablespoons toasted coconut shavings Freshly ground black pepper

Directions:

In a huge soup pot on moderate heat, melt the coconut oil. Place the cashews and sauté for a couple of minutes. Take off from the pan and save for later. Place the peppers, garlic, and onion, and sauté for minimum 6 minutes. Then put the ginger and carrots, and sauté for minimum 3 minutes, or until the carrots and squash start to become tender. Stir in the cabbage, green beans, broth, coconut milk, and salt, flavor with pepper. Simmer for fifteen minutes. Remove the heat. Mix in the bean sprouts and coconut shavings. Pour into soup bowls and serve instantly.

448. Cream of Mushroom Soup

Time To Prepare: twenty minutes Time to Cook: thirty minutes Yield: Servings 6

Ingredients:

5 cups mushrooms (cut) 1 tablespoon sherry 3 tablespoons butter 3 tablespoons flour 1 cup half-and-half Salt Ground black pepper 1½ cups chicken broth ½ cup onion (chopped) 1/8 teaspoon dried thyme

Directions:

Cook mushrooms with onion and thyme in the broth until soft. Puree the mixture. Whisk some flour in a pan of melted butter. Put in half-and-half, vegetable puree, and seasoning. Boil until it becomes thick. Put in sherry.

449. Creamy Broccoli Soup

Time To Prepare: fifteen minutes Time to Cook: 4 hours Yield: Servings 7

Ingredients:

¼ teaspoon ground black pepper ½ teaspoon paprika powder ½ teaspoon salt ⅔ cup heavy whipping cream 1 pinch cayenne pepper 1 red onion, roughly chopped 1 tablespoon olive oil 2 cups chicken broth 20 ounces (567 g) broccoli, cut into stalks and florets 3 garlic cloves, chopped 3 tablespoons butter ounces (99 g) Cheddar cheese, shredded

Directions:

Warm 1 tablespoon of butter and olive oil in a deep cooking pan, then fry the broccoli stalks and chopped onion on moderate heat for five minutes until soft. Put in the garlic and keep frying for a couple of minutes until mildly browned, then drizzle with cayenne pepper, paprika, salt, and ground black pepper. Cook for another one minutes. Pour over the chicken broth. Cover the lid and leave to simmer for five minutes. Take away the cooked vegetables from the deep cooking pan to a food processor and process. Lightly ladle the soup into the food processor while processing until creamy. Melt the rest of the butter in the deep cooking pan, and fry the broccoli florets for five minutes until tender and soft. Pour the soup from the food processor into the deep cooking pan. Blend to mix thoroughly. If the soup is too thick, you can put in some water to make it thinner. Bring the soup to its boiling point, then reduce the heat and bring to a simmer using low heat for about three minutes. Put in the Cheddar cheese and heavy whipping cream and cook for a couple of minutes more until the cheese melts. Take away the soup from the deep cooking pan and serve warm.

450. Creamy Leek Soup

Time To Prepare: two minutes Time to Cook: 8 minutes Yield: Servings 4

Ingredients:

½ cup heavy cream ½ cup Monterey-Jack cheese, shredded ½ cup tomato purée ½ pound chorizo, cut 1 bay leaf 1 cup leeks, chopped 1 green chili, deseeded and finely chopped 1 tablespoon sesame oil 2 chicken bouillon cubes 2 cloves garlic, minced 4 cups water

Directions:

Push the "Sauté" button to heat up your Instant Pot. Once hot, heat the oil and sauté the leeks until soft. Now, mix in chorizo, garlic, and green chili; carry on cooking until aromatic. Next, put in water, tomato puree, heavy cream, bouillon cubes, and bay leaf. Secure the lid. Choose "Manual" mode and High pressure; cook for about six minutes. Once cooking is complete, use a natural pressure release; cautiously remove the lid. Next, press the "Sauté" button and put in the cheese; allow it to simmer until the cheese is melted and thoroughly heated

451. Creamy Pumpkin Puree Soup

Time To Prepare: ten minutes Time to Cook: forty-five minutes Yield: Servings 3

Ingredients:

1 cup Heavy Cream 1 cup Pumpkin puree 2 cups Chicken broth 2 tbsp. Olive oil 4-5 Garlic cloves Salt and black pepper to taste

Directions:

In the Instant Pot, put in all ingredients. Secure the lid and cook for forty minutes on Meat/Stew mode on High. When ready, press Cancel and do a quick pressure release. Move to a blender and blend thoroughly. Pour into serving bowls to serve

452. Creamy Turmeric Cauliflower Soup

Time To Prepare:ten minutes Time to Cook: fifteen minutes Yield:Servings 4

Ingredients:

¼ cup finely chopped fresh cilantro ¼ teaspoon freshly ground black pepper ¼ teaspoon ground cumin ½ teaspoon salt 1 (1¼-inch) piece fresh ginger, peeled and cut 1 cup full-fat coconut milk 1 garlic clove, peeled 1 leek, white part only, thinly cut 1½ teaspoons turmeric 2 tablespoons extra-virgin olive oil 3 cups cauliflower florets 3 cups vegetable broth

Directions:

In a large pot, heat the oil on high heat. Put in the leek, and sauté until it just starts to brown, three to four minutes. Put in the cauliflower, garlic, ginger, turmeric, salt, pepper, and cumin and sauté to lightly toast the spices, one to two minutes. Pour the broth then bring to its boiling point. Reduce the heat and cook until the cauliflower is soft about five minutes. Use an immersion blender to purée the soup in the pot until the desired smoothness is achieved. Stir in the coconut milk and cilantro, heat through, before you serve.

453. Detox Cabbage Soup

Time To Prepare: ten minutes Time to Cook: thirty-five minutes Yield: Servings 4

Ingredients:

1 tbs. freshly grated ginger root 2 big carrot 1 cup whole canned tomatoes with juice 1 whole head of cabbage 1 tbs. freshly grated turmeric root 3 celery stalks with leaves Enough water to immerse the vegetables 2 medium Russet potatoes Sea salt & black pepper to taste ½ medium onion 1/4 cup extra virgin olive oil

Directions:

Heat the oil in a large pot on moderate heat for a couple of minutes. Put in the celery, onions, ginger, carrots & turmeric, then sauté on medium until translucent. Sprinkle with salt & pepper to taste. With the heat still on moderate, dice the potatoes & generally slash the cabbage at that point put in to the pot alongside the whole tomatoes & juice. While they cook, break separated the tomatoes using a fork or blade. Fill the pot with sufficient water to simply cover the cabbage. Cover with a top & heat to the point of boiling. When bubbling, evacuate the top & cook for around thirty minutes or until the potatoes & cabbage are fork delicate. Put in the ice chest for as long as 5 days & in the cooler for as long as three months

454. French Caramelized Onion Soup

Time To Prepare: five minutes Time to Cook: ten minutes Yield: Servings 4

Ingredients:

½ stick butter, softened 4 cups chicken stock ½ teaspoon dried basil Kosher salt and ground black pepper, to taste ½ cup Swiss cheese, freshly grated 3/4 pound yellow onions, cut

Directions: Push the "Sauté" button to heat up your Instant Pot. Once hot, melt the butter and sauté the onions until caramelized and soft. Put in chicken stock, basil, salt, and black pepper. Secure the lid. Choose "Manual" mode and High pressure; cook for about ten minutes. Once cooking is complete, use a quick pressure release; cautiously remove the lid. Ladle the soup into separate bowls and top with grated cheese. Enjoy

455. Garlic Mushroom & Beef Soup

Time To Prepare: ten minutes Time to Cook: forty minutes Yield: Servings 6

Ingredients:

½ cup heavy cream ½ cup whipped cream cheese 1 pound beef chuck, cubed 1 tablespoon coconut oil, for cooking 1 yellow onion, chopped 1½ cups cremini mushrooms 2 cloves garlic, chopped 6 cups beef broth Salt & pepper, to taste

Directions:

Put in the coconut oil to a frying pan and brown the beef. Once cooked, put in the beef to the base of a stockpot with all of the ingredients minus the heavy cream. Mix thoroughly. Heat to a simmer and whisk again until the cream cheese is mixed uniformly into the soup. Cook for half an hour Warm the heavy cream, and then put in to the soup

456. Golden Chickpea And Vegetable Soup

Time To Prepare: fifteen minutes Time to Cook: twenty minutes Yield: Servings 6

Ingredients:

1 ½ cup Diced celery 1 ½ cup Sliced leeks 1 cup cooked chickpeas 1 cup diced carrots 1 cup Torn curly kale leaves 1 tbsp. Grated ginger 2 cloves minced garlic 2 cups Cauliflower florets 2 tbsp. Curry powder 2 tbsp. Minced organic parsley 2 tsp. Coconut oil 4 cups Bone broth

Directions:

Warm the coconut oil in a pot and put in the garlic and ginger. Sauté for one minute before you put in the turmeric and curry powder and sautéing for one more minute. Throw in celery, leeks, carrots, and cauliflower, continuously stirring for approximately one minute. Put in the bone broth and chickpeas. Cover the pot and leave to boil. Reduce the heat and allow it to simmer for minimum fifteen minutes. Turn off heat and put in parsley and kale, leaving the heat to cook the leaves. Drizzle salt and pepper. Serve

457. Green Blast Soup

Time To Prepare:ten minutes Time to Cook: twenty minutes Yield:Servings 4

Ingredients:

¼ cup chopped cashews (not necessary) ¼ cup extra-virgin olive oil ¼ teaspoon freshly ground black pepper 1 bunch Swiss chard, crudely chopped 1 fennel bulb, trimmed and thinly cut 1 garlic clove, peeled 1 teaspoon salt 2 leeks, white parts only, thinly cut 2 tablespoons apple cider vinegar 3 cups vegetable broth 4 cups crudely chopped kale 4 cups crudely chopped mustard greens

Directions:

In a large pot, heat the oil on high heat. Put in the leeks, fennel, and garlic and sauté until tender, for approximately five minutes. Put in the Swiss chard, kale, and mustard greens and sauté until the greens wilt, two to three minutes. Pour the broth then bring to its boiling point. Reduce the heat to a simmer and cook until the vegetables are completely tender and soft about five minutes. Mix in the vinegar, salt, pepper, and cashews (if using). Use an immersion blender to purée the soup in the pot until the desired smoothness is achieved before you serve

458. Hamburger & Tomato Soup

Time To Prepare: ten minutes Time to Cook: 4 hours Yield: Servings 6

Ingredients:

½ cup beef broth ½ cup no-sugar added marinara sauce ½ cup shredded cheddar cheese 1 pound lean ground beef 1 yellow onion, chopped 2 cloves garlic, chopped Salt & pepper, to taste

Directions: Put in all the ingredients to a slow cooker minus the shredded cheese and cook on high for 4 hours. Mix in the cheese before you serve

459. Hearty Root Vegetable Soup

Time To Prepare: five minutes Time to Cook: ten minutes Yield: Servings 4

Ingredients:

1 bay leaf 1 carrot, cut 1 celery, diced 1 garlic clove, minced 1 parsnip, cut 1 tablespoon fresh parsley, roughly chopped 1 teaspoon fresh sage 2 cups cauliflower, cut into little florets 4 cups chicken stock 4 tablespoons olive oil Kosher salt and freshly ground black pepper, to taste

Directions:

Simply drop all of the above ingredients into your Instant Pot. Secure the lid. Choose "Manual" mode and High pressure; cook for about ten minutes. Once cooking is complete, use a natural pressure release; cautiously remove the lid. Taste, calibrate the seasonings and serve instantly. Enjoy!

460. Italian Beef Soup

Time To Prepare: ten minutes Time to Cook: 4 hours Yield: Servings 6

Ingredients:

½ cup diced tomatoes ½ cup shredded mozzarella cheese 1 cup beef broth 1 cup heavy cream 1 pound lean ground beef 1 tablespoon Italian seasoning 1 yellow onion, chopped 2 cloves garlic, chopped Salt & pepper, to taste

Directions:

Put in all the ingredients to a slow cooker minus the heavy cream and mozzarella cheese. Cook on high for 4 hours. Warm the heavy cream, and then put in the warmed cream and cheese to the soup. Stir thoroughly before you serve.

461. Sugars Italian Summer Squash Soup

Time To Prepare:ten minutes Time to Cook: fifteen minutes Yield:Servings 4

Ingredients:

½ cup shredded carrot 1 cup shredded yellow squash 1 cup shredded zucchini 1 garlic clove, minced 1 small red onion, thinly cut 1 tablespoon finely chopped fresh chives 1 teaspoon salt 2 tablespoons finely chopped fresh basil 2 tablespoons pine nuts 3 cups vegetable broth 3 tablespoons extra-virgin olive oil

Directions:

In a large pot, heat the oil using high heat. Put in the onion and garlic and sauté until tender, five to seven minutes. Put in the zucchini, yellow squash, and carrot and sauté until tender, one to two minutes. Pour the broth and salt then bring to its boiling point. Reduce the heat and cook until the vegetables are soft, one to two minutes. Mix in the basil and chives and serve, sprinkled with the pine nuts

462. Lamb Stew

Time To Prepare: five minutes Time to Cook: 8 hours Yield: Servings 6

Ingredients:

1 lamb stock cube 1 onion, roughly chopped 2 pounds (907 g) boneless lamb, cut into cubes 2 tablespoons olive oil, plus more for greasing the frying pan 2 teaspoons dried rosemary 3 cups water 4 garlic cloves, finely chopped From the cupboard: Salt and freshly ground black pepper, to taste

Directions:

Position the lamb into a mildly greased nonstick frying pan, and cook using high heat for a couple of minutes or until browned. Grease a slow cooker with olive oil, then put in the cooked lamb, stock cube, rosemary, onion, garlic, salt, black pepper, and 3 cups of water. Blend to blend well. Place the slow cooker lid on and cook on LOW for eight hours. Take away the cooked lamb stew from the slow cooker and serve warm.

463. Lebanese Lentil Soup

Time To Prepare: fifteen minutes Time to Cook: 60 minutes Yield: Servings 6

Ingredients:

1 cup brown lentils 1 lemon juiced 1 medium onion 1 tablespoon olive oil 2 medium carrots 2 teaspoons cinnamon 2 teaspoons cumin 3 stalks celery 4 cloves garlic 4 cups chicken broth low sodium 4 cups water 8 cups spinach salt& pepper to taste

Directions:

Over moderate heat, heat oil in a soup pot, Put in & cook carrots, celery & onions until become soft for seven minutes, put in pepper & salt to taste. Stir cumin, cinnamon & garlic heat it for 30-60 minutes. Put in lentils & heat for a couple of minutes to slightly toast. Pour in the lemon juice, water & chicken broth, then bring the pot to its boiling point. When lentils are soft, decrease the heat to low & simmer, approximately 30-45 minutes. Before you serve, mix in the spinach, cook until the color is green, now served to put in pepper, lemon juice & salt

464. Lemon Chicken Soup

Time To Prepare: ten minutes Time to Cook: 4 hours Yield: Servings 4

Ingredients:

¼ cup freshly squeezed lemon juice 1 yellow onion, chopped 2 boneless, skinless chicken breasts 2 cloves garlic, chopped 2 tablespoons chives, chopped 6 cups chicken broth Salt & pepper, to taste

Directions: Put in all the ingredients to a slow cooker and cook on high for 4 hours. Once cooked, shred the chicken and stir back into the soup

465. Minestrone Soup with Quinoa

Time To Prepare: ten minutes ime to Cook: twenty minutes Yield: Servings 6

Ingredients:

½ cup quinoa, washed well ½ red bell pepper, diced ½ teaspoon salt 1 (14 oz.) can cannellini beans, drained and washed well 1 (14 oz.) can diced tomatoes with its juice 1 bay leaf 1 cup packed kale, stemmed and meticulously washed 1 medium white onion, diced 1 small zucchini, diced 1 tablespoon freshly squeezed lemon juice 1 tablespoon ghee 2 carrots, chopped 2 celery stalks, diced 2 garlic cloves, minced 2 teaspoons dried rosemary 2 teaspoons dried thyme 5 cups vegetable broth Freshly ground black pepper

Directions: In a huge soup pot on moderate heat, put in the ghee, garlic, onion, carrots, and celery, and sauté for about three minutes. Put in the zucchini and red bell pepper, and sauté for a couple of minutes. Mix in the broth, tomatoes, beans, kale, quinoa, lemon juice, rosemary, thyme, bay leaf, and salt, and flavor with black pepper. Put it to a simmer, reduce the heat temperature, cover, and cook for fifteen minutes, or until the quinoa is cooked. Take away the bay leaf and discard it. Serve hot.

466. Mushroom And Thyme Soup

TimeTo Prepare:five minutes Time to Cook: twenty minutes Yield:Servings 4

Ingredients:

¼ cup butter 12 ounces (340 g) wild mushrooms, chopped 2 garlic cloves, minced 2 teaspoons thyme leaves 4 cups vegetable broth 5 ounces (142 g) crème fraiche From the cupboard: Salt and freshly ground black pepper, to taste

Directions: Place the butter in a deep cooking pan and melt on moderate heat. Put in the minced garlic and cook for a minutes or until aromatic. Put in the chopped mushrooms, and drizzle with salt and black pepper. Stir to blend and cook for about ten minutes or until the mushrooms are soft. Put in the vegetable broth and bring the soup to its boiling point. Stir continuously. Reduce the heat and simmer the soup for about ten minutes or until it becomes slightly thick. Pour the soup in a blender, and pulse until smooth, then fold in the crème fraiche. Move the soup in a big container and top with thyme leaves before you serve.

467. Pork Stew

Time To Prepare: five minutes Time to Cook: 8 hours Yield: Servings 6

Ingredients:

1 onion, finely chopped 1 teaspoon dried mixed spices (homemade or store-bought) 2 pounds (907 g) pork loin, cut into cubes 2 tablespoons olive oil 3 cups chicken stock 4 garlic cloves, crushed From the cupboard: Salt and freshly ground black pepper, to taste

Directions:

Grease the insert of the slow cooker with olive oil. Combine the pork, chicken stock, onion, dried mixed spices, garlic, salt, and black pepper in the slow cooker. Place the slow cooker lid on and cook on LOW for eight hours. Ladle the stew in a big container and serve warm.

468. Pumpkin, Coconut & Sage

Soup Time To Prepare: fifteen minutes Time to Cook: thirty minutes Yield: Servings 6

Ingredients:

1 cup canned pumpkin 1 cup full-fat coconut milk 1 teaspoon freshly chopped sage 2 cloves garlic, chopped 6 cups vegetable broth Pinch of salt & pepper, to taste

Directions:

Put in all the ingredients minus the coconut milk to a stockpot on moderate heat and bring to its boiling point. Reduce to a simmer and cook for half an hour Put in the coconut milk and stir

469. Red Lentil Dal

Time To Prepare:ten minutes Time to Cook: twenty minutes Yield:Servings 6

Ingredients:

½ teaspoon salt 1 (14-ounce) can unsweetened coconut milk 1 bay leaf 1 cup red dried lentils, sorted and washed well 1 medium tomato, diced 1 medium white onion, diced 1 tablespoon coconut oil 1 teaspoon ground cumin 1 teaspoon ground ginger 1 teaspoon ground turmeric 1 teaspoon mustard seeds 1 teaspoon sesame seeds 2 garlic cloves, minced 2 tablespoons chopped fresh cilantro leaves 3 cups vegetable broth Dash ground cinnamon

Directions: In a huge soup pot using high heat, combine the broth, lentils, and bay leaf, and place to its boiling point. Lessen the heat to moderate-low and simmer for about twenty minutes, or until the lentils are cooked. In the meantime, in a moderate-sized deep cooking pan on moderate heat, sauté the onion and garlic in the coconut oil for a couple of minutes. Put in the tomato, sesame seeds, ginger, cumin, turmeric, mustard seeds, salt, and cinnamon. Cook, regularly stirring, for five minutes. Mix in the coconut milk, then put it to a simmer. Remove and discard the bay leaf. Put in the coconut milk mixture to the lentils together with the cilantro, and stir until blended. Serve alone or over rice if you wish.

470. Rich Onion And Beef Stew

Time To Prepare: five minutes Time to Cook: 10 hours Yield: Servings 6

Ingredients:

1 beef stock cube 1 teaspoon dried mixed herbs (such as Italian seasoning) 2 onions, roughly chopped 2 pounds (907 g) boneless stewing beef, cut into cubes 3 cups water 3 tablespoons olive oil, divided 5 garlic cloves, crushed From the cupboard: Salt and freshly ground black pepper, to taste

Directions: Grease the insert of the slow cooker with 2 tablespoons of olive oil. Coat a nonstick frying pan with the rest of the olive oil. Heat the oil in the frying pan on moderate to high heat, then put the beef in the frying pan and sear for a couple of minutes or until medium-rare. Shake the frying pan continuously to sear the beef cubes uniformly. Position the cooked beef in the slow cooker, then put in the stock cube, mixed herbs, garlic, onions, salt, black pepper, and water. Stir to mix thoroughly. Place the slow cooker lid on and cook on LOW for ten hours. Ladle the stew in a big container and serve warm.

471. Russian Cabbage Soup

Time ToPrepare: ten minutes Time to Cook: twenty minutes Yield:Servings 6

Ingredients:

½ big head cabbage, shredded ½ teaspoon salt 1 (14 oz.) can diced tomatoes with its juice 1 bay leaf 1 big potato, peeled and diced 1 celery stalk, diced 1 medium white onion, diced 1 tablespoon ghee 2 carrots, shredded 3 garlic cloves, minced 6 cups vegetable broth Freshly ground black pepper

Directions:

In a huge soup pot using high heat, mix the broth, bay leaf, and potato, and bring to its boiling point. Lower the heat to low and simmer for fifteen minutes. In the meantime, in a moderate-sized deep cooking pan on moderate heat, heat the ghee. Place the onion and garlic, and sauté for five minutes. Put in the carrots, celery, and cabbage, and cook for a couple of minutes, stirring frequently. Move to the soup pot. Mix in the tomatoes and salt, and flavor with pepper. Mix thoroughly and carry on simmering until all ingredients have become tender and cooked, approximately five minutes. Take off and discard the bay leaf, and serve instantly

472. Slow Cooker Lamb & Cauliflower Soup

Time To Prepare: ten minutes Time to Cook: 4 hours Yield: Servings 6

Ingredients:

½ teaspoon cracked black pepper ½ teaspoon salt 1 cauliflower head, cut into florets 1 cup heavy cream 1 pound ground lamb 1 tablespoon freshly chopped thyme 1 yellow onion, chopped 2 cloves garlic, chopped 5 cups beef broth

Directions:

Put in the ground lamb and cauliflower to the base of a stockpot. Put in in the rest of the ingredients minus the heavy cream, and cook on high for 4 hours. Warm the heavy cream before you put in to the soup. Use an immersion blender to combine the soup until creamy.

473. Sugars Spicy Cabbage Turmeric Coconut Soup

TimeTo Prepare: ten minutes Time to Cook: twenty minutes Yield:Servings 4

Ingredients:

½ teaspoon black pepper ½ teaspoon salt 1 head white cabbage 1 teaspoon cumin powder 1/4 cup coconut milk 2 cloves garlic 2 tablespoons coconut oil 2 teaspoons turmeric powder 3 cups vegetable/chicken stock

Directions:

Heat the oil in a frying pan on moderate heat. Put in the cabbage & garlic & sauté until the cabbage is delicate. Put in the stock, bubble, spread, & stew for about twenty minutes. Turn off the heat, including the coconut milk & flavors. Blend until the desired smoothness is achieved & season to taste. Serve, gulp & appreciate!

474. Spicy Ramen Noodles

Time To Prepare: fifteen minutes Time to Cook: 0 minutes Yield: Servings 4

Ingredients:

¼ cup chopped fresh cilantro ¼ cup cut scallion ¼ cup thinly cut cucumber 1 tablespoon coconut aminos 1 tablespoon freshly squeezed lime juice 1 tablespoon grated peeled fresh ginger 1 tablespoon raw honey 1 teaspoon chili powder 2 tablespoons rice vinegar 2 tablespoons sesame oil 2 tablespoons sesame seeds 8 ounces buckwheat noodles or rice noodles, cooked

Directions:

In a big serving container, meticulously mix the noodles, sesame seeds, cucumber, scallion, cilantro, sesame oil, vinegar, ginger, coconut aminos, honey, lime juice, and chili powder. Split among 4 soup bowls and serve at room temperature

475. Sweet Potato and Black Bean Chili

Time To Prepare: ten minutes Time to Cook: twenty minutes Yield: Servings 8

Ingredients:

¼ teaspoon cayenne pepper ¼ teaspoon dried oregano ½ teaspoon ground cinnamon 1 (28-ounce) can diced tomatoes with their juice 1 green bell pepper, diced 1 red bell pepper, diced 1 red onion, diced 1 tablespoon chili powder 1 tablespoon freshly squeezed lime juice 1 teaspoon cocoa powder 1 teaspoon ground cumin 1 teaspoon salt 2 cups vegetable broth 2 tablespoons avocado oil 3 cups black beans, drained and washed well 3 cups cooked sweet potato cubes 5 garlic cloves, minced

Directions:

In a huge soup pot on moderate heat, warm the avocado oil. Place the onion and garlic, and sauté for a couple of minutes. Mix in the red bell pepper and the green bell pepper, and sauté for approximately 3 minutes until tender. Put in the sweet potato, beans, broth, tomatoes, lime juice, chili powder, cocoa powder, cumin, salt, cinnamon, cayenne pepper, and oregano, then stir until blended. Put to a simmer, and cook for fifteen minutes. Serve instantly

476. Tex-Mex Chicken Soup

Time To Prepare: ten minutes Time to Cook: 1 hour Yield: Servings 4

Ingredients:

¼ cup roasted pumpkin seeds 1 teaspoon paprika powder 1 yellow onion, chopped 1¾ cups coconut cream 12 ounces (340 g) boneless chicken thighs 2 tablespoons coconut oil 3 tablespoons Tex-Mex seasoning 4 tablespoons lime juice Fresh cilantro, chopped Salt and ground black pepper, to taste

Directions: Cook the chicken thighs in a pot of water, covered, for thirty minutes or until the chicken is completely fork-soft. Move the chicken to a container and reserve the chicken broth until ready to use. Warm the coconut oil in a nonstick frying pan on moderate heat, then put in the onion and drizzle with Tex-Mex seasoning, salt, and pepper. sauté for five minutes until the onion is translucent. Pour over the reserved chicken broth and coconut cream. Bring them to a simmer for about twenty minutes or until it becomes thick. Put in the chicken, pumpkin seeds, paprika powder, lime juice, and cilantro to the soup. Stir to blend well before you serve.

477. Thai Winter Vegetable Soup

Time To Prepare: 60 minutes Time to Cook: 6 hours Yield: Servings 12

Ingredients:

½ Of Lemon Juice 1 Lime Juice 1 Piece Ginger (Peeled, Grated) 1 Teaspoon Cumin 14 Ounce Coconut Milk 14 Ounce Peeled Italian Plum Tomatoes 2 Large Onions (Peeled, Quartered) 2 Stalks Lemongrass (Split) 3 Carrots (Peeled, Chopped) 3 Cloves Garlic (Peeled, Chopped) 3 Red Bell Peppers (Quartered, Seeded) 4 Large Sweet Potatoes (Peeled, Cut) 4 Tablespoons Cilantro (Chopped) Ground Black Pepper Optional: 1 Green Chili Pepper (Chopped) Salt

Directions:

Cook the vegetables with ginger and chili before pouring in coconut milk. Mix in cilantro, cumin, lemon juice, and seasoning, cooking for around six hours. Remove lemongrass and blend until thick. Put in lime juice, seasoning, and cilantro to serve.

478. Tomato Bisque Soup

Time To Prepare: ten minutes Time to Cook: forty minutes Yield: Servings 6

Ingredients:

1 cup heavy cream 1 teaspoon freshly chopped thyme 2 tablespoons butter 3 cloves garlic, chopped 3 cups canned whole, peeled tomatoes 4 cups chicken broth Salt & black pepper, to taste

Directions: Put in the butter to the bottom of a stockpot. Put in in all the rest of the ingredients minus the heavy cream. Bring to its boiling point, and then simmer for forty minutes. Warm the heavy cream, and then mix into the soup.

479. Tuscan Style Soup

Time To Prepare: three minutes Time to Cook: five minutes Yield: Servings 4

Ingredients:

½ cup leeks, cut 1 carrot, trimmed and grated 1 zucchini, shredded 1/4 teaspoon ground black pepper 2 cups broth, if possible homemade 2 cups water 2 garlic cloves, minced 2 tablespoons butter, melted 4 cups broccoli rabe, broken into pieces Sea salt, to taste

Directions:

Push the "Sauté" button to heat up your Instant Pot; now, melt the butter. Cook the leeks for approximately 2 minutes or until tender. Put in minced garlic and cook an additional 40 seconds. Put in the rest of the ingredients. Secure the lid. "Manual" mode and Low pressure; cook for about three minutes. Once cooking is complete, use a quick pressure release; cautiously remove the lid. Enjoy

480. Vegetarian Garlic, Tomato & Onion Soup

Time To Prepare: fifteen minutes Time to Cook: thirty minutes Yield: Servings 6

Ingredients:

½ cup full-fat unsweetened coconut milk 1 bay leaf 1 teaspoon Italian seasoning 1 yellow onion, chopped 1½ cups canned diced tomatoes 3 cloves garlic, chopped 6 cups vegetable broth Fresh basil, for serving Pinch of salt & pepper, to taste

Directions:

Put in all the ingredients minus the coconut milk and fresh basil to a stockpot on moderate heat and bring to its boiling point. Reduce to a simmer and cook for half an hour Take away the bay leaf, and then use an immersion blender to combine the soup until the desired smoothness is achieved. Mix in the coconut milk. Decorate using fresh basil before you serve.

481. White Velvet Cauliflower Soup

Time ToPrepare: ten minutes Time to Cook: twenty minutes Yield:Servings 6

Ingredients:

1 head cauliflower, chopped into 1-inch pieces 1 small celery root, peeled, cut into 1-inch pieces 1 small white onion, diced 1 tbsp. avocado oil 2 scallions, cut 2 tbsp. ghee 3 garlic cloves, minced 4 cups vegetable broth

Directions:

In a huge soup pot on moderate heat, heat the avocado oil. Place the onion and garlic, and sauté for five minutes. Place the celery root and cauliflower. Raise the heat to moderate-high, then continue to sauté for minimum five minutes, or until the cauliflower starts to brown and caramelize the sides. Mix in the broth and ghee and place it to its boiling point. Lessen the heat to moderate-low and simmer for about ten minutes. Take away the pot from the heat. Use an immersion blender to or in batches in a standard blender, purée the soup until creamy. Serve instantly, sprinkled with the scallions.

482. Sugars Zesty Broccoli Soup

TimeTo Prepare: ten minutes Time to Cook: twenty minutes Yield:Servings 4

Ingredients:

½ teaspoon freshly squeezed lemon juice ½ teaspoon lemon zest ½ teaspoon salt 1 carrot, chopped 1 celery stalk, diced 1 head broccoli, roughly chopped 1 medium white onion, diced 1 tablespoon ghee 3 cups vegetable broth 3 garlic cloves, minced Freshly ground black pepper

Directions:

In a huge soup pot on moderate heat, melt the ghee. Place the onion and garlic, and sauté for five minutes. Put in the broccoli, carrot, and celery, and sauté for a couple of minutes. Mix in the broth, salt, lemon juice, and lemon zest, and flavor with pepper. Heat to a simmer, and cook for minimum ten minutes. Serve instantly.

483. Carrot Soup

Yield: 8 servings Preparation Time: fifteen minutes Cooking Time: 1 hour 40 minutes

Ingredients:

2 pounds carrots, peeled and cut into slices • 7 tablespoons extra-virgin essential olive oil, divided • 2 large fennel bulbs, sliced • Salt, to taste • ¼ cup pumpkin seeds • 1 medium yellow onion, chopped • 6 garlic cloves, minced • 1 tablespoon fresh ginger, grated • 1 tablespoon ground turmeric • ½ teaspoon red pepper cayenne • 2 tablespoons fresh lime juice • 1½ cups coconut milk • 4-6 cups water • ¼ cup scallion (green part), minced

Directions:

1. Preheat the oven to 375 degrees F. 2. In a baking sheet, place the carrot and drizzle with 2 tablespoons of oil. 3. Roast approximately one hour. 4. Remove the carrots from oven and make aside. 5. Now, raise the temperature of oven to 400 degrees F. 6. In a skillet, heat 3 tablespoons of oil on medium heat. 7. Add fennel bulbs and pinch of salt and sauté for about 4-5 minutes. 8. Transfer the fennel bulb onto a baking sheet and roast approximately 20-a half-hour. 9. Meanwhile, heat a nonstick skillet on medium heat. Keep aside. 10. Add pumpkin seeds and stir fry for around 3-4 minutes or till toasted. Keep aside. 11. Meanwhile in a very soup pan, heat remaining oil on medium heat. 12. Add onion and sauté for around 12 minutes. 13. Add garlic and sauté for approximately 1 minute. 14. In a blender, add onion mixture, carrots, ginger, spices, lime juice and coconut milk and pulse till well combined. 15. Add required amount of water and pulse till smooth. 16. Return the soup in the pan on medium heat. 17. Bring to some boil and cook approximately 3-5 minutes. 18. Serve hot with all the topping of fennel and pumpkin seeds.

484. Curried Carrot & Sweet Potato Soup

Yield: 5 servings Preparation Time: fifteen minutes Cooking Time: 37 minutes

Ingredients:

2 teaspoons olive oil • ½ cup shallots, chopped • 1½ cups carrots, peeled and sliced into ¼-inch size • 3 cups sweet potato, peeled and cubed into ½-inch size • 1 tablespoon fresh ginger, grated • 2 teaspoons curry powder • 3 cups Fat-free chicken broth • Salt, to taste

Directions:

1. In a sizable soup pan, heat oil on medium heat. 2. Add shallots and sauté for approximately 3 minutes. 3. Add carrot, sweet potato, ginger and curry powder and sauté for around 3-4 minutes. 4. Add broth and bring to a boil. 5. Reduce heat to low. 6. Cover and simmer approximately 25-thirty minutes. 7. Stir in salt and black pepper and remove from heat. 8. Keep aside to cool down the slightly. 9. In a blender, add soup in batches and pulse till smooth. 10. Serve immediately.

485. Pumpkin Soup

Yield: 2 servings Preparation Time: quarter-hour Cooking Time: 18 minutes

Ingredients:

2 teaspoons coconut oil • 1 brown onion, chopped • 1 (¾-inch) fresh turmeric piece • 1 (¾-inch) fresh galangal piece • 1 long red chili, seeded and chopped • 2 tablespoons fresh cilantro, chopped • 4 kefir lime leaves • 3 cups pumpkin, peeled and cubed • 1 teaspoon fresh lime peel piece • 1 large garlic oil, chopped • 4 cups vegetable broth • 2 tablespoons fish sauce • ½ cup coconut cream • 2 tablespoons fresh lime juice

Directions:

In a substantial soup pan, heat oil on medium heat. 2. Add onion, turmeric, galangal, red chili, cilantro and lime leaves and sauté for approximately 2-3 minutes. 3. Add pumpkin, lime peel, garlic, broth and fish sauce and convey to your boil 4. Reduce the heat to low. 5. Cover and simmer approximately quarter-hour. 6. Remove from heat whilst aside to chill slightly. 7. Discard the turmeric, galangal and lemon peel. 8. In a blender, add soup mixture with coconut cream and lemon juice in batches and pulse till smooth.

486. Butternut Squash Soup

Yield: 4 servings Preparation Time: quarter-hour Cooking Time: twenty minutes

Ingredients:

1 small butternut squash, peeled, seeded and cubed • 2 tablespoons coconut oil, melted • Salt, to taste • 4 cups reduced-sodium vegetable broth, divided • 14-ounces coconut milk • 1 small shallot, sliced thinly • 2 lemongrass stalks, cut into 6-inch pieces • 3 tablespoons fresh ginger, grated • ½ of Serrano pepper, chopped • 1 cup fresh mushrooms, sliced • Freshly ground black pepper, to taste • 2 tablespoons fresh lime juice • Chopped fresh cilantro, for garnishing

Directions:

1. Preheat the oven to 400 degrees F. 2. Place the butternut squash in a baking sheet. 3. Drizzle with oil and sprinkle with salt and roast approximately 12-quarter-hour. 4. Remove from oven whilst aside to chill completely. 5. In a big soup pan, add 3 cups from the broth, coconut milk, shallot, lemongrass, ginger and Serrano pepper and bring to a boil. 6. Reduce the warmth to simmer. 7. In a blender, add roasted butternut squash and remaining broth and pulse till smooth. 8. Add squash puree and mushrooms in simmering broth and stir to combine. 9. Simmer for about 5 minutes. 10. Stir in salt, black pepper and lime juice and take away from heat. 11. Serve hot with all the garnishing of cilantro.

487. Cauliflower & Zucchini

Yield: 4-6 servings Preparation Time: quarter-hour Cooking Time: 45 minutes

Ingredients:

2-3 cups cauliflower, chopped into large pieces • 2 tablespoons coconut oil, divided • 1 medium yellow onion, chopped • 1 tablespoon garlic, minced • 1 teaspoon fresh ginger, minced • 1 teaspoon dried ginger • 1½ teaspoons ground coriander • Salt and freshly ground black pepper, to taste • 1½ pound zucchini, peeled and chopped • 4 cups chicken broth • ½ cup coconut milk • Chopped chives, for garnishing

Directions:

1. Preheat the oven to 375 degrees F. 2. Place the cauliflower in a baking sheet and drizzle with 1 tablespoon of oil 3. Roast approximately half an hour, stirring once in the middle way. 4. Meanwhile in a large soup pan, heat remaining oil on medium heat. 5. Add onion and sauté approximately 5 minutes. 6. Add garlic, ginger, coriander, salt and black pepper and sauté for around 1 minute. 7. Add zucchini and cook for around 1 minute. 8. Add broth and produce to your boil. 9. Reduce the temperature to simmer. 10. Add the cauliflower and stir to combine. 11. Simmer approximately quarter-hour. 12. Remove in the heat and stir in coconut milk. 13. With an immersion blender, puree the soup completely. 14. Serve hot with the topping of chives.

488. Kabocha Squash Soup

Yield: 8 servings Preparation Time: quarter-hour Cooking Time: 65 minutes

Ingredients:

1 (4-5-pound) kabocha squash, stemmed, peeled, seeded and chopped • Coconut oil, as required • 1 large sweet onion, chopped • 6-10 garlic cloves, chopped • 6 cups chicken broth • 1 (14-ounce) can coconut milk • ¼ teaspoon ground cumin • ¼ teaspoon ground ginger • ¼ teaspoon ground turmeric • Pinch of freshly ground white pepper • Salt and freshly ground black pepper, to taste • Pumpkin seeds, for garnishing

Directions:

Preheat the oven to 350 degrees F. 2. Place the squash into a baking sheet and drizzle with a few melted oil 3. Roast for around 30-45 minutes or till 10der. 4. Remove from oven and make aside. 5. In a substantial soup pan, heat some oil on medium heat. 6. Add onion and garlic and sauté for around 4-5 minutes. 7. Add squash and remaining ingredients and simmer approximately 10-15 minutes. 8. Remove from heat and by having an immersion blender, puree the soup completely. 9. Serve hot using the topping of pumpkin seeds.

489. Mixed Veggie Soup

Yield: 4 servings Preparation Time: twenty or so minutes Cooking Time: 31 minutes

Ingredients:

1 tbsp extra virgin olive oil • ½ of small onion, chopped • 1 tablespoon fresh ginger herb, chopped finely • 2-3 garlic cloves, minced • ¼ teaspoon ground turmeric • 2 celery stalks, chopped • ½ head of cauliflower, chopped • 2 small potatoes, peeled and chopped • 2 large carrots, peeled and chopped • 1 medium zucchini, chopped • Salt and freshly ground black pepper, to taste • 2 tablespoons fresh lemon juice • ¼-½ teaspoon cayenne • 4 cups vegetable broth

Directions:

1. In a substantial soup pan, heat oil on medium heat. 2. Add onion, ginger, garlic and turmeric and sauté for approximately 4-5 minutes. 3. Add vegetables, salt and black pepper and cook, stirring occasionally approximately 5-7 minutes. 4. Stir in fresh lemon juice. 5. Add red pepper cayenne and broth and produce to a boil. 6. Simmer, covered for about 10-15 minutes. 7. Remove from heat and with an immersion blender, puree the soup completely. 8. Return the soup in pan on medium-low heat and simmer for around 3-4 minutes or till heated completely. 9. Serve immediately.

490. Tangy Mushroom Soup

Yield: 3-4 servings Preparation Time: quarter-hour Cooking Time: 15-twenty minutes

Ingredients:

For Soup: • 4 cups low-sodium vegetable broth • 1 cup button mushrooms, sliced • 1 cup cherry tomatoes, chopped • ½ of white onion, sliced • 3 slices lemongrass • 3 pieces fresh ginger • 5 fresh kaffir lime leaves • 5 Thai chile peppers, seeded and mashed • ¼ cup fresh lime juice • 2 tablespoons tamari For Garnishing: • 1 cu bean sprouts • ¼ cup scallion, chopped • ½ cup fresh cilantro, chopped

Directions:

1. In a sizable pan, add broth on medium-high heat. 2. Bring with a boil reducing the temperature to medium. 3. Add remaining soup ingredients and again bring to some gentle simmer. 4. Simmer approximately 15-20 min. 5. Remove from heat and discard lemongrass, ginger and lime leaves. 6. Serve hot while using ingredients of garnishing.

491. Tomatoes & Quinoa Soup

Yield: 4 servings Preparation Time: 15 minutes Cooking Time: 22 minutes

Ingredients:

5 tablespoons extra-virgin coconut oil • 1 brown onion, chopped • 1 (3-inch) piece fresh ginger, chopped • 4 garlic cloves, chopped • 2 teaspoons ground cumin • 1 teaspoon ground turmeric • 1 teaspoon dried sage • 1 teaspoon dried thyme • 1/8 teaspoon red pepper cayenne • Salt and freshly ground black pepper, to taste • 1½ cups quinoa • 4 tomatoes, chopped • 1 red bell pepper, seeded and chopped • 3 celery stalks, chopped • ¾ cup fresh cilantro, chopped and divided • 6 cups water • 2 tablespoons fresh lemon juice • 2 tablespoons extra-virgin extra virgin olive oil • 1 avocado, peeled, pitted and sliced • 1 lemon, cut into 4 wedges

Directions:

In a big soup pan, heat coconut oil on medium heat. 2. Add onion, ginger and garlic and sauté for around 4 minutes. 3. Add cumin, turmeric, sage and thyme and sauté for about 1 minute. 4. Add cayenne pepper, salt and black pepper and sauté approximately 2 minutes. 5. Add quinoa, tomatoes, bell pepper, celery, ¼ cup of cilantro, and water and produce with a boil on high heat. 6. Reduce the warmth to medium-low 7. Simmer, covered for around quarter-hour. 8. Stir in remaining cilantro and lemon juice and remove from heat. 9. Transfer the soup into serving bowls and drizzle with organic olive oil. 10. Serve hot using the garnishing of avocado lemon wedges.

492. Sweet Potato, Spinach & Lentil

Yield: 4 servings Preparation Time: quarter-hour Cooking Time: 31 minutes

Ingredients:

1 tbsp extra virgin olive oil • 1 large onion, minced • 6 garlic cloves, minced • 1½ teaspoons garam masala • ½ teaspoon ground turmeric • 2 pinches red pepper flakes, crushed • 4 cups vegetable broth • 1 cup lentil • 2 sweet potatoes, peeled and cubed into ½-inch size • 4 cups fresh spinach, chopped

Directions:

1. In a substantial soup pan, heat oil on medium heat. 2. Add onion and garlic and sauté for approximately 2-4 minutes. 3. Stir in garam masala, turmeric and red pepper flakes and sauté approximately 2 minutes. 4. Add broth and lentil and provide with a boil. 5. Reduce heat to low and simmer, covered approximately fifteen minutes. 6. Stir in sweet potatoes and simmer approximately 10 min. 7. Stir in spinach and simmer for approximately 3-5 minutes. 8. Stir in salt and serve hot.

493. Barley, Beans & Veggie Soup

Yield: 6 servings Preparation Time: 20 minutes Cooking Time: 48 minutes

Ingredients:

3 tablespoons extra virgin olive oil • ¼ cup pearl barley • 1 onion, chopped • 2 celery stalks, chopped • 2 carrots, peeled and chopped • 1 garlic clove, minced • ½ teaspoon ground turmeric • ½ teaspoon curry powder • Salt and freshly ground black pepper, to taste • 6 cups chicken broth • 1 small sweet potato, peeled and chopped • 1 (14-ounce) can diced tomatoes, drained • 1 (19-ounce) can mixed beans, rinsed and drained

Directions: 1. In a substantial soup pan, heat oil on medium heat. 2. Add barley, onion, celery, carrots, garlic, turmeric and curry powder and sauté for around 6-8 minutes. 3. Add salt, black pepper and broth and bring to a boil. 4. Reduce the heat and simmer, covered for approximately 30 minutes. 5. Stir in the remaining ingredients and again bring to some boil. 6. Simmer, covered for around 10 minutes. 7. Serve hot.

494. Black Beans Soup

Yield: 4 servings Preparation Time: 15 minutes Cooking Time: 30-45 minutes

Ingredients:

2 (15-ounce) cans black beans, rinsed and drained • 1 (14½-ounce) can diced tomatoes • 1 cup vegetable broth • 1 (14-ounce) can coconut milk • 2 scallions, chopped • 2 minced garlic cloves • 1 tablespoon ground cumin • 1 tablespoon ground ginger • 1 tablespoon ground turmeric • Salt, to taste

Directions: 1. In a large soup pan, mix together all ingredients except salt on medium-high heat. 2. Bring to your boil and reduce the heat. 3. Simmer for approximately 30-45 minutes. 4. Stir in salt and serve hot.

495. Chicken & Veggies Soup

Yield: 10-12 servings Preparation Time: quarter-hour Cooking Time: 33 minutes

Ingredients:

1½ tablespoons extra virgin olive oil • 1 large onion, chopped • 2 large potatoes, peeled and chopped • 4 parsnips, peeled and chopped • 1-2 zucchinis, chopped • 1 cup fresh peas, shelled • 2 large raw chicken breasts • 2 teaspoons ground cumin • 1 tablespoon ground turmeric • 4 cups chicken broth • 6 cups water • Chopped fresh cilantro, for garnishing

Directions:

1. In a large soup pan, heat oil on medium heat. 2. Add onion and sauté approximately 3 minutes. 3. Stir in vegetables and cook for around 5 minutes. 4. Stir in remaining ingredients and produce with a boil. 5. Reduce the heat to medium-low. 6. Simmer for around 10-fifteen minutes 7. Remove the chicken breasts from soup with forks, shred them 8. Return the shredded chicken into soup and simmer for approximately 10 min. 9. Serve hot while using garnishing of cilantro.

496. Beef, Mushroom & Broccoli Soup

Yield: 8 servings Preparation Time: 15 minutes Cooking Time: 13 minutes

Ingredients:

8 cups beef broth • 2-3 cups broccoli, chopped • 8-ounces mushrooms, sliced • 1 bunch scallion, chopped (reserve dark green part for garnishing) • 1 (1-inch) piece fresh ginger, minced • 5 garlic cloves, minced • 1 pound cooked beef, sliced thinly • ½ teaspoon red pepper flakes, crushed • 3 tablespoons coconut aminos • 1 lemon, sliced

Directions:

1. In a soup pan, add broth and provide to a boil. 2. Add broccoli and cook for approximately 2 minutes. 3. Stir in mushroom, scallions, ginger and garlic and simmer for around 7-8 minutes. 4. Stir in beef, red pepper flakes and coconut aminos minimizing heat to low. 5. Simmer approximately 2-3 minutes. 6. Serve hot while using garnishing of reserved green part of scallion and lemon slices.

497. Mixed Veggies Stew

Yield: 4 servings Preparation Time: fifteen minutes Cooking Time: 21 minutes

Ingredients:

2 tablespoons coconut oil • 1 large onion, chopped • 1 teaspoon ground turmeric • 1 teaspoon ground cumin • Salt and freshly ground black pepper, to taste • 1-2 cups water, divided • 1 cup cabbage, shredded • 1 bunch broccoli, chopped • 2 large carrots, peeled and sliced • 2 teaspoons fresh ginger, grated

Directions:

1. In a large soup pan, melt coconut oil on medium heat. 2. Add onion and sauté approximately 5 minutes. 3. Stir in spices and sauté for about 1 minute. 4. Add 1 cup of water and convey to some boil. 5. Simmer approximately 10 min. 6. Add vegetables and enough water that covers the 50 % of vegetables mixture. 7. Simmer, covered for about 10-fifteen minutes, stirring occasionally. 8. Serve hot.

498. Chicken & Tomato Stew

Yield: 6-8 servings Preparation Time: fifteen minutes Cooking Time: 31 minutes

Ingredients:

2 tablespoons olive oil • 1 onion, chopped • ½ tablespoon fresh ginger, grated finely • 1 tablespoon fresh garlic, minced • 1 teaspoon ground turmeric • 1 teaspoon ground cumin • 1 teaspoon ground coriander • 1 teaspoon paprika • 1 teaspoon red pepper cayenne • 6 skinless, boneless chicken thighs, trimmed and cut into 1-inch pieces • 3 Roma tomatoes, chopped • 1 (14-ounce) coconut milk • Salt and freshly ground black pepper, to taste • 1/3 cup fresh cilantro, chopped

Directions:

In a substantial pan, heat oil on medium heat. 2. Add onion and sauté for around 8-10 minutes. 3. Add ginger, garlic and spices and sauté for approximately 1 minute. 4. Add chicken and cook for around 4-5 minutes. 5. Add tomatoes, coconut milk, salt and black pepper and brig to gentle simmer. 6. Reduce the heat to low and simmer, covered for around 10-15 minutes or till desired doneness. 7. Stir in cilantro and take away from heat.

499. Beef & Squash Stew

Yield: 4-6 servings Preparation Time: fifteen minutes Cooking Time: 60 minutes 17 minutes

Ingredients:

1½ tablespoons coconut oil, divided • 2-3 pound stew meat, trimmed and cubed into 1½-inch size • 1 onion, chopped • 1 (2-inch) piece fresh ginger, minced • 5 garlic cloves, minced • 2 cups bone broth • 1 butternut squash, peeled and cubed • ¼ teaspoon ground cinnamon • 2 pears, cored and chopped • 1 cup fresh mushrooms, sliced • 1 tablespoon fresh thyme, chopped

Directions:

1. In a big heavy bottomed pan, heat 1 tablespoon of oil on medium-high heat 2. Add beef and sear for around 8-10 minutes or till browned completely. 3. With a slotted spoon, transfer the beef in to a bowl. 4. Now, decrease the heat to medium. 5. Add onion and sauté for approximately 5 minutes. 6. Add ginger and garlic and sauté for about 2 minutes. 7. Add cooked beef and broth and provide with a boil. 8. Reduce the warmth to low and simmer, covered approximately 15 minutes. 9. Stir in squash, cinnamon and salt and simmer, covered for around fifteen minutes. 10. Stir in pears and simmer, covered for approximately half an hour. 11. Meanwhile in the small skillet, heat the remainder oil on high heat. 12. Add mushrooms and cook for approximately 5 minutes or till browned. 13. Serve the stew with the topping f mushrooms and thyme.

500. Haddock & Potato Stew

Yield: 4 servings Preparation Time: 15 minutes Cooking Time: 13 minutes

Ingredients:

2 large Yukon Gold potatoes, sliced into ¼-inch size • 1 tbsp olive oil • 1 (2-inch) piece fresh ginger, chopped finely • 1 (16-ounce) can whole tomatoes, crushed • ½ cup water • 1 cup clam juice • ¼ teaspoon red pepper flakes, crushed • Salt, to taste • 1½ pound boneless haddock, cut into 2inch pieces • 2 tablespoons fresh parsley, chopped

Direction:

1. Arrange a steamer basket in a big pan of water and produce to your boil. 2. Place the potatoes in steamer basket and cook, covered approximately 8 minutes. 3. Meanwhile in the pan, heat oil on medium heat. 4. Add ginger and sauté for about 1 minute. 5. Add tomatoes and cook, stirring continuously approximately 2 minutes. 6. Add water, clam juice, red pepper flakes and produce to a boil. 7. Simmer for around 5 minutes, stirring occasionally. 8. Gently, stir in haddock pieces and simmer, covered for about 5 minutes or till desired doneness. 9. In serving bowls, divide potatoes and top with haddock mixture. 10. Garnish with parsley and serve.

501. Black-Eyed Beans Stew

Yield: 4-5 servings Preparation Time: 15 minutes Cooking Time: 120 minutes 20 min

Ingredients:

2 cups dried black eyed beans, soaked for overnight, rinsed and drained • 2 medium onions, chopped and divided • 1 (4-inch) piece fresh ginger chopped • 4 garlic cloves, chopped • ¼ cup essential olive oil • 2 scotch bonnet peppers • 2 (14-ounce) cans plum tomatoes • ½-¾ cup water • 1 vegetable bouillon cube • Salt, to taste

Directions:

In a big pan of boiling water, add beans and cook, covered approximately 60-90 minutes or till bens become soft. 2. In a blender, add 1 onion, ginger and garlic and pulse till a puree forms. 3. In a big pan, heat oil on medium heat. 4. Add onion and sauté for around 2-5 minutes. 5. Stir in 5 tablespoons of onion puree and cook for approximately 5 minutes. 6. Meanwhile in blender, add bonnet peppers and tomatoes and pulse till smooth. 7. Add tomato mixture and stir to blend. 8. Reduce the warmth to low and simmer, covered for about 30 minutes, stirring occasionally. 9. Stir in beans, cube and salt and simmer for approximately 10 minutes.

502. Lentil Stew

Yield: 4 servings Preparation Time: quarter-hour Cooking Time: 50 minutes

Ingredients:

1 cup dry lentils, rinsed and drained • 1 cup potato, peeled and chopped • ½ cup celery, chopped • ½ cup carrot, peeled and chopped • ½ cup onion, chopped • 1 garlic cloves, minced • 1 (14½-ounce) peeled Italian tomatoes, chopped • 1 tablespoon dried basil, crushed • 1 tablespoon dried parsley, crushed • Freshly ground black pepper, to taste • 3½ cups chicken broth

Directions:

1. In a big pan, add all ingredients and stir to blend. 2. Bring with a boil on high heat. 3. Reduce heat to low and simmer, covered approximately 45-50 minutes, stirring occasionally.

503. Chilled Tomato & Bell Pepper Soup

Yield: 4-6 servings Preparation Time: 25 minutes Cooking Time: 20 seconds

Ingredients:

8 ripe Roma tomatoes • 1 small red bell pepper, seeded and chopped roughly • 1 small green bell pepper, seeded and chopped roughly • 1 medium cucumber, peeled, seeded and chopped roughly • 1 small red onion, chopped roughly • 3 large garlic cloves, chopped • 1 fresh long red chili, seeded and chopped roughly • 2 teaspoons fresh orange zest, grated finely • 1 cup fresh tomato juice • ¾ cup olive oil • 2-3 tablespoons fresh orange juice • 2 tablespoons apple cider vinegar treatment • 1 cup chilled water • 1 teaspoon salt • ½ freshly ground black pepper

Directions:

1. In a sizable pan of boiling water, add tomatoes and boil for 20 seconds or till your skin actually starts to crack. 2. Drain well and rinse under cold water. Then peel skin of tomatoes. Cut the tomatoes and discard the seeds. 3. In a substantial food processor, add tomatoes add tomatoes and remaining all ingredients and pulse till smooth. 4. Refrigerate to relax for about 1 hour before serving.

504. Chilled Spinach & Cucumber Soup

Yield: 2 servings Preparation Time: 15 minutes

Ingredients:

2 medium cucumbers, peeled seeded and chopped • 2 cups fresh spinach • 1 small avocado, peeled, pitted and chopped • ½ of jalapeño, seeded and chopped • 1cup mixed fresh herbs • 1 cup water • 1 tablespoon fresh lime juice • 1 tablespoon essential olive oil

Directions:

1. In a substantial mixer, add all ingredients and pulse till smooth. 2. Refrigerate to chill for around a couple of hours before serving.

505. Chilled Pineapple Soup

Yield: 4 servings Preparation Time: fifteen minutes

Ingredients:

1 under ripe pineapple, peeled, cored and chopped • ½ cup cucumber, peeled, seeded and chopped finely • ½ cup red bell pepper, seeded and chopped finely • ¼ cup red onion, chopped finely • 1 tablespoon fresh cilantro, chopped finely • ¼ of serrano Chile, seeded and minced • 2 tablespoons fresh lime juice • ½ teaspoon salt

Directions:

1. In a blender, add pineapple and pulse till pureed. 2. Strain the puree in a very bowl. 3. Stir in remaining ingredients. Cover and chill for approximately 120 minutes before serving.

506. Creamy Carrot Soup

Yield: 2-3 servings Preparation Time: fifteen minutes Cooking Time: 25 minutes

Ingredients:

1. 3 cups homemade vegetable broth 2. 1½ cups fennel bulb, chopped 3. 3 cups carrots, peeled and chopped 4. 2 garlic cloves, minced 5. 1 cup full- Fat coconut milk 6. Salt, to taste 7. 4-ounces pancetta, chopped 8. ½ cup pine nuts, toasted and chopped

Directions: 1. In a big soup pan, add broth and vegetables and produce with a boil on high heat. 2. Reduce heat to medium-low. Simmer for about 15-twenty minutes. 3. Stir in coconut milk and simmer for approximately 3-5 minutes. Stir in salt and remove from heat. 4. Meanwhile heat a nonstick skillet on medium-high heat. 5. Add pancetta and cook for around 8-10 minutes or till crispy. 6. Serve this soup hot with the topping of cooked pancetta and pine nuts.

507. Chicken & Veggie Soup

Yield: 4 servings Preparation Time: twenty minutes Cooking Time: 28-30 minutes

Ingredients:

2 tablespoons coconut oil • 1 bunch scallion, sliced thinly • 2-inch piece fresh ginger, minced • 4 garlic cloves, minced • 1 cup shiitake mushrooms, sliced • 1 large carrot, peeled and shredded • 1 red bell pepper, seeded and chopped • 1 jalapeño pepper, chopped • 14-ounces coconut milk • 4 cups chicken broth • 1 tablespoon red bat fish sauce • 1 pound skinless, boneless chicken breasts • Fresh cilantro, as required • 1 teaspoon fresh lime zest, grated finely • Salt and freshly ground black pepper, to taste

Directions: 1. In a large soup pan, heat oil on medium heat. 2. Add scallion, ginger and garlic and sauté for around 2-3 minutes. 3. Add mushrooms, carrot, bell pepper and jalapeño pepper and sauté for approximately 5 minutes. 4. Add broth, coconut milk, fish sauce and chicken and convey to your boil. 5. Reduce the heat to low. Simmer for about 15 minutes. 6. Transfer the chicken right into a plate and chop into small chunks. 7. Add chopped chicken, cilantro, lime zest, salt and black pepper and simmer for 5 minutes more.

508. Roasted Veggies Soup

Yield: 4-6 servings Preparation Time: twenty minutes Cooking Time: 30 minutes

Ingredients:

2½ pounds zucchini, cut into 1-inch pieces • ½ of yellow onion, chopped • 1 leek, chopped • 3 garlic cloves, peeled • 2 tablespoons coconut oil, melted • 2½ cups water • ½ cup raw cashews, soaked for 3 hours • Salt and freshly ground black pepper, to taste

Directions: 1. Preheat the oven to 400 degrees F. Line a baking sheet using a parchment paper. 2. Arrange zucchini, onion, leek and garlic onto prepared baking sheet. 3. Roast for about twenty minutes. Remove from oven and cool slightly. 4. In a blender, add roasted veggies, water and cashews and pulse till smooth. 5. Transfer the pureed mixture in a soup pan on medium heat. 6. Simmer for around 5 minutes. Stir in salt and black pepper and take away from heat. 7. Serve hot.

509. Shrimp & Snow Peas Soup

Yield: 8 servings Preparation Time: fifteen minutes Cooking Time: 8-10 min

Ingredients:

4 teaspoons coconut oil • 4 medium scallions (white and green part), sliced thinly • 2-inch piece fresh ginger herb, sliced thinly • 8 cups homemade chicken broth • ¼ teaspoon red boat fish sauce • ¼ cup coconut aminos • 1/8 teaspoon freshly ground white pepper • 1 pound shrimp, peeled and deveined • 1 (5-ounce) can sliced bamboo shoots, drained • ½ pound snow peas, cleaned • 1 tablespoon sesame oil, toasted

Directions: 1. In a big soup pan, heat oil on medium heat. 2. Add white portion of scallion and ginger and sauté for approximately 2 minutes. 3. Add broth, fish sauce, coconut aminos and white pepper and bring to a boil. 4. Stir in shrimp, bamboo shoots and snow peas. 5. Reduce the warmth to low. Simmer for around 2-3 minutes. 6. Stir in sesame oil and green portion of scallion and remove from heat. 7. Serve hot.

510. Spicy Leek Soup With Poached Eggs

Yield: 6-8 servings Preparation Time: quarter-hour Cooking Time: 10 minutes

Ingredients:

2 tablespoons coconut oil • 1 large leek, sliced • 4 carrots, peeled and sliced • 6 garlic cloves, minced • 6-8 cups chicken broth • ¾ teaspoon dried oregano, crushed • ½ teaspoon paprika • Pinch of red pepper flakes, crushed • 2 teaspoons unrefined salt • 6-8 organic eggs

Directions:

1. In a substantial soup pan, heat oil on medium heat. 2. Add leeks and sauté approximately 3-4 minutes. 3. Add carrots and cook approximately 4-5 minutes. 4. Add garlic and sauté for about 1 minute. 5. Add broth, oregano and spices and convey with a boil. Reduce the heat to low. 6. Simmer approximately 10 minutes. 7. Meanwhile inside a frying pan, add 1-2-inch water and bring to your gentle simmer. Stir in most salt. 8. Carefully, crack eggs in pan and cook approximately 3-4 minutes on medium-low heat. 9. With a slotted spoon, place 1 egg in each bowl. 10. Divide the soup in bowls evenly and serve.

511. Sweet Potato Soup

Time To Prepare: twenty minutes Time to Cook: thirty minutes Yield: Servings 8

Ingredients:

1 13.66-ounce can lite coconut milk 1 big zucchini, cut width-wise 1 garlic clove 1 liter low-sodium vegetable stock 1 tablespoon sweet yellow curry powder 1 teaspoon black pepper 1 teaspoon cayenne pepper 1 teaspoon turmeric 1 white onion 2 moderate-sized white potatoes, 3 moderate-sized sweet potatoes, 3/4 tablespoons salt 4 cups of hot water 4 tablespoons olive oil A pinch of cinnamon A pinch of cloves

Directions:

Prepare every one of your vegetables by cutting, cleaning & cubing. Put in a safe spot. To a large pot, include 4 tablespoons of additional virgin olive oil. Allow it to heat up swiftly; at that point, include your white onion. Allow it to sweat for minimum five minutes on low warmth. Put in all your flavoring & garlic. Give it a decent mix; at that point, including the potatoes. Allow these cook on moderate heat for around five minutes to get a pleasant darker shading. Continue blending to abstain from consuming. Put in your stalk & water, warm it to the point of boiling & then stew for around 20-twenty-five minutes. Part of the way through the stewing procedure, include your zucchini. After 20-twenty-five minutes, include your coconut milk. Before pouring the soup to the blender, do a fork content to guarantee your potatoes are cooked. Use your blender to purée the soup. Embellishment with lemon juice, dark pepper & herbs & flavors of your preference.

512. Beef And Veggie Soup

Time To Prepare: ten minutes Time to Cook: twenty minutes Yield: Servings 8

Ingredients:

½ cup heavy whipping cream ½ cup onion, chopped 1 (8 ounces / 227 g) package cream cheese, softened 1 pound (454 g) ground beef 1 tablespoon ground cumin 1 teaspoon chili powder 2 (10 ounces / 284 g) cans diced tomatoes and green chiles 2 (14.5 ounces / 411 g) cans beef broth 2 cloves garlic, minced 2 teaspoons salt, or to taste

Directions:

Position the ground beef, chopped onion, and garlic in a pot, stir until blended well. Cook on moderate to high heat for five to seven minutes or until the beef is thoroughly browned. Stir continuously. Discard the grease extract from the beef, then put in chili powder and cumin, and cook for an extra two minutes. Stir continuously. Put in the cream cheese to the pot and cook for three to five minutes more, then fold in the tomatoes and green chiles, beef broth, heavy whipping cream, and salt, and cook for about ten minutes to cook through. Keep stirring during the cooking. Serve the soup in a big serving container. Allow to stand for a couple of minutes before you serve

513. Broccoli Soup with Gorgonzola Cheese

Time To Prepare: ten minutes Time to Cook: thirty minutes Yield: Servings 4

Ingredients:

½ cup 18% cream 1 big broccoli, divided into little roses 1 flat teaspoon of sweet pepper 1 onion, diced 1 tablespoon of chopped fresh basil 1 tablespoon of chopped parsley 1 tablespoon of oil 150 g Gorgonzola cheese, diced 2 potatoes, peeled and diced 4 tablespoons of almond flakes roasted in a dry pan 5 garlic cloves, chopped 750 ml broth a pinch of sugar pumpkin oil (not necessary) salt and pepper

Directions: In a big deep cooking pan, warm the oil on moderate heat, put the onion and garlic, and fry it until the vitrified glass onion. Then put the broccoli with potatoes, pour the broth and cook for approximately fifteen-twenty minutes until the vegetables become tender. Put in basil, parsley, sugar, pepper, and pepper to taste. Put in cheese and cream, and when the cheese dissolves, blend with a blender until the desired smoothness is achieved. Sprinkle with salt and pepper if required. Serve the soup sprinkled with almond flakes and sprinkled with pumpkin oil.

514. Buffalo Sauce And Turkey Soup

Time To Prepare: five minutes Time to Cook: ten minutes Yield: Servings 4

Ingredients:

⅓ cup buffalo sauce 2 cups turkey, cooked, shredded 3 tablespoons butter, melted 4 cups chicken broth 4 ounces (113 g) cream cheese 4 tablespoons cilantro, chopped From The Cupboard: Salt and freshly ground black pepper, to taste

Directions: Place the buffalo sauce, cream cheese, and melted butter in a blender, and process until the desired smoothness is achieved. Pour the buffalo sauce mixture in a deep cooking pan, and put in the chicken broth. Heat the soup using high heat until hot and nearly boil off but not boil. Keep stirring during the heating. Put in the shredded turkey, and drizzle with salt and black pepper. Cook for five minutes or until the desired smoothness is achieved. Stir continuously. Ladle the soup into a big container and top with chopped cilantro before you serve.

515. Cannellini Bean Soup

Time To Prepare: twenty-five minutes Time to Cook: thirty minutes Yield: Servings 6

Ingredients:

1 bunch red Swiss chard 1 cannellini beans 1 clove garlic (minced) 1 onion (chopped) 1 tablespoon extra-virgin olive oil 1/4 teaspoon nutmeg (grated) 1/8 teaspoon red pepper flakes (crushed) 2 ounces Parmesan cheese rind 2 slices smoked bacon (chopped) 2 tablespoons chopped sun-dried tomatoes 5 big sage leaves (minced) 5 leaves basil (chopped) 6 cups chicken broth

Directions: Cook the bacon with garlic, onion, nutmeg, and red pepper flakes for five minutes. Pour in beans, chicken broth, sun-dried tomatoes, and Parmesan cheese rind, simmering for about ten minutes. Put in the cut chard and chard leaves into the soup. Simmer and then put in into bowls with a sprinkle of oil and Parmesan cheese

516. Carrot, Ginger & Turmeric Soup

Time To Prepare: fifteen minutes Time to Cook: forty minutes Yield: Servings 8

Ingredients:

1/4 cup full-fat unsweetened coconut milk 3/4 pound carrots, peeled and chopped 1 sweet yellow onion, chopped 1 teaspoon ground turmeric 2 cloves garlic, chopped 2 teaspoons grated ginger 6 cups vegetable broth Pinch of sea salt & pepper, to taste

Directions: Put in all the ingredients minus the coconut milk to a stockpot on moderate heat and bring to its boiling point. Reduce to a simmer and cook for forty minutes or until the carrots are soft. Use an immersion blender and blend the soup until the desired smoothness is achieved. Mix in the coconut milk. Enjoy immediately and freeze any remainings.

517. Cauliflower, Coconut Milk, And Shrimp Soup

Time To Prepare: five minutes Time to Cook: 2 hours and fifteen minutes Yield: Servings 4

Ingredients:

1 (13.5-ounce / 383-g) can unsweetened full-fat coconut milk 1 cup shrimp, peeled, deveined, tail off, and cooked 1 cup water 2 cups riced cauliflower 2 tablespoons chopped fresh cilantro leaves, divided 2 tablespoons red curry paste From the cupboard: Salt and freshly ground black pepper, to taste

Directions:

Put in the riced cauliflower, red curry paste, coconut milk, 1 tablespoon cilantro, water, then drizzle with salt and black pepper. Combine the mixture to blend well. Place the slow cooker lid on and cook on HIGH for about two hours. Place the shrimp on a clean working surface, then drizzle salt and black pepper to season. Place the shrimp in the slow cooker and cook for fifteen minutes more. Move the soup into a big container and top with the rest of the cilantro leaves before you serve

518. Sugars Cheesy Broccoli Soup

Time To Prepare: five minutes Time to Cook: twenty minutes Yield: Servings 4

Ingredients:

1 cup broccoli, cut into florets 1 cup chicken broth 1 cup heavy whipping cream 1 cup shredded Cheddar cheese, plus more for topping 2 tablespoons butter From the cupboard: Salt and freshly ground black pepper, to taste

Directions: Place the butter in a deep cooking pan, and melt on moderate heat. Put in and sauté the broccoli for four to five minutes or until tender. Stir in the chicken broth and heavy whipping cream over the broccoli, and drizzle with salt and black pepper. Cook for approximately fifteen minutes or until the soup is smooth and thickened. Keep stirring during the cooking. Lower the heat to low and gently fold in the Cheddar cheese. Keep stirring until well blended. Ladle the soup into a big container. Spread more cheese over the soup before you serve

519. Cheesy Tomato And Basil Soup

Time To Prepare:five minutesTime to Cook: fifteen minutesYield:Servings 12

Ingredients:

¼ teaspoon ground black pepper 1 tablespoon dried basil 1 teaspoon dried oregano 1 teaspoon salt 2 (14 ounces / 397 g) canned whole tomatoes, diced 2 garlic cloves, minced 2 tablespoons coconut oil 4 cups chicken broth 4 ounces (113 g) red onions, finely diced 5 ounces (142 g) grated Parmesan cheese, plus more for decoration 8 ounces (227 g) cream cheese, softened Fresh basil, chopped, for decoration

Directions: Grease a nonstick frying pan with coconut oil, and sauté the onions, basil, oregano, and garlic in the frying pan for about four minutes or until aromatic. Put in the cream cheese and fully whisk until no clump, then fold in the chicken broth, and put in the cheese, tomatoes, salt, and pepper. Stir to blend well. Cover the lid and bring them to a simmer on moderate heat for eight minutes. Move the soup into a blender, then blitz until it becomes thick. Lightly pour the soup into a big serving container and sprinkle with Parmesan cheese and basil as decorate.

520. Chicken And Kale Soup

Time To Prepare: five minutes Time to Cook: 4 hours Yield: Servings 4

Ingredients:

1 (7-ounce / 198-g) bunch kale, trimmed and chopped 1 big chicken breast, cut into little strips 2 tablespoons olive oil 3 tablespoons fresh ginger, grated 6 cups chicken stock 6 garlic cloves, finely chopped From the cupboard: Salt and freshly ground black pepper, to taste

Directions: Grease the insert of the slow cooker with olive oil. Combine the chicken breast, stock, kale, ginger, garlic, ginger, salt, and black pepper in the slow cooker. Place the slow cooker lid on and cook on HIGH for 4 hours. Ladle the stew in a big container and serve warm

521. Chicken Tortilla Soup

TimeToPrepare:ten minutesTimetoCook:twenty minutesYield:Servings 8-10

Ingredients:

1 teaspoon cayenne pepper or to taste 2 cups onions, chopped 2 teaspoons chili powder 2 teaspoons cumin powder 2 teaspoons dried oregano 2 teaspoons garlic powder 4 cups carrots, cut 4 cups celery, cut 4 cups water 4 teaspoons olive oil 6 cups rotisserie chicken, skinless, chopped or shredded 8 cloves garlic, minced 8 cups chicken broth 8 medium tomatoes, chopped Avocado, peeled, pitted, chopped For the topping: Use any (not necessary) Fresh cilantro, chopped Greek yogurt Pepper powder to taste Salt to taste Tortilla chips, crumbled

Directions:

Put a soup pot on moderate heat. Put in oil. When the oil is warmed, put the onion and celery and sauté until slightly soft. Put in garlic and sauté for a few seconds until aromatic. Stir in the tomatoes and cook until tender. Remove the heat. Move into a blender. Put in water and blend until the desired smoothness is achieved. Put back the mixed mixture into the pot. Put in the remaining ingredients and stir. If it's beginning to boil, reduce the heat then simmer until vegetables are tender. Ladle into soup bowls before you serve.

522. Clear Clam Chowder

Time To Prepare:ten minutes Time to Cook: fifteen minutes Yield:Servings 4

Ingredients:

¼ teaspoon freshly ground black pepper ½ teaspoon dried thyme ½ teaspoon salt 1 (10-ounce) can clams 1 (8-ounce) bottle clam juice 1 small red onion, cut into ¼-inch dice 2 celery stalks, thinly cut 2 cups vegetable broth 2 garlic cloves, cut 2 medium carrots, cut into ½-inch pieces 2 tablespoons unsalted butter

Directions:

In a large pot, melt the butter on high heat. Put in the carrots, celery, onion, and garlic and sauté until slightly softened two to three minutes. Pour the broth and clam juice, then bring it to its boiling point. Reduce the heat and cook until the carrots are soft, three to five minutes. Mix in the clams and their juices, thyme, salt, and pepper, heat through for two to three minutes, before you serve

523. Coconut Curried Ban-Apple Soup

Time To Prepare: ten minutes Time to Cook: 10-fifteen minutes Yield: Servings 4

Ingredients:

¼ cup toasted coconut, for decoration 1 big potato 1 Granny Smith apple 1 celery heart 1 cup coconut milk 1 ripe banana 1 sweet onion 1 teaspoon curry powder 1 teaspoon salt 2 cups Basic Vegetable Stock or low-sodium canned vegetable stock 2 tablespoons chopped fresh cilantro, for decoration

Directions:

Place the vegetable stock in a soup pot. Peel the banana and potato, cut them, and place them in the soup pot. Core the apple, cut it, and put in it to the soup pot. Cut the celery heart and onion and put in them to the soup pot. Put the soup to its boiling point, then reduce the heat and simmer for ten to fifteen minutes. Put in the coconut milk, curry powder, and salt. Place the hot soup in a blender and purée. Serve the soup hot. Decorate using toasted coconut and cilantro.

524. Creamy & Culture Tomato Sauce

Time To Prepare: ten minutes Time to Cook: fifteen-twenty minutes Yield: Servings 6

Ingredients:

⅛ teaspoon dried thyme ⅛ teaspoon freshly ground black pepper ¼ cup tomato paste ¼ teaspoon chili powder ½ cup plain whole-milk yogurt ½ teaspoon salt 1 small onion, chopped 1 tablespoon ghee 1 teaspoon dried basil 1 teaspoon dried oregano 2 (14-ounce) cans diced tomatoes with their juice 2 cups vegetable broth 3 garlic cloves, chopped

Directions:

In a huge soup pot on moderate heat, melt the ghee. Place the onion and garlic, and sauté for five minutes. Stir in the basil, oregano, salt, chili powder, pepper, and thyme. Place the tomatoes, broth, and tomato paste, and stir until blended. Heat to a simmer, turn the heat to low, and cook for five to ten minutes. Take away the pot from the heat. With an immersion blender (or in batches in a standard blender), purée the mixture in the pot until you have the desired consistency. Put in the yogurt. Blend for a minute more. Serve instantly.

525. Creamy Celery And Chicken Broth

Time To Prepare: five minutes Time to Cook: twenty minutes Yield: Servings 4

Ingredients:

¼ cup celery, chopped ½ cup coconut cream 1 onion, chopped 2 chicken breasts, chopped 3 tablespoons butter 4 cups water From The Cupboard: Salt and freshly ground black pepper, to taste

Directions:

Place the butter in a deep cooking pan, and melt on moderate heat. Put in and sauté the celery and onion for about three minutes or until the onion is translucent. Put in the chicken, salt, black pepper, and water, and simmer for fifteen minutes. Keep stirring during the simmering. Mix in the coconut cream. Pour the soup in a big container and serve warm.

526. Sugars Creamy Parsnip Soup

Time To Prepare: twenty-five minutes Time to Cook: 60 minutes Yield: Servings 10

Ingredients:

1 big onion (diced) 1 cup whole milk 1 tablespoon brown sugar 1 tablespoon butter 1 tablespoon olive oil 1 teaspoon ground ginger ½ teaspoon ground allspice ½ teaspoon ground cardamom ½ teaspoon ground nutmeg 1/4 teaspoon cayenne pepper 2 pounds parsnips (peeled, cut) 3 carrots (peeled, cut) 3 cloves garlic (minced) 3 stalks celery (diced) 4 cups chicken stock Ground black pepper Salt

Directions: Preheat your oven to 425 F. Toss the parsnips and carrots with oil and seasoning in a container. Put them over a baking sheet. Roast in oven until for half an hour Cook the onion and celery in oil till golden brown, approximately seven minutes. Put in butter, brown sugar, garlic, and the parsnips and carrots, cooking for about ten minutes. Season and stir. Put in the chicken stock to its boiling point until soft. Puree the soup. Put in milk and cream and simmer some more before you serve with seasoning.

527. Creamy Turkey Soup

Time To Prepare: fifteen minutes Time to Cook: 4 hours Yield: Servings 7

Ingredients:

1 carrot, chopped 1 cup cream cheese 1 pound turkey breast, cubed 1 stalk celery, chopped 1 teaspoon freshly chopped rosemary 3 cloves garlic, chopped 5 cups chicken broth Salt & black pepper, to taste

Directions:

Put in all the ingredients minus the cream cheese to the base of a slow cooker. Cook on high for 4 hours. Mix in the cream cheese until well blended.

528. Crock-Pot Turkey Taco Soup

Time To Prepare: ten minutes Time to Cook: 4 hours Yield: Servings 6

Ingredients:

1 cup canned diced tomatoes (no sugar added) 1 cup whipped cream cheese 1 pound ground turkey 1 tablespoon chili powder 1 teaspoon cumin 1 teaspoon garlic powder 1 teaspoon onion powder 1 yellow onion, chopped 5 cups chicken bone broth (you can also use regular chicken broth)

Directions:

Put in all the ingredients to the base of a Crock-Pot minus the cream cheese and cover with the chicken broth. Set on high and cook for 4 hours putting in in the cream cheese at the 3.5 hour mark. Stir thoroughly before you serve.

529. Fennel and Pear Soup

Time To Prepare: fifteen minutes Time to Cook: twenty minutes Yield: Servings 4

Ingredients:

⅛ Teaspoon ground nutmeg ¼ cup freshly squeezed lemon juice ¼ cup honey ¼ teaspoon freshly ground black pepper 1 teaspoon finely chopped fresh tarragon 1 teaspoon salt 2 fennel bulbs, trimmed and slice into ½-inch dice 2 shallots, halved 2 tablespoons extra-virgin olive oil 4 cups vegetable broth 4 pears, cored and slice into ½-inch dice

Directions:

In a large pot, heat the oil on high heat. Put in the pears, fennel, and shallots, and sauté until the pears and fennel barely start to brown, approximately five minutes. Pour the broth, then bring to its boiling point. Reduce the heat to a simmer, then cook, once in a while stirring, until the fennel is soft, 5 to 8 minutes. Stir in the lemon juice, honey, salt, pepper, and nutmeg. Use an immersion blender to purée the soup in the pot until the desired smoothness is achieved. Drizzle with the tarragon before you serve.

530. Sugars Garlic and Lentil Soup

Time To Prepare: fifteen minutes Time to Cook: fifteen minutes Yield: Servings 4

Ingredients:

¼ cup chopped walnuts (not necessary) ¼ teaspoon freshly ground black pepper 1 (fifteen-ounce) can lentils, drained and washed 1 small white onion, cut into ¼-inch dice 1 tablespoon minced or grated orange zest 1 teaspoon ground cinnamon 1 teaspoon salt 2 garlic cloves, thinly cut 2 medium carrots, thinly cut 2 tablespoons extra-virgin olive oil 2 tablespoons finely chopped fresh flat-leaf parsley 3 cups vegetable broth

Directions:

In a large pot, heat the oil using high heat. Put in the carrots, onion, and garlic and sauté until tender, five to seven minutes. Place the cinnamon, salt, and pepper and stir to uniformly coat the vegetables, one to two minutes. Pour the broth then bring to its boiling point. Reduce the heat to a simmer, put in the lentils and cook until they are thoroughly heated about one minute. Mix in the orange zest and serve, sprinkled with the walnuts (if using) and parsley

531. Garlicky Chicken Soup

Time To Prepare:ten minutes Time to Cook: fifteen minutes Yield:Servings 6

Ingredients:

¼ teaspoon black pepper ½ cup whipped cream cheese 1 tablespoon butter for cooking 1 teaspoon salt 1 teaspoon thyme 2 boneless, skinless chicken breasts 3 cloves garlic, chopped 4 cups chicken broth

Directions: Preheat a stockpot on moderate heat with the butter. Put in the chicken and brown until completely thoroughly cooked. Turn off the heat. Shred the chicken and put in it back to the stockpot together with the rest of the ingredients minus the cream cheese. Heat to a simmer. Put in in the cream cheese and whisk until there are no more clumps. Simmer for about ten minutes before you serve.

532. Greek Split Pea Soup

Time To Prepare: fifteen minutes Time to Cook: 2 hours Yield: Servings 6

Ingredients:

1 pinch dried marjoram 1 potato (diced) 1½ pounds ham bone 2 onions (cut) 2 quarts cold water 2-1/4 cups dried split peas 3 carrots, (chopped) 3 stalks celery (chopped) Ground black pepper Salt

Directions:

Simmer the peas in a pot for a couple of minutes and then soak for an hour. Put in ham bone, onion, marjoram, and seasoning. Boil for 1½hours. Remove bone and meat. Put in the meat (diced) to the soup. Put the rest of the vegetables and cook until soft.

533. Gut-Healing Bone Broth

Time To Prepare:fifteen minutes Time to Cook: 8 to one day Yield:Servings 4

Ingredients:

1 medium onion, chopped 1 tablespoon apple cider vinegar 2 bay leaves 2 celery stalks, chopped 2 pounds beef marrow bones 3 medium carrots, chopped 4 garlic cloves Filtered water, to cover

Directions: In a 6-quart slow cooker, mix the bones, garlic, carrots, celery, onion, bay leaves, and vinegar. Cover with filtered water. Set the cooker on low and simmer for minimum 8 hours and up to one day. Skim off and discard any foam that forms on the surface. Ladle the broth through a fine-mesh sieve or cheesecloth to strain out the solids. Pour into airtight glass containers. The broth can be placed in the fridge for maximum one week; just boil it again before use. To freeze, let the broth fully cool and then fill jars up to an inch below the top to allow for expansion, and keep for four to 5 months.

534. Harvest Stew

Time To Prepare: fifteen minutes Time to Cook: 60 minutes Yield: Servings 6

Ingredients:

¼ cup flour ½ cup cut carrots ½ cup diced celery ¾ cup diced onions 1 bay leaf 1 leek, cleaned and diced 1 potato, peeled and diced 1 pound stewing beef cubes 2 cups diced zucchini 2 tablespoons olive oil 2 tablespoons Worcestershire sauce 2 tomatoes, chopped 3 sprigs fresh thyme 3 turnips, diced 4 cups low-sodium beef broth 6 garlic cloves, peeled Salt and pepper, to taste

Directions: Brown the beef cubes in olive oil. Dust the flour on the meat and stir to coat and spread. Put in the onions, carrots, celery, leek, garlic, zucchini, potato, turnips, tomatoes, bay leaf, thyme sprigs, and beef broth. Put to its boiling point, then reduce the heat and simmer for 60 minutes. Take away the bay leaf and thyme sprigs. Put in the Worcestershire sauce, salt, and pepper. Serve hot.

535. Sugars Hungarian Lentil Soup

Time To Prepare: fifteen minutes Time to Cook: 2 hours Yield: Servings 8

Ingredients:

7 Cups Chicken Stock 3 Carrots (Diced) 2 Stalks Celery (Diced) 1 Teaspoon Garlic (Minced) 2 Bay Leaves 1 Sprig Fresh Parsley (Chopped) 2 Tablespoons Olive Oil 2 Large Onions (Cubed) Salt Ground Black Pepper 1½ Cups Lentils (Soaked, Rinsed, Drained) ½ Teaspoon Paprika ½ Cup Grated Parmesan Cheese 3½ Cups Crushed Tomatoes 3/4 Cup White Wine

Directions:

Sauté onions in oil until shiny and put in garlic, paprika, celery, and carrots, cooking for about ten minutes. Mix in tomatoes, chicken stock, lentils, bay leaves, seasoning, and wine to boil. Cook until the lentils are soft. Top with parsley and Parmesan before you serve

536. Italian Modena Soup

Time To Prepare: two minutes Time to Cook: 8 minutes Yield: Servings 4

Ingredients:

½ cup Parmigiano-Reggiano cheese, shaved ½ teaspoon crushed chili 1 cup water 1 onion, chopped 1 tablespoon Italian seasonings 16 ounces Cotechino di Modena, cut 2 cups tomatoes, purée 2 tablespoons olive oil 3 cups roasted vegetable broth Sea salt and ground black pepper, to taste

Directions:

Push the "Sauté" button to heat up your Instant Pot. Once hot, heat the oil and sauté the onions until soft and translucent. Now, put in the sausage and cook an additional three minutes, Mix in tomatoes, broth, water, sea salt, black pepper, crushed chili, and Italian seasonings. Secure the lid. Choose "Manual" mode and High pressure; cook for five minutes. Once cooking is complete, use a quick pressure release; cautiously remove the lid. Top with shaved Parmigiano-Reggiano cheese and serve warm

537. Kumara & Chickpea Soup

Time To Prepare: twenty-five minutes Time to Cook: thirty-five minutes Yield: Servings 6

Ingredients:

1 bay leaf 1 onion (chopped) 1 teaspoon dried basil 1 tomato (chopped) ½ teaspoon dried thyme 1/4 teaspoon paprika 2 cloves garlic (minced) 2 cups kumara (peeled, chopped) 2 tablespoons olive oil 200g garbanzo beans 3 cups chicken broth Ground black pepper Mixed vegetables Salt

Directions:

Sauté onion, garlic, and sweet potatoes in oil for five minutes. Put in broth, bay leaf, herbs, and seasoning. Boil until soft. Put in tomato, beans, and chickpeas, simmering some more before you serve.

538. Lamb Taco Soup

Time To Prepare: ten minutes Time to Cook: 4-6 hours minutes Yield: Servings 6

Ingredients:

½ teaspoon cayenne pepper 1 cup diced tomatoes 1 cup shredded cheddar cheese 1 green bell pepper, chopped 1 pound ground lamb 1 teaspoon ground coriander 1 teaspoon ground cumin 1 teaspoon paprika 1 yellow onion, chopped 2 cloves garlic, chopped 4 cups beef broth Salt & pepper, to taste

Directions:

Put in all the ingredients to a slow cooker minus the shredded cheese and cook on high for four to 6 hours. Mix in the shredded cheese before you serve

539. Leek, Chicken and Spinach Soup

Time To Prepare:ten minutes Time to Cook: fifteen minutes Yield:Servings 4

Ingredients:

¼ teaspoon freshly ground black pepper 1 tablespoon thinly cut fresh chives 1 teaspoon salt 2 cups shredded rotisserie chicken 2 leeks, white parts only, thinly cut 2 teaspoons grated or minced lemon zest 3 tablespoons unsalted butter 4 cups baby spinach 4 cups chicken broth

Directions:

In a large pot, melt the butter on high heat. Put in the leeks and sauté until tender and starting to brown, three to five minutes. Put in the spinach, broth, salt, and pepper and bring to its boiling point. Reduce the heat and cook till the spinach wilts, one to two minutes. Place the chicken and cook until warmed through one to two minutes. Drizzle with the chives and lemon zest before you serve

540. Mediterranean Stew

Time To Prepare: ten minutes Time to Cook: fifteen minutes Yield: Servings 4

Ingredients:

1 (19-ounce) can cannellini beans, drained and washed 1 (fifteen½-ounce) can chickpeas, drained and washed 1 cup Basic Vegetable Stock or low-sodium canned vegetable stock 1 teaspoon dried oregano 1 teaspoon red pepper, crushed or to taste 1½ cups artichoke hearts, quartered 2 cups roasted tomatoes 3 cloves garlic, crushed and minced 3 tablespoons olive oil 4 tablespoons grated Parmesan cheese Chopped Italian parsley, for decoration Chopped sun-dried tomatoes, for decoration Crumbled feta cheese, for decoration Fresh oregano leaves, for decoration Freshly ground black pepper, to taste Garlic-seasoned croutons, for decoration Salt, to taste

Directions:

Warm the olive oil in a huge deep cooking pan on moderate heat and sauté the garlic for two to three minutes or until golden. Lower the heat to moderate-low. Mix in the chickpeas, cannellini beans, roasted tomatoes, artichoke hearts, stock, Parmesan cheese, crushed red pepper, oregano, salt, and pepper. Cook and stir for approximately ten minutes. Serve in separate bowls, garnishing as you wish.

541. Moong Daal

Time To Prepare: fifteen minutes Time to Cook: thirty minutes Yield: Servings 6

Ingredients:

½ Cup Tomatoes (Diced) ½ Dried Red Chili Pepper ½ Teaspoon Ginger Root (Grated) ½ Teaspoon Ground Turmeric 1 Pinch Asafoetida 1 Teaspoon Cumin Seed 1 Teaspoon Jalapeno (Diced) 1/4 Cup Cilantro (Chopped) 2 Cloves Garlic (Chopped) 2 Teaspoons Vegetable Oil 2½ Cups Moong Dal (Rinsed) 2½ Cups Water 3 Teaspoons Lemon Juice Salt

Directions:

Soak daal for thirty minutes before boiling in water with salt until thick. Put in ginger, jalapeno, tomato, lemon juice, and turmeric. Heat cumin seed and red Chile pepper in a pan before you put in asafoetida powder and garlic. Combine with split peas and serve with cilantro.

542. Onion, Kale and White Bean Soup

Time To Prepare: fifteen minutes Time to Cook: twenty-five minutes Yield: Servings 4

Ingredients:

⅛ Teaspoon red pepper flakes (not necessary) ¼ cup extra-virgin olive oil ¼ teaspoon freshly ground black pepper 1 (fifteen½-ounce) can white beans, drained and washed 1 big onion, thinly cut 1 teaspoon finely chopped fresh rosemary 1 teaspoon salt 2 garlic cloves, thinly cut 3 cups stemmed kale leaves cut into ½-inch pieces 4 cups vegetable broth

Directions:

In a large pot, heat the oil on high heat. Lower the heat to moderate, and put in the onion, garlic, salt, pepper, and red pepper flakes (if using). Sauté until the onion is golden, approximately ten minutes. Put in the kale, and sauté until wilted, one to two minutes. Pour the broth then bring to its boiling point. Lower the heat to simmer, and cook until the kale is tender about five minutes. Put in the beans and rosemary. Cook until the beans are warmed through minimum two to three minutes before you serve.

543. Pumpkin And Sausage Soup

Time To Prepare: five minutes Time to Cook: 33 minutes Yield: Servings 4

Ingredients:

½ cup heavy whipping cream ½ cup pumpkin puree ½ teaspoon dried sage ½ teaspoon ground dried thyme ½ teaspoon red chili pepper flakes (not necessary) 1 garlic clove, minced 1 moderate-sized red onion, minced 1 pinch salt 1 small red bell pepper, diced 2 cups chicken broth 2 tablespoons butter, melted pounds (680 g) fresh sausage

Directions:

Sauté the sausage in a nonstick frying pan on moderate to high heat for a minutes, then put in the onion and bell pepper. Continue sautéing for about six minutes until the sausage is mildly browned and the onion is translucent. Fold in the chili pepper flakes, thyme, sage, minced garlic, and salt, then put in the pumpkin puree, chicken broth, and heavy whipping cream. Reduce the heat and bring them to a simmer using low heat for fifteen minutes or until it becomes thick. Pour the cooked soup into a big serving container and put in the butter. Stir to mix thoroughly before you serve.

544. Quick Miso Soup with Wilted Greens

Time To Prepare: ten minutes Time to Cook: five minutes Yield: Servings 4

Ingredients:

½ teaspoon fish sauce 1 cup cut mushrooms 1 cup fresh baby spinach, meticulously washed 3 cups filtered water 3 cups vegetable broth 3 tablespoons miso paste 4 scallions, cut

Directions:

In a huge soup pot on high heat, put in the water, broth, mushrooms, and fish sauce, and bring to its boiling point. Turn off the heat. In a small container, combine the miso paste with ½ cup of heated broth mixture to dissolve the miso. Mix the miso mixture back into the soup. Mix in the spinach and scallions. Serve instantly.

545. Ribollita

Time To Prepare: forty-five minutes Time to Cook: 195 minutes Yield: Servings 12

Ingredients:

½ Cup Olive Oil 1 Bunch Kale (Trimmed, Chopped) 1 Bunch Swiss Chard (Trimmed, Chopped) 1½ Cups Cabbage (Chopped) 12½ Inch-Thick Slices French Bread (Toasted) 2 Bay Leaves 2 Cups Dry Cannellini Beans (Rinsed) 2 Onions (Diced) 2 Potatoes (Peeled, Cut) 3 Carrots (Peeled, Sliced) 3 Large Stalks Celery (Chopped) 32 Ounce Chicken Broth 4 Cups Water 4 Sage Leaves 5 Cloves Garlic (Minced) Grated Parmesan Cheese Ground Black Pepper Ounce Tomatoes (Diced) Salt

Directions:

Boil beans in water for minimum five minutes and cool for 70 minutes. Boil beans, garlic, sage leaves, bay leaves, and salt in chicken broth until soft. Discard the leaves from half of the mixture. Combine the remaining until the desired smoothness is achieved. Set aside. Cook onions in oil, putting in carrots, potatoes, cabbage, celery, Swiss chard, and kale, tomatoes, and seasoning for about twenty minutes. Put in the pureed bean and cook for forty minutes before you put in the rest of the mixture. Put in toasted bread slices. Heat the soup for about twenty minutes. Serve with Parmesan cheese and olive oil.

546. Roasted Butternut Squash Apple Soup

Time To Prepare: ten minutes Time to Cook: forty minutes Yield: Servings 4

Ingredients:

1 butternut squash 1 celery rib 1 cup water 1 small onion 1/4 teaspoon cinnamon 1/4 teaspoon ginger 1/4 teaspoon nutmeg 2 red, sweet apples 3 cups low-sodium chicken/vegetable stock 4 tablespoons olive oil Salt & pepper to taste

Directions:

Preheat your oven to 400°F. Put diced apple on a one-sheet pan & put the diced butternut squash on the second sheet pan. Allow season to squash olive oil & put in pepper & salt. Stir get everything mix thoroughly. Put in apple with one tablespoon olive oil & stir to coat. Apple & Roast squash for around half an hour, until browned. Heat olive oil (remaining 1 ½ tablespoons) in a big stockpot. Sauté celery & onion for around seven minutes, until soft. Put in Pepper & salt to taste. Put in vegetable or chicken stock & water & bring to a simmer. Once the apple & squash are roasted, put in them to the pot. Put in cinnamon, nutmeg & ginger. Now blend the soup until the desired smoothness is achieved. Season pepper & salt to taste. Serve with desired toppings

547. Saffron and Salmon Soup

Time To Prepare: ten minutes Time toCook: twenty minutes Yield:Servings 4

Ingredients:

¼ cup extra-virgin olive oil ¼ tsp. freshly ground black pepper ¼ tsp. saffron threads ½ cup dry white wine 1 lb. salmon fillets, cut into 1-inch pieces 1 tsp. salt 2 cups baby spinach 2 garlic cloves, thinly cut 2 leeks, white parts only, thinly cut 2 medium carrots, thinly cut 2 tablespoons chopped scallions, both white and green parts 2 tablespoons finely chopped fresh flat-leaf parsley 4 cups vegetable broth

Directions:

In a large pot, heat the oil using high heat. Put in the leeks, carrots, and garlic and sauté until tender, five to seven minutes. Pour the broth then bring to its boiling point. Reduce the heat to a simmer then put in the salmon, salt, pepper, and saffron. Cook until the salmon is thoroughly cooked, minimum 8 minutes. Put in the spinach, wine, scallions, and parsley and cook until the spinach has wilted, one to two minutes, before you serve

548. Spicy Asian-Style Soup

Time To Prepare: ten minutes Yield: Servings 4

Ingredients:

½ cup soy milk ½ pound asparagus, diced 1 bay leaf 1 cup celery, diced 1 shallot, diced 1 tablespoon coconut aminos 1 teaspoon Taco seasoning 1/4 teaspoon freshly ground black pepper 2 chicken bouillon cubes 2 cloves garlic, diced 2 cups Crimini mushrooms 2 tablespoons butter, softened 4 cups water Sea salt and black pepper, to taste

Directions:

Push the "Sauté" button to heat up your Instant Pot. Once hot, melt the butter; then, sweat the shallot until tender. Mix in garlic; cook an additional 40 seconds, stirring regularly. Put in the rest of the ingredients. Secure the lid. Choose "Manual" mode and High pressure; cook for seven minutes. Once cooking is complete, use a quick pressure release; cautiously remove the lid. Ladle into separate bowls and serve warm. Enjoy!

549. Spicy Lime-Chicken "Tortilla-Less" Soup

TimeTo Prepare: ten minutes Time to Cook: twenty minutes Yield:Servings 6

Ingredients:

¼ teaspoon cayenne pepper ½ teaspoon salt 1 (14 oz.) can diced tomatoes, and it's juice 1 (4oz.) can diced green chiles 1 avocado, cut 1 jalapeño pepper, seeded and minced 1 medium white onion, diced 1 pound shredded cooked chicken 1 tablespoon avocado oil 1 teaspoon chili powder 1 teaspoon ground cumin 3 garlic cloves, minced 3 tablespoons freshly squeezed lime juice 6 cups chicken broth or vegetable broth Fresh cilantro, for decoration Freshly ground black pepper

Directions:

In a huge soup pot on moderate heat, heat the avocado oil. Put in the garlic, onion, and jalapeño pepper, and sauté for five minutes. Mix in the broth, chicken, tomatoes, green chiles, lime juice, chili powder, cumin, salt, and cayenne pepper, and flavor with black pepper. Put it to a simmer, and cook for about ten minutes. Serve hot, topped with slices of avocado and decorated with cilantro.

550. Spicy Seafood Stew

TimeTo Prepare: ten minutes Time to Cook: twenty minutes Yield:Servings 6

Ingredients:

¼ cup freshly squeezed lime juice ½ cup chopped fresh cilantro ½ cup chopped yellow onion ½ cup coconut milk ½ cup diced green pepper ½ cup thinly cut scallions ¾ pound medium-size shrimp, shelled and deveined ¾ pound skinless firm-fleshed fish fillets, (cod, center-cut salmon, or halibut) 1 tablespoon minced garlic 1 teaspoon hot pepper sauce 2 tablespoons olive oil 3 cups canned peeled, chopped tomatoes, undrained Seasoned salt, to taste

Directions:

Warm the oil in a huge nonstick frying pan on moderate to high heat. Put in the onions, green pepper, garlic, and tomatoes. Put to a simmer while stirring once in a while, then cook for three to four minutes. Put in the coconut milk, pepper sauce, lime juice, and seasoned salt. Set to a simmer and cook for minimum 2 minutes. Put in the fish and stir, being cautious not to break apart the fillets. Cook till the fish is thoroughly cooked, approximately eight minutes. Put in the shrimp and cook until opaque and thoroughly cooked, approximately five minutes. To serve, use a slotted spoon to take equal amounts of the fish and shrimp to 4 shallow serving bowls. Place the sauce over the seafood and decorate with scallions and cilantro. Serve hot

551. Sweet Potato and Corn Soup

Time To Prepare:ten minutes Time to Cook: twenty minutes Yield:Servings 4

Ingredients:

¼ cup extra-virgin olive oil or coconut oil ¼ teaspoon freshly ground black pepper 1 cup broccoli florets 1 cup coconut milk or almond milk 1 cup frozen corn kernels 1 cup thinly cut mushrooms 1 medium zucchini, cut into ¼-inch dice 1 small onion, cut into ¼-inch dice 1 teaspoon salt 2 cups peeled sweet potatoes cut into ¼-inch dice 2 tablespoons finely chopped fresh flat-leaf parsley 4 cups vegetable broth

Directions:

In a large pot, heat the oil on high heat. Put in the zucchini, broccoli, mushrooms, and onion and sauté until tender, 5 to 8 minutes. Pour the broth and sweet potatoes and place it to its boiling point. Lower the heat to a simmer and cook until the sweet potatoes are soft, five to seven minutes. Put in the corn, coconut milk, parsley, salt, and pepper. Cook on low heat up to the corn is thoroughly heated before you serve.

552. Thai Chicken Noodle Soup

Time To Prepare: ten minutes Time to Cook: ten minutes Yield: Servings 2-3

Ingredients:

6 cups low-sodium chicken broth 1 stalk lemongrass, minced 1 bay leaf 1 tablespoon ginger, grated 1 big carrot, cut 1 cup broccoli florets, trimmed 1 cup mushrooms, quartered ½ teaspoon. cayenne pepper 3 cloves garlic, minced 2 Tablespoon. gluten-free soy sauce Salt and black pepper (to taste) a handful of fresh cilantro, chopped 1-2 fresh chicken breasts, chopped 1/4 cup fresh lime juice 1/4 cup coconut milk 8-10 oz. gluten-free flat Thai rice noodles

Directions:

Boil noodles in accordance with package directions, or until firm to the bite. Drain and save for later. Pour chicken broth in a big pot and bring to its boiling point using high heat. Put in chicken, broccoli, mushrooms, lemongrass, ginger, carrot, bay leaf. Turn heat to high and let the broth boil for a minute. Cover the pot and decrease the heat to moderate. Simmer the soup for 6 more minutes. While the soup is simmering, mix in cayenne, garlic, lime juice, and soy sauce. Turn heat to low and put in the coconut milk; stir thoroughly. Put cooked noodles into bowls. Pour soup over the noodles, then drizzle with cilantro.

553. Tomato And Basil Soup

Time To Prepare:five minutes Time to Cook: fifteen minutes Yield:Servings 4

Ingredients:

¼ cup chopped fresh basil leaves ¼ cup heavy whipping cream 1 (14.5-ounce / 411-g) can diced tomatoes 2 ounces (57 g) cream cheese 4 tablespoons butter From the cupboard: Salt and freshly ground black pepper, to taste

Directions:

Position the diced tomatoes in a food processor. Process until the desired smoothness is achieved. Melt the butter in a deep cooking pan on moderate heat. Put in the tomato purée, cream, and cheese. Cook for about ten minutes or until well blended. Keep stirring during the cooking. Drizzle with chopped basil leaves, salt, and black pepper. Keep cooking for another five minutes or until the desired smoothness is achieved and the soup has become thick. Stir continuously. Ladle the soup into a big container and serve warm.

554. Turkey Meatball Soup

Time To Prepare: fifteen minutes Time to Cook: fifteen minutes Yield: Servings 6

Ingredients:

For the Meatballs: ¼ teaspoon red pepper flakes ½ teaspoon dried oregano ½ teaspoon salt 1 pound ground turkey 1 tablespoon Dijon mustard 1 tablespoon ghee 1 teaspoon dried basil 1 teaspoon garlic powder Freshly ground black pepper For the Soup: ½ teaspoon dried thyme 1 bay leaf 1 medium white onion, diced 2 carrots, diced 2 cups shredded kale leaves, stemmed and meticulously washed 2 garlic cloves, minced 6 cups vegetable broth

Directions:

To make the Meatballs: In a moderate-sized container, put the turkey, mustard, basil, garlic powder, oregano, salt, and red pepper flakes, and flavor with pepper. With your hands, combine the ingredients until they are well blended. Put in the ghee to a stockpot on moderate to high heat. Roll the meat mixture into 1-inch balls and layer across the bottom of the pot. Cook for minimum 2 minutes per side, until almost thoroughly cooked. Move the meatballs to a plate. To make the Soup: To the stockpot, put in the onion, carrots, garlic, and thyme. Cook for approximately 2 minutes, slowly stirring, until the onions are translucent. Put in the broth, kale, bay leaf, and meatballs. Put to a simmer, lessen the heat to moderate-low and simmer for approximately fifteen minutes until the meatballs are thoroughly cooked, and the kale has tenderized. Remove and discard the bay leaf. Serve hot.

555. Sugars Vegetable Beef Soup

Time To Prepare: ten minutes Time to Cook: 4-6 hours Yield: Servings 6

Ingredients:

½ cup diced tomatoes 1 pound lean ground beef 1 teaspoon freshly chopped rosemary 1 teaspoon freshly chopped thyme 1 yellow onion, chopped 1 zucchini, diced 2 cloves garlic, chopped 2 stalks celery, chopped 4 cups beef broth Salt & pepper, to taste

Directions:

Put in all the ingredients to a slow cooker and cook on high for four to 6 hours. Stir thoroughly before you serve

556. Wedding Soup

Time To Prepare: fifteen minutes Time to Cook: 60 minutes Yield: Servings 6

Ingredients:

¼ bunch fresh parsley, chopped ¾ pound lean ground beef 1 cup rough chopped fresh spinach with stems removed 1 egg or ¼ cup egg substitute 1 yellow onion, chopped 2 quarts Rich Poultry Stock or low-sodium canned chicken stock 2 sprigs fresh basil, chopped 3 cloves garlic, minced 3 slices Italian bread, toasted 3 sprigs fresh oregano, chopped 4 ounces fresh grated Parmesan cheese Freshly cracked black pepper, to taste

Directions: Preheat your oven to 375°F. Wet the toasted Italian bread with water, then squeeze out all the liquid. In a big container, combine the bread, beef, egg, onion, garlic, parsley, oregano, basil, pepper, and half of the Parmesan. Form the mixture into 1- to two-inch balls; put in a baking dish and cook for twenty minutes to half an hour. Take off from the oven and drain using paper towels. Steam the spinach firm to the bite. In a big stockpot, mix the stock, spinach, and meatballs; simmer for half an hour Ladle the soup into serving bowls then top with the rest of the cheese

557. Wholesome Cabbage Soup

Time To Prepare: two minutes Time to Cook: 8 minutes Yield: Servings 4

Ingredients:

½ pound Capocollo, chopped ½ teaspoon cayenne pepper 1 bay leaf 1 celery stalk, chopped 1 cup tomatoes, puréed 1 cup water 1 onion, chopped 1 parsnip, chopped 1 pound cabbage, cut into wedges 2 cups broth, if possible homemade Coarse sea salt and ground black pepper, to your preference

Directions: Put in all of the above ingredients to your Instant Pot. Secure the lid. Choose "Manual" mode and High pressure; cook for about three minutes. Once cooking is complete, use a quick pressure release; cautiously remove the lid. Ladle into four soup bowls and serve hot. Enjoy!

558. Zucchini And Chicken Broth

Time To Prepare: twenty minutes Time to Cook: twenty minutes Yield: Servings 2

Ingredients:

¾ cup coconut milk 1 big zucchini, thinly cut 1 pound (454 g) boneless, skinless chicken breasts, cut into little pieces 1 tablespoon fresh parsley or fresh cilantro, finely chopped 2 cups water 2 garlic cloves, minced 2 tablespoons olive oil, divided 2 white onions, finely chopped 3 tablespoons green curry paste Salt and ground black pepper, to taste

Directions: Sprinkle 1 tablespoon of olive oil in a deep cooking pan and warm on moderate heat. Reduce the heat and cook the onions and garlic in the deep cooking pan using low heat for three to four minutes until translucent. Then put the curry paste, coconut milk, parsley and water into the deep cooking pan. Bring them to a simmer for about three minutes. Put in the chicken pieces and simmer for another six minutes until the chicken is thoroughly cooked. In the meantime, warm the rest of the olive oil in a nonstick frying pan, then sauté the zucchini in the frying pan for about three minutes. Drizzle with salt and ground black pepper and sauté for another two minutes until tender. Put in the cooked zucchini into the chicken broth and serve warm.

559. Carrot & Ginger Soup

Yield: 4 servings Preparation Time: fifteen minutes Cooking Time: 30 minutes

Ingredients:

1 tablespoon coconut oil • 1 medium brown onion chopped • 2 minced garlic cloves • 1 long red chili, chopped • 1 (1/3-inch) fresh turmeric piece, peeled and sliced • 1 (¾-inch) fresh galangal piece, peeled and sliced • 1 (¾-inch) fresh ginger piece, peeled and sliced • 4 cups carrots, peeled and chopped • 2 lemongrass stalks • 2 cups water • 2 cups vegetable broth • Coconut cream, as required

Directions:

1. In a substantial soup pan, heat oil on medium heat. 2. Add onion and sauté for about 5 minutes. 3. Add garlic, red chili, turmeric and sauté for approximately 5 minutes. 4. Add carrots, lemongrass stalks, water and broth and produce to some boil. 5. Reduce the warmth to low and simmer for about 15-20 minutes. 6. Remove from heat and aside to chill slightly. 7. Discard the lemongrass stalks. 8. In a blender, add soup in batches and pulse till smooth. 9. Serve immediately with the topping of coconut cream.

560. Creamy Broccoli Soup

Yield: 3-4 servings Preparation Time: 15 minutes Cooking Time: 35 minutes

Ingredients:

1 tablespoon virgin coconut oil • 1 celery stalk, chopped • ½ cup white onion, chopped • Salt, to taste • 1 teaspoon ground turmeric • 2 minced garlic cloves • 1 large head broccoli, cut into florets • ¼ teaspoon fresh ginger, grated • 1 bay leaf • 1/8 teaspoon cayenne pepper • Freshly ground black pepper, to taste • 5 cups vegetable broth • 1 small avocado, peeled, pitted and chopped • 1 tablespoon fresh lemon juice

Directions:

1. In a substantial soup pan, heat oil on medium heat. 2. Add celery, onion and several salt and sauté for around 3-4 minutes. 3. Add turmeric and garlic and sauté for approximately 1 minute. 4. Add desired mount of salt and remaining ingredients except avocado and lemon juice and provide with a boil 5. Reduce heat to medium-low. 6. Cover and simmer for about 25-thirty minutes. 7. Remove from heat and keep aside to cool down the slightly. 8. In a blender, add soup and avocado in batches and pulse till smooth. 9. Serve immediately with the drizzling of freshly squeezed lemon juice.

561. Butternut Squash Soup

Yield: 6 servings Preparation Time: fifteen minutes Cooking Time: 33 minutes a few seconds

Ingredients:

3 tablespoons extra virgin olive oil • 1 large onion, chopped finely • 1 cup raw cashews • 1 garlic herb, minced • 2 tablespoons fresh ginger, minced • 1 (2-pound) butternut squash, peeled and cubed into ½-inch size • 2 teaspoons ground coriander • 2 tsps. ground cumin • 1 teaspoon ground turmeric • 1 teaspoon curry powder • Freshly ground black pepper and salt, to taste • 5 cups vegetable broth • 1 cup coconut milk

Directions:

In a large soup pan, heat oil on medium heat. 2. Add onion and sauté for approximately 5 minutes. 3. Add cashews and sauté for around 3 minutes. 4. Add garlic and ginger and sauté approximately 30 seconds. 5. Add remaining ingredients except coconut milk and bring to some boil 6. Reduce the temperature to low. 7. Cover and simmer for around 20-25 minutes. 8. Remove from heat and make aside to cool down the slightly. 9. In a blender, add soup mixture with coconut milk in batches and pulse till smooth. 10. Serve immediately.

562. Soup

Yield: 2 servings Preparation Time: 15 minutes Cooking Time: 46 minutes

Ingredients:

2 teaspoons essential olive oil • ½ cup onion, chopped • 1 large head cauliflower, cut into small florets • 1 (1-inch) piece fresh ginger, chopped • Salt and freshly ground black pepper, to taste • 3 cups chicken broth

Directions:

1. In a big soup pan, heat oil on medium heat. 2. Add onion and sauté for approximately 1 minute. 3. Add cauliflower and cook, covered approximately 10 min, stirring occasionally. 4. Add remaining ingredients and provide with a boil 5. Reduce the warmth to low. 6. Cover and simmer for approximately 30 minutes. 7. Remove from heat and make aside for cooling slightly. 8. In a blender, add soup mixture in batches and pulse till smooth. 9. Return the soup inside the pan on low heat. 10. Simmer for approximately 4-5 minutes or till heated completely. 11. Serve immediately.

563. Cauliflower & Apple Soup

Yield: 5 servings Preparation Time: 15 minutes Cooking Time: 42 minutes

Ingredients:

½ cup pistachios • 2 tablespoons extra-virgin olive oil • 2 cups carrots, peeled and sliced • 1 large onion, chopped • 1 teaspoon fresh ginger, minced • 1 tablespoon garlic, minced • 3 cups cauliflower, cut into small florets • 3 cups apples, cored and chopped roughly • 1 teaspoon ground cumin • 1 tablespoon ground cinnamon • ¼ teaspoon paprika • 1/8 teaspoon allspice • Salt and freshly ground black pepper, to taste • 2 cups low-sodium vegetable broth • 7 tablespoons water • Chopped fresh cilantro, for garnishing

Directions:

1. Preheat the oven to 400 degrees F. 2. Place the pistachios in to a baking sheet and bake for about 5-7 minutes or till toasted. 3. Transfer the pistachios in a very pan of water on medium heat. 4. Bring to some gentle boil and simmer for about 35 minutes. 5. Meanwhile in a substantial soup pan, heat oil on medium heat. 6. Add carrot, onion, ginger and garlic and sauté for around 2 minutes. 7. Add cauliflower, apples and spices and cook, stirring occasionally for around 5 minutes. 8. Add broth and produce to your boil, then simmer, covered for about 20 minutes. 9. Remove from heat and keep aside for cooling slightly. 10. Drain the pistachios and transfer into a higher speed blender, then pulse till creamy and smooth. 11. Add the soup mixture in batches and pulse till smooth. 12. Serve immediately while using garnishing of cilantro.

564. Collard Greens Soup

Yield: 6 servings Preparation Time: fifteen minutes Cooking Time: 50 minutes

Ingredients:

2 tablespoons olive oil • 1 large onion, chopped • Salt, to taste • 2 large leeks, sliced • 2 tablespoons fresh ginger, minced • 1 bunch collard greens, chopped • 8 cups chicken broth • 1 tablespoon fresh lemon juice

Directions:

In a substantial soup pan, heat oil on low heat. 2. Add onion and salt and cook for approximately twenty minutes. 3. Stir in leeks and cook approximately 10 minutes. 4. Stir in ginger and greens and cook for approximately 5 minutes. 5. Add broth and provide to a boil on medium heat. 6. Cook approximately 10 min. 7. Remove from heat and make aside to chill slightly. 8. In a blender, add the soup mixture and pulse till smooth. 9. Return the soup in pan on medium heat. 10. Cook approximately 5 minutes. 11. Stir in freshly squeezed lemon juice and serve hot.

565. Citrus Acorn Squash Soup

Yield: 3-4 servings Preparation Time: 10 minutes Cooking Time: an hour 5 minutes

Ingredients:

1 large acorn squash, halved and seeded • ½ teaspoon essential olive oil • Salt and freshly ground black pepper, to taste • 1 teaspoon fresh orange zest, grated finely • ¾ teaspoon ground ginger • 2 pinches of cayenne pepper • 2 cups vegetable broth • ¼ cup fresh orange juice • ¼ cup coconut milk • 1 tablespoon coconut aminos • Fresh pomegranate seeds, for garnishing

Directions:

1. Preheat the oven to 400 degrees F. Line a baking sheet with foil paper. 2. Coat the squash halves with oil evenly and sprinkle with salt and black pepper. 3. Arrange the squash halves, cut side up within the prepared baking sheet. 4. Roast approximately one hour. 5. Remove from oven and allow it to go cool slightly. 6. Scoop the flesh from roasted squash and transfer right into a blender. 7. Add remaining all ingredients except pomegranate seeds and pulse till smooth. 8. Transfer the soup in a very pan on medium heat. 9. Cook approximately 3-5 minutes or till heated completely. 10. Serve hot while using garnishing of pomegranate seeds.

566. Butternut Squash & Lentil Soup

Yield: 6-8 servings Preparation Time: 15 minutes Cooking Time: 60 minutes 40 minutes

Ingredients:

1 medium butternut squash, halved and seeded • 2/3 cup celery, divided • ¼ cup onion, chopped and divided • 3 teaspoons garlic, minced and divided • 2 teaspoons dried parsley, crushed and divided • 2 teaspoons dried basil, crushed and divided • 2 fresh thyme pieces, divided • Salt, to taste • 2 tablespoons extra-virgin essential olive oil • ½ cup carrot, peeled and chopped • 1 medium tomato, chopped • 1 teaspoon ground turmeric • 1 bay leaf • 1 teaspoon freshly squeezed lemon juice • 1 vegetable bouillon cube • 6 cups water, divided • ½ cup split red lentil, soaked and drained • Freshly ground black pepper, to taste

Directions:

1. Preheat the oven to 375 degrees F. Line a baking sheet with foil paper. 2. Arrange the squash halves within the prepared baking sheet, cut side up. 3. Place about ¼ cup from the celery, 2 tablespoons of onion, 1 teaspoon garlic, 1 teaspoon of every dried herbs, 1 thyme piece and salt. 4. Roast for around 50-60 minutes or till squash becomes 10der. 5. Remove from heat whilst aside to cool completely. 6. Chop the three cups of flesh and aside. 7. Meanwhile in a soup pan, heat oil on medium-low heat. 8. Add carrot, remaining celery, onion and garlic and sauté for approximately 5-7 minutes. 9. Add tomato, turmeric, bay leaf, fresh lemon juice, bouillon cube, remaining herbs and 1 cup of water and simmer, covered for around 15 minutes. 10. In the center way, add 1 cup of more water. 11. Stir in lentils, squash and remaining water and provide to some boil. 12. Reduce heat to low. 13. Cover partially and simmer approximately 30-40 minutes. 14. Remove through the heat and by having an immersion blender, puree the soup completely. 15. Serve hot together with your desired topping.

567. Tomato & Lentil Soup

Yield: 4 servings Preparation Time: fifteen minutes Cooking Time: 33 minutes

Ingredients:

2 garlic cloves, peeled • 2 tablespoons extra-virgin extra virgin olive oil • 1 large yellow onion, sliced • 1 cup red lentils • 2 carrots, peeled and chopped • 1 (28-ounce) can tomatoes • 2 teaspoons ground coriander • 2 teaspoons ground cumin • 1 teaspoon ground ginger • Salt and freshly ground black pepper, to taste • 6 cups vegetable broth

Directions:

Crush the garlic cloves whilst in a very bowl for about 5-10 min. 2. In a large soup pan, heat oil on medium heat. 3. Add onion and sauté for approximately 3 minutes. 4. Add lentils, carrots, tomatoes, spices and broth and bring to some boil. 5. Simmer, covered for around 25 minutes. 6. Stir in garlic and simmer approximately 5 minutes more. 7. Remove from heat and having an immersion blender, puree the soup completely. 8. Serve immediately.

568. Carrot & Lentil Soup

Yield: 2 servings Preparation Time: 15 minutes Cooking Time: a half-hour

Ingredients:

For Soup: • 6 carrots, peeled and sliced • 3 tablespoons olive oil, divided • 1 tablespoon herbs de Provence • Salt and freshly ground black pepper, to taste • ¼ cup split red lentils • 1 teaspoon mustard seeds • 1 teaspoon ground cumin • 1 teaspoon ground turmeric • 3 garlic cloves, chopped • 1/3 cup coconut milk • 1½ cups water For Topping: • 1 tbsp organic olive oil • 12 chestnut mushrooms, sliced thinly • 1 (14-ounce) can cannellini beans, drained • 2 minced garlic cloves • 1 tablespoon mixed dried herbs

Directions:

1. Preheat the oven to 355 degrees F. 2. Arrange the carrot slices inside a baking dish in the single layer. 3. Drizzle with 1 tablespoon of oil and sprinkle with herbs de Provence, salt and black pepper. 4. Roast for around 25 minutes. 5. Meanwhile in a very pan of boiling water, add lentils and cook for approximately 10 min. 6. Drain well. 7. In a sizable frying pan, heat remaining oil on medium heat. 8. Add mustard seeds, cumin and turmeric and sauté for approximately 30 seconds. 9. In a blender, add carrots, lentils, mustard seeds mixture, coconut milk and water and pulse till smooth. 10. Transfer the soup mixture inside a pan on medium heat and cook approximately 4-5 minutes or till heated completely. 11. For mushroom mixture inside same frying pan, of spices, heat oil on medium heat. 12. Add mushrooms, beans, garlic and herbs and sauté for about 3-4 minutes. 13. Transfer soup in serving bowls and top with mushroom mixture and serve.

569. Carrot Soup with Chickpeas

Yield: 4 servings Preparation Time: fifteen minutes Cooking Time: thirty minutes

Ingredients:

1 (15-ounce) can chickpeas, drained • ½ teaspoon ground allspice • ½ teaspoon ground cinnamon • 1 teaspoon extra virgin olive oil • 2 tablespoons coconut oil • 2-3 teaspoons fresh ginger, chopped finely • 2 garlic cloves, chopped finely • 1 teaspoon ground turmeric • 5 cups carrots, peeled and chopped • 1½ cups vegetable broth • Freshly ground black pepper and salt, to taste • ½ cup coconut milk

Directions:

1. Preheat the oven to 375 degrees F. 2. In a bowl, add chickpeas, allspice, cinnamon and olive oil and toss to coat well. 3. Transfer a combination in to a baking dish and bake approximately 30 minutes. 4. In a substantial soup pan, melt coconut oil on medium heat. 5. Add ginger, garlic and turmeric and sauté for approximately 5 minutes. 6. Add remaining ingredients except coconut milk and produce with a boil. 7. Reduce the temperature and simmer approximately 20-25 minutes. 8. Stir in coconut milk and take off from heat. 9. With an immersion blender, puree the soup completely. 10. Serve immediately with all the topping of chickpeas.

570. Veggies & Quinoa Soup

Yield: 4-6 servings Preparation Time: fifteen minutes Cooking Time: 43 minutes

Ingredients:

2 tablespoons extra-virgin essential olive oil • 1 medium shallot, chopped • 1 medium onion, chopped • 2 medium turnips, peeled and chopped • 5 large carrots, peeled and chopped • 2 teaspoons fresh ginger, minced • ½ cup uncooked quinoa • 3 cups water • 3 cups vegetable broth • ½ teaspoon ground turmeric • ¼ tsp cayenne • Salt and freshly ground black pepper, to taste

Directions:

1. In a large soup pan, heat oil on medium-high heat. 2. Add shallot, onion, turnips and carrots and sauté for about 5-7 minutes. 3. Stir in ginger and sauté for approximately 1 minute. 4. Stir in remaining ingredients and bring to some boil. 5. Reduce the heat to low and simmer, covered for around 20-a half-hour. 6. Remove from heat and make aside to chill slightly. 7. In an increased speed blender, add soup mixture in batches and pulse till smooth. 8. Return the soup in pan on medium heat. 9. Simmer approximately 4-5 minutes or till heated completely.

571. Halibut, Quinoa & Veggies Soup

Yield: 8-10 servings Preparation Time: 15 minutes Cooking Time: 1 hour 10 min

Ingredients:

2 cups onions, chopped • 1 cup celeriac root, chopped • 2 garlic cloves, chopped • 2 tablespoons fresh ginger herb, chopped finely • 1 cup shiitake mushrooms, sliced • 1 cup quinoa • 8 cups vegetable broth • 14-ounces halibut fillets • 6 cups fresh baby spinach • 1cup fresh cilantro, chopped • 1 cup coconut milk • Salt, to taste • 2 scallions, chopped

Directions:

1. In a sizable soup pan, onions, celeriac root, garlic, ginger root, mushrooms, quinoa and broth and provide to your boil. 2. Reduce heat to low and simmer, covered approximately 45 minutes. 3. Arrange the halibut fillets over soup mixture. 4. Simmer, covered for around quarter-hour. 5. Stir in remaining ingredients except scallions and simmer for around 5 minutes. 6. Serve hot using the garnishing of scallions.

572.   Butternut Squash & Chickpeas Stew

Yield: 6 servings Preparation Time: quarter-hour Cooking Time: 36 minutes

Ingredients:

1 tbsp olive oil • 1 medium sweet onion, chopped • 1½ teaspoons fresh ginger, grated • 2 minced garlic cloves • ½ tablespoon coconut sugar • ¼ teaspoon ground cumin • ¾ teaspoon ground cinnamon • 1-2 teaspoons red chili flakes, crushed • 3½ cups butternut squash, peeled and chopped • Salt and freshly ground black pepper, to taste • 1½ cups water, divided • Salt and freshly ground black pepper, to taste • ¼ cup creamy natural almond butter • 1½ cups cooked chickpeas • 3 cups fresh kale, trimmed and chopped • ½ cup raw almonds, chopped

Directions:

1. In a big soup pan, heat oil on medium heat. 2. Add onion and cook, covered for about 5 minutes, stirring occasionally. 3. Stir in ginger, garlic, coconut sugar and spices and sauté approximately 1 minute. 4. Add squash and stir to mix well. 5. Add 1¼ glasses of water, salt and black pepper and bring with a boil. 6. Reduce heat to low. 7. In a bowl, mix together remaining water and peanut butter. 8. Add peanut butter mixture in pan and stir to mix. 9. Simmer, covered for approximately twenty minutes. 10. Stir in chickpeas, kale and almonds and simmer for around 10 min more.

573.   Root Veggies Stew

Yield: 6-8 servings Preparation Time: fifteen minutes Cooking Time: 33 minutes

Ingredients:

2 tablespoons coconut oil • 1 large sweet onion, chopped • 1 medium parsnips, peeled and chopped • 3 tablespoons tomato paste • 2 large garlic cloves, minced • ½ teaspoon ground cinnamon • ½ teaspoon ground ginger • 1 teaspoon ground cumin • ¼ tsp red pepper cayenne • Salt, to taste • 2 medium carrots, peeled and chopped • 2 medium purple potatoes, peeled and chopped • 2 medium sweet potatoes, peeled and chopped • 4 cups vegetable broth • 2 tablespoons freshly squeezed lemon juice • 2 cups fresh kale, kale, trimmed and chopped • ¼ cup fresh cilantro leaves, chopped • Slivered almonds, for garnishing

Directions:

In a sizable soup pan, melt coconut oil on medium-high heat. 2. Add onion and sauté for approximately 5 minutes. 3. Add parsnip and sauté for approximately 3 minutes. 4. Stir in tomato paste, garlic and spices and sauté approximately 2 minutes. 5. Add carrots, potatoes and sweet potatoes and stir to mix well. 6. Add broth and produce with a boil and reduce the temperature to medium-low. 7. Simmer for about twenty or so minutes. 8. Stir in freshly squeezed lemon juice and kale and simmer approximately 2-3 minutes. 9. Serve using the garnishing of cilantro and almonds.

574. Chicken, Chickpeas & Olives Stew

Yield: 10-12 servings Preparation Time: quarter-hour Cooking Time: 60 minutes 9 minutes

Ingredients:

6 pound skinless, boneless grass-fed chicken thighs, trimmed • Salt and freshly ground black pepper, to taste • ¼ cup extra-virgin essential olive oil • 3 large yellow onions, sliced thinly • 8 garlic cloves, crushed • 3 small red chiles, stemmed • 2 fresh bay leaves • 1 tablespoon ground turmeric • 2 teaspoon ground coriander • 2 teaspoons ground cumin • 2 (3-inch) cinnamon sticks • 4 teaspoons fresh lemon zest, grated finely • ½ cup fresh lemon juice, divided • 4 cups low-sodium chicken broth • 2 cups small green olives, pitted • 2 cups canned chickpeas, rinsed and drained • 3 tablespoons fresh cilantro, chopped

Directions:

1. Sprinkle the chicken thighs with salt and black pepper evenly. 2. In a sizable pan, heat oil on medium-high heat. 3. Add the chicken thighs in 4 batches and cook for around 3 minutes from each party. 4. Transfer the chicken into a bowl and make aside. 5. Reduce the warmth to medium and sauté the onion for about 5-6 minutes. 6. Add garlic, red chiles, bay leaves and spices and sauté for about 1 minute. 7. Add lemon zest, 1/3 cup with the lemon juice and broth and produce to your boil. 8. Reduce the warmth to medium-low and simmer, covered approximately a half-hour. 9. Stir inside the cooked chicken, olives and chickpeas and boost the heat to medium-high. 10. Cook, stirring occasionally for about 6-8 minutes. 11. Stir in remaining fresh lemon juice, salt and black pepper and remove from heat. 12. Serve hot while using garnishing of cilantro.

575. Baked Lamb Stew

Yield: 4 servings Preparation Time: 15 minutes Cooking Time: 1 hour 10 minutes

Ingredients:

For Lamb Marinade: • 3 large garlic cloves, minced • 1 tablespoon fresh ginger, minced • 1 lemongrass stalk, minced • 2 tablespoons coconut aminos • 2 tablespoons tapioca starch • Salt and freshly ground black pepper, to taste • 2-3 pound boneless lamb shoulder, trimmed and cubed into 2-inch pieces For Stew: • 2 tablespoons coconut oil • 4 shallots, minced • 2 Thai chilies, minced • 2 tablespoons tomato paste • 4 large tomatoes, chopped • 4 carrots, peeled and chopped • 1 butternut squash, peeled and cubed • 2 star anise • 1 cinnamon stick • 1 teaspoon Chinese 5-spice powder • 2½ cups hot beef broth

Directions:

1. For lamb marinade in a substantial glass bowl, add all ingredients and mix well. 2. Cover and refrigerate to marinate for around 2-8 hours. 3. Preheat the oven to 325 degrees F. 4. In an oven proof casserole dish, heat oil on medium-high heat. 5. Add lamb and cook for around 4-5 minutes. 6. Reduce heat to medium. 7. Add shallots and chilies and cook for around 2-3 minutes. 8. Stir in tomato paste and tomatoes and cook approximately 1-2 minutes. 9. Add remaining ingredients and stir to combine well. 10. Cover the casserole dish and immediately, transfer into oven. 11. Bake for approximately one hour or till desired doneness.

576. Adzuki Beans & Carrot Stew

Yield: 4 servings Preparation Time: quarter-hour Cooking Time: 1 hour 18 minutes

Ingredients:

2 tablespoons extra virgin olive oil • 1 large yellow onion, chopped • 5 (½-inch) fresh ginger slices • Salt, to taste • 3 cups water • 1 cup dried adzuki beans, soaked for overnight, rinsed and drained • 4 large carrots, peeled and sliced into ¾-inch pieces • 2 tablespoons brown rice vinegar • 3 tablespoons tamari • ½ cup fresh parsley, minced

Directions:

In a sizable pan, heat oil on medium heat. 2. Add onion, ginger and salt and sauté for around 2-3 minutes. 3. Add water and beans and convey to a boil. 4. Reduce heat to low and simmer, covered for around 45 minutes. 5. Arrange carrot slices over beans and simmer, covered for around 20-thirty minutes. 6. Stir in vinegar and tamari and remove from heat. 7. Discard te ginger slices before serving. 8. Serve hot with garnishing of parsley.

577. Creamy Chickpeas Stew

Yield: 4-6 servings Preparation Time: fifteen minutes Cooking Time: 56 minutes

Ingredients:

¼ cup coconut oil • 1 medium yellow onion, chopped • 2 teaspoons fresh ginger, chopped finely • 2 minced garlic cloves • 1 teaspoon ground cumin • 1 teaspoon ground coriander • ¾ teaspoon ground turmeric • ¼ teaspoon yellow mustard seeds • ¼ tsp cayenne • 1 (19-ounce) can chickpeas, rinsed and drained • 2 large sweet potatoes, peeled and cubed into 1-inch size • 1 pound fresh kale, trimmed and chopped • 5 cups vegetable broth • Salt, to taste • 1 cup coconut milk • ¼ cup red bell pepper, seeded and julienned • 2 tablespoons fresh cilantro, chopped

Directions:

1. In a substantial pan, heat oil on medium heat. 2. Add onion and sauté for around 3 minutes. 3. Add ginger and garlic and sauté for about 2 minutes. 4. Add spices and sauté for around 1 minute. 5. Add chickpeas, sweet potato, kale and broth and bring with a boil on medium-high heat. 6. Reduce the temperature to medium-low and simmer, covered for about 35 minutes. 7. Stir in coconut milk and simmer for about fifteen minutes or till desired thickness of stew. 8. Serve hot with garnishing of bell pepper and cilantro.

578. Lentil & Quinoa Stew

Yield: 4-6 servings Preparation Time: fifteen minutes Cooking Time: 34 minutes

Ingredients:

1 tablespoon coconut oil • 3 carrots, peeled and chopped • 3 celery stalks, chopped • 1 yellow onion, chopped • 4 garlic cloves, minced • 1 (26½-ounce) can chopped tomatoes • 1 cup red lentils, rinsed and drained • ½ cup quinoa • 1½ teaspoons ground cumin • ½ teaspoon ground turmeric • ½ teaspoon ground ginger • Salt, to taste • 5 cups water • 2 cups fresh kale, chopped

Directions:

1. In a large pan, heat oil on medium heat. 2. Add celery, onion and carrot and sauté for approximately 8 minutes. 3. Add garlic and sauté approximately 1 minute. 4. Add remaining ingredients except kale and provide to your boil. 5. Reduce the temperature to low and simmer, covered approximately twenty minutes. 6. Stir in kale and simmer for around 4-5 minutes. 7. Serve hot.

579. Chilled Peas Soup

Yield: 4 servings Preparation Time: 10 min Cooking Time: 20 seconds

Ingredients:

½ tablespoons coconut oil • 1 large shallot, minced • 10 fresh mint leaves • 2 cups homemade chicken broth • 1 pound frozen baby peas • Salt and freshly ground black pepper, to taste

Directions:

In a medium pan, heat oil on medium-high heat. 2. Add shallots and sauté for about 1 minute. 3. Add mint and broth and convey with a boil. 4. Stir in peas and again bring to a boil. 5. Reduce heat to medium-low. Simmer approximately 4 minutes. 6. Season with salt and black pepper and take away from heat. Let it cool slightly. 7. Transfer the soup inside a blender and pulse till smooth. 8. Refrigerate to sit back for around an hour before serving.

580. Chilled Fruit Soup

Yield: 4 servings Preparation Time: fifteen minutes

Ingredients:

For Soup: • 2 pounds fresh strawberries, hulled and sliced • ½ of medium watermelon, seeded and chopped For Raspberry Sauce: • 6-ounce fresh raspberries • ¼ cup coconut milk • 1 teaspoon fresh lemon zest, grated finely • 1 tablespoon freshly squeezed lemon juice

Directions:

1. In a bowl, add watermelon and strawberries. With a hand blender, blend till an even and creamy mixture forms. 2. Refrigerate to chill. 3. In a bowl, add raspberries and mash having a fork completely. 4. Add remaining ingredients and stir to mix well. Refrigerate to sit back. 5. Divide the soup in serving bowls. Top with raspberry sauce and serve.

581. Creamy Cauliflower Soup

Yield: 4-6 servings Preparation Time: fifteen minutes Cooking Time: 22-25 minutes

Ingredients:

1 tablespoon extra-virgin extra virgin olive oil • 1 medium onion, chopped • 4 garlic cloves, minced • Salt, to taste • 1 medium head cauliflower, cut into 1-inch pieces • 4 ½-5½ cups water • 1 avocado, peeled, pitted and chopped • 2-3 cups mixed greens • Freshly ground black pepper, to taste • Fresh chopped parsley, for garnishing

Directions:

1. In a substantial soup pan, heat oil on medium heat. 2. Add onion and sauté for approximately 4-5 minutes. 3. Add garlic and pinch of salt and sauté approximately 2-3 minutes. 4. Stir in cauliflower and ad water. Bring with a boil on high heat. 5. Reduce the heat to low. Simmer for about 10 minutes. 6. Stir in avocado and greens and simmer for about 3 minutes. 7. Remove from heat and cool slightly. 8. In a blender, transfer the soup in batches and pulse till smooth. 9. Add the soup within the pan on medium heat. Cook for around 3-4 minutes. 10. Stir in salt and black pepper and take off from heat. 11. Serve with all the garnishing of parsley.

582. Green Veggie Soup

Yield: 6 servings Preparation Time: 20 min Cooking Time: 25 minutes

Ingredients:

2 tablespoons ghee (clarified butter) • 3-4 garlic cloves, minced • 4 leeks (white part), chopped roughly • 2 medium heads broccoli, chopped roughly • ½ of small head cauliflower, chopped roughly • 4 celery sticks, chopped roughly • 8 cups homemade vegetable broth • 2-3 cups fresh baby spinach • 1 cup fresh parsley, chopped • Freshly ground black pepper, to taste • Pinch of ground nutmeg • 1 tablespoon coconut cream

Directions:

In a big soup pan, heat oil on medium heat. 2. Add garlic and leeks and sauté for approximately 4-5 minutes. 3. Add broccoli, cauliflower and celery and sauté for approximately 5 minutes. 4. Add broth and convey with a boil. Reduce heat to low. Simmer for approximately 10-fifteen minutes. 5. Stir in spinach and parsley and remove from heat. 6. With an immense blender, blend till pureed. Stir in nutmeg and black pepper. 7. Top using the dollop of coconut cream and serve.

583. Mushroom Soup

Yield: 4 servings Preparation Time: twenty minutes Cooking Time: half an hour

Ingredients:

½-ounce dried porcini mushrooms • 2 tablespoons ghee (clarified butter) • 1 celery stalk, chopped • 1 large leek (pale part), chopped • 1 small sweet potato, peeled and chopped • 15 medium crimini mushrooms, sliced roughly • 3 garlic cloves, minced • 1 tablespoon dried thyme, crushed • 3 cups homemade chicken broth • ½ teaspoon Dijon mustard • 1 tablespoon red boat fish sauce • 2 bay leaves • 1 teaspoon fresh lemon zest, grated finely • ½ teaspoon freshly ground black pepper • 3 tablespoons almond butter • 1 tablespoon fresh lemon juice

Directions:

1. In a bowl, soak porcini mushrooms in boiling water. Keep aside for about 15-twenty or so minutes. 2. Strain the mushrooms, reserving ½ cup of liquid. Then chop the mushrooms. 3. In a sizable soup pan, heat ghee on medium heat. 4. Add celery and leek and sauté for about 5-7 minutes. 5. Add sweet potato, cremini mushrooms, garlic and thyme and sauté for approximately 1-2 minutes. 6. Add broth, mustard, fish sauce, bay leaves, lemon zest, black pepper and cremini mushrooms with reserved liquid and convey to a boil. 7. Reduce the temperature to low. Cover and simmer for about quarter-hour. 8. Uncover and simmer for 5 minutes more. 9. Stir in almond butter and lemon juice and serve hot.

584. Chicken & Asparagus Soup

Yield: 8 servings Preparation Time: 20 min Cooking Time: 20 min

Ingredients:

1 tablespoon coconut oil • 1 onion, chopped • 2 cups mushrooms, sliced thinly • 1 celery stalk, chopped • 2 cups grass-fed boneless chicken, chopped • 15-20 fresh asparagus spears, trimmed and chopped • 6-8 cups homemade chicken broth • 14-ounce coconut milk • 2 cups fresh spinach, chopped • Salt and freshly ground black pepper, to taste

Directions:

1. In a big soup pan, heat oil on medium heat. 2. Add onion, mushrooms and celery and sauté for approximately 5 minutes. 3. Add chicken, asparagus and broth and bring to a boil. 4. Reduce heat to low. Simmer for around 10 min. 5. Stir in coconut milk and spinach and bring to your boil on high heat. 6. Reduce the temperature to low. Simmer for around 3-4 minutes. 7. Stir in salt and black pepper and take off from heat. 8. Serve hot.

585. Zucchini & Squash Soup

Yield: 4 servings Preparation Time: quarter-hour Cooking Time: 12-quarter-hour

Ingredients:

2 tablespoons coconut oil • 1 small onion, chopped • 3 garlic cloves, minced • 1 teaspoon ground cumin • 1½ pounds yellow squash, chopped • 3 cups zucchini, chopped • 2 tablespoons jalapeño peppers, chopped finely • 4 cups homemade vegetable broth • 1 cup coconut milk • 3 tablespoons fresh lemon juice • ¼ cup fresh cilantro, chopped • 2 tablespoons nutritional yeast • Avocado slices, for garnishing

Directions:

1. In a large soup pan, heat oil on medium heat. 2. Add onion and sauté approximately 4-5 minutes. 3. Add garlic and cumin and sauté approximately 1 minute. 4. Add squash and zucchini and sauté for about 3-4 minutes. 5. Add jalapeño peppers and broth and convey to your boil. Immediately, turn off heat. 6. Keep, covered approximately 10 minutes. 7. Stir in coconut milk, fresh lemon juice, cilantro and nutritional yeast and again bring with a boil. 8. Serve hot while using topping of avocado slices.

SEAFOOD

586. Shrimp with Fruit & Bell Pepper

Yield: 4-6 servings Preparation Time: 15 minutes Cooking Time: 12 minutes

Ingredients:

½ cup onion, sliced thinly • 1 teaspoon coconut oil • 1½ pound shrimp, peeled and deveined • ½ of red bell pepper, seeded and sliced thinly • 1 mango, peeled, pitted and sliced • 8-ounce can of pineapple tidbits with unswee10ed juice • 1 cup coconut milk • 1 tablespoon red curry paste • 2 tablespoons fish sauce • 2 tablespoons fresh cilantro, chopped

Directions:

1. Heat a nonstick pan on medium-high heat. 2. Add onion and sauté for approximately 3-4 minutes. 3. With a spoon, push the onion to side in the pan. 4. Add coconut oil and shrimp and cook for about 2 minutes per side. 5. Add peppers and cook for approximately 3-4 minutes. 6. Add remaining ingredients except cilantro and simmer for approximately 5 minutes. 7. Serve hot using the sprinkling of cilantro.

587. Shrimp with Asparagus

Yield: 4 servings Preparation Time: fifteen minutes Cooking Time: 11 minutes

Ingredients:

2 tablespoons coconut oil • 1 bunch asparagus, peeled and chopped • 1 pound shrimp, peeled and deveined • 4 garlic cloves, minced • ½ teaspoon ground ginger • 2 tablespoons fresh lemon juice • 2/3 cup chicken broth

Directions:

1. In a big skillet, melt coconut oil on medium-high heat. 2. Add all ingredients except broth and cook for around 2 minutes, without stirring. 3. Stir and cook for around 5 minutes. 4. Add broth and cook for around 2-4 minutes. 5. Serve hot.

588. Pan Fried Squid

Yield: 2 servings Preparation Time: quarter-hour Cooking Time: 13 minutes

Ingredients:

1 teaspoon organic olive oil • ¼ of yellow onion, sliced • 1 pound squid, cleaned and cut into rings • ¼ teaspoon ground turmeric • Salt, to taste • 1 organic egg, bea10

Directions: 1. In a skillet, heat oil on medium-high heat. 2. Add onion and sauté for about 4-5 minutes. 3. Add squid rings, turmeric and salt and toss to coat well. 4. Reduce the temperature to medium-low and simmer for approximately 5 minutes. 5. Add bea10 eggs and cook, stirring continuously approximately 2-3 minutes. 6. Serve hot.

589. Scallops with Veggies

Yield: 1 serving Preparation Time: 15 minutes Cooking Time: 9 minutes

Ingredients:

½ cup unsalted vegetable broth, divided • 1/3 cup carrot, peeled and chopped • ¾ cup celery chopped • 1 cup green beans, trimmed and chopped • ¾ of green apple, cored and chopped • ½ teaspoon fresh ginger herb, grated finely • 1 teaspoon ground cardamom • 1 teaspoon extra virgin olive oil • 4-ouces sea scallops • 1 tablespoon walnuts, chopped

Directions: 1. In a skillet, heat 3 tablespoons of broth and cook for approximately 4-5 minutes. 2. Stir in green beans, apple, ginger, cardamom and remaining broth and cook approximately 3-4 minutes. 3. Meanwhile in the frying pan, heat oil and cook the scallops for around 2-4 minutes per side. 4. Divide veggie mixture in serving plates. 5. Top with squid and serve.

590. Spicy Scallops

Yield: 3-4 servings Preparation Time: quarter-hour Cooking Time: 13 minutes

Ingredients:

2 tablespoons coconut milk • ½ cup shallot, minced • ¼ cup tomato paste • 2 teaspoons fresh ginger paste • 2 teaspoons garlic paste • ½ teaspoon garam masala • ¼ teaspoon ground cinnamon • ¼ teaspoon ground cumin • Pinch of red pepper cayenne • Salt, to taste • 1 pound sea scallops • 8-ounce plain Greek yogurt, whipped • Chopped fresh cilantro, for garnishing

Directions:

1. In a large skillet, melt coconut oil on medium-high heat 2. Add shallots and sauté approximately 2-3 minutes. 3. Add remaining ingredients except scallops, yogurt and cilantro and cook for about 3-5 minutes. 4. Stir in scallops and yogurt and cook approximately 5 minutes. 5. Serve hot using the garnishing of cilantro.

591. Spicy Kingfish

Yield: 2 servings Preparation Time: fifteen minutes Cooking Time: 10 min

Ingredients:

1 teaspoon dried unswee10ed coconut • 1 teaspoon cumin seeds • 1 teaspoon fennel seeds • 1 teaspoon peppercorns • 10 curry leaves • ½ teaspoon ground turmeric • 1½ teaspoons fresh ginger, grated finely • 1 garlic herb, minced • Salt, to taste • 1 tablespoon fresh lime juice • 4 (4-ounce) kingfish steaks • 1 tbsp olive oil • 1 lime wedge

Directions:

1. Heat a surefire skillet on low heat. 2. Add coconut, cumin seeds, fennel seeds, peppercorns and curry leaves and cook, stirring continuously for about 1 minute. 3. Remove in the heat and let it cool completely. 4. In a spice grinder, add the spice mixture and turmeric and grind rill powdered finely. 5. Transfer the mixture in to a large bowl with ginger, garlic, salt and lime juice and mix well. 6. Add fish fillets and cat while using mixture evenly. 7. Refrigerate to marinate approximately 3 hours. 8. In a big nonstick skillet, heat oil on medium heat. 9. Add the fish fillets and cook for approximately 3-5 minutes per side or till desired doneness. 10. Transfer onto a paper towel lined plate to drain. 11. Serve with lime wedges.

592. Spicy Salmon

Yield: 4 servings Preparation Time: quarter-hour Cooking Time: 7 minutes

Ingredients:

Salt, to taste • 2 small onions, chopped • 2 large garlic cloves, chopped • 1 (1-inch) piece fresh ginger, chopped • 1 teaspoon ground turmeric • 2 teaspoons red chili powder • Salt and freshly ground black pepper, to taste • 2 tablespoons fresh lemon juice • 4 salmon steaks • Coconut oil, as required for shallow frying

Directions:

In a food processor, add all ingredients except salmon and oil and pulse till smooth. 2. Transfer the mix right into a bowl. 3. Add steaks and coat with marinade generously. 4. Refrigerate to marinate for overnight. 5. In a large skillet, melt coconut oil on medium-high heat. 6. Add salmon fillet, skin-side up and cook for approximately 4 minutes. 7. Flip the medial side and cook for approximately 3 minutes. 8. Transfer onto a paper towel lined plate to drain. 9. Serve with lemon wedges.

593. Salmon with Cabbage

Yield: 4 servings Preparation Time: fifteen minutes Cooking Time: 10 minutes

Ingredients: • 1 (1-inch) piece fresh ginger, grated finely • 2 tablespoons taw honey • 1 tablespoon freshly squeezed lemon juice • 1 tablespoon Dijon mustard • 4 tablespoons organic olive oil, divided • 4 (8-ounce) salmon fillets • 1 small head cabbage, sliced thinly • 1 garlic clove, minced • 1 tablespoon sesame seeds • Freshly ground black pepper, to taste • 4 scallions, chopped

Directions:

1. In a bowl, mix together ginger, honey, fresh lemon juice and Dijon mustard. Keep aside. 2. In a sizable nonstick skillet, heat 1 tablespoon of oil on medium-high heat. 3. Add salmon and cook for around 3-4 minutes per side. 4. Place the honey mixture over salmon fillets evenly and immediately remove from heat. 5. Cover and make aside till serving. 6. Meanwhile in another skillet, heat 2 tablespoons of oil on medium heat. 7. Add cabbage and stir fry for approximately 3-4 minutes. 8. Add remaining oil and stir fry for around 5 minutes. 9. Add garlic, sesame seeds and black pepper and cook for about 1 minute. 10. Place salmon over cabbage and serve with garnishing of scallion.

594. Basa with Mushroom & Bell Pepper

Yield: 2 servings Preparation Time: quarter-hour Cooking Time: 18 minutes

Ingredients:

1 (8-ounce) basa fish fillet, cubed • ¼ teaspoon ginger paste • ¼ teaspoon garlic paste • 1 teaspoon red chili powder • Salt, to taste • 1 tablespoon coconut vinegar • 1 tablespoon extra-virgin organic olive oil, divided • ½ cup fresh mushrooms, sliced • 1 small onion, quartered • ¼ cup red bell pepper, seeded and cubed • ¼ cup yellow bell pepper, seeded and cubed • 2-3 scallions, chopped • 1 teaspoon fish sauce

Directions:

1. In a bowl, mix together fish, ginger, garlic, chili powder and salt whilst aside for around twenty minutes. 2. In a nonstick skillet, heat 1 teaspoon of oil on medium-high heat. 3. Sear the fish for about 5-6 minutes or till golden coming from all sides. 4. In another skillet, heat remaining oil on medium heat. 5. Add mushrooms and onion and stir fry for about 5-7 minutes. 6. Add bell pepper and fish and stir fry for about 2 minutes. 7. Add scallion and fish sauce and stir fry for bout 1-2 minutes. 8. Serve hot.

595. Snapper with Carrot & Broccoli

Yield: 2 servings Preparation Time: quarter-hour Cooking Time: 6 minutes

Ingredients:

2½ tbsp essential olive oil, divided • 1 teaspoon red curry paste • Salt, to taste • 2 skinless snapper fillets • 2 teaspoons coconut oil, divided • ½ tablespoon fresh ginger, sliced thinly • 10 baby carrots, peeled and halved • 1 tablespoon fish sauce • 1½ tablespoons freshly squeezed lemon juice, divided • 1 teaspoon organic honey • 2 cups broccoli florets • Freshly ground black pepper, to taste • 1 garlic cloves, minced

Directions:

In a bowl, mix together 2 tablespoons of essential olive oil, curry paste and salt. 2. Add snapper fillets and rub with oil mixture evenly. Keep aside for about 5-10 min. 3. In a small skillet, melt 1 teaspoon of coconut oil on medium heat. 4. Add ginger and carrots and stir fry for around 2 minutes. 5. Add fish sauce, 1 tablespoon of fresh lemon juice, honey and black pepper and stir fry approximately 2-3 minutes. 6. Meanwhile in another skillet, heat remaining olive oil on medium heat. 7. Add snapper fillets and cook for about 3 minutes from both sides. 8. Drizzle with remaining lemon juice. 9. Meanwhile in a pan of boiling water add broccoli and cook for around 2 minutes. 10. Drain well. 11. In a similar pan, melt remaining coconut oil on medium heat. 12. Add garlic and sauté for around 1 minute. 13. Add broccoli and toss to coat well. 14. Serve snapper fillets with carrots and broccoli.

596. Steamed Snapper Parcel

Yield: 2 servings Preparation Time: fifteen minutes Cooking Time: 10 min

Ingredients:

2 tablespoons garlic, minced • 1 tablespoon fresh turmeric, grated finely • 1 tablespoon fresh ginger, grated finely • 2 tablespoons fresh lime juice • 2 tablespoons coconut aminos • 2 tablespoons essential olive oil • 1 bunch fresh cilantro, chopped • 2 (6-ounce) snapper fillets

Directions:

1. In a food processor, add garlic, turmeric, ginger, lime juice, coconut aminos and extra virgin olive oil and pulse till smooth. 2. Transfer a combination in the bowl with cilantro and mix well. 3. Add snapper fillets and coat using the mixture generously. 4. Place each fish fillet in the foil paper and wrap the paper to create a parcel. 5. Arrange a steamer basket inside a pan of boiling water. 6. Place the parcels in steamer basket. 7. Cover and steam for about 10 min.

597. Broiled Sweet & Tangy Salmon

Yield: 3 servings Preparation Time: quarter-hour Cooking Time: 12 minutes

Ingredients:

2 garlic cloves, crushed • 2 tablespoons fresh ginger grated finely • 2 tablespoons organic honey • 2 tablespoons coconut aminos • 2 tablespoons fresh lime juice • 3 tablespoons olive oil • 3 tablespoons sesame oil • 2 tablespoons black sesame seeds • 1 tablespoon white sesame seeds • 1 pound boneless salmon fillets • 1/3 cup scallion, chopped

Directions:

1. In a baking dish, mix together all ingredients except the salmon. And scallion. 2. Add salmon and coat with mixture generously. 3. Refrigerate to marinate for about 40-45 minutes. 4. Preheat the broiler of oven and arrange the rack inside top in the oven. 5. Place the baking dish inside the oven and broil for approximately 10-12 minutes. 6. In serving platter, put the salmon and top with all the pan sauce. 7. Serve while using garnishing of scallion.

598. Baked parsley Salmon

Yield: 3-4 servings Preparation Time: fifteen minutes Cooking Time: twenty or so minutes

Ingredients:

16-24-ounce salmon fillets • 2 tablespoons coconut oil, melted • 3 tablespoons fresh parsley, minced • ¼ teaspoon ginger powder • Salt, to taste

Directions: 1. Preheat the oven to 400 degrees F. Grease a substantial baking dish. 2. Arrange the salmon fillets into prepared baking dish in a single layer. 3. Drizzle with coconut oil and sprinkle with parsley, ginger powder and salt. 4. Bake for about 15-twenty or so minutes.

599. Baked Crispy Cod

Yield: 2-4 servings Preparation Time: quarter-hour Cooking Time: fifteen minutes

Ingredients:

1 green bell pepper, seeded and sliced • 2 large eggs • 1/3 cup blanched almond flour • ¼ teaspoon dried dill weed, crushed • ½ teaspoon garlic powder • 1/8 teaspoon ground turmeric • Freshly ground black pepper, to taste • 1½ pound cod fillets • Chopped fresh chives, for garnishing

Directions: 1. Preheat the oven to 350 degrees F. Line a large rimmed baking dish with parchment paper. 2. Arrange the bell pepper slices into prepared baking dish. 3. In a shallow dish, crack the eggs and brat well. 4. In another shallow dish, mix together almond flour, dill weed, garlic powder, turmeric and black pepper. 5. Coat the cod fillets in egg and then roll into flour mixture evenly. 6. Place the cod fillets over bell pepper slices. 7. Bake for approximately fifteen minutes. 8. Serve with all the garnishing of chives.

600. Grilled Sweet & Tangy Salmon

Yield: 4 servings Preparation Time: 15 minutes Cooking Time: 15 minutes

Ingredients:

1 scallion, chopped • 1 teaspoon garlic powder • 1 teaspoon ground ginger • ¼ cup organic honey • 1/3 cup fresh orange juice • 1/3 cup coconut aminos • 1½ pound salmon fillets

Directions:

1. In a zip lock bag, add all ingredients and seal the bag. 2. Shake the bag to coat the mix with salmon. 3. Refrigerate for around thirty minutes, flipping occasionally. 4. Preheat the grill to medium heat. Grease the grill grate. 5. Remove the salmon from your bag, reserving the marinade. 6. Grill for around 10 minutes. 7. Coat the fillets with reserved marinade and grill for 5 minutes more.

601. Grilled Spicy Salmon

Yield: 6-8 servings Preparation Time: fifteen minutes Cooking Time: 6-10 min

Ingredients:

½ tablespoon ground ginger • ½ tablespoon ground coriander • ½ tablespoon ground cumin • ½ teaspoon paprika • ¼ tsp red pepper cayenne • Salt, to taste • 1 tablespoon fresh orange juice • 1 tablespoon coconut oil, melted • 1½-2 pound salmon fillets

Directions:

1. In a big bowl, add all ingredients except salmon and mix till a paste forms. 2. Add salmon and coat with mixture generously. 3. Refrigerate to marinate for approximately thirty minutes. 4. Preheat the propane gas grill to high heat using the lid closed not less than 10 minutes. 5. Grease the grill grate make the salmon fillets, skin-side down. 6. Cover with all the lid and grill approximately 3 minutes. 7. Flip the medial side and cover while using lid and grill for around 3 minutes more.

602. Rockfish Curry

Yield: 8 servings Preparation Time: 15 minutes Cooking Time: a half-hour

Ingredients:

2 pound rockfish • ¾ teaspoon ground turmeric, divided • Salt, to taste • 2 tablespoons coconut oil • 12 pearl onions, halved • 2 medium red onions, sliced thinly • 2 Serrano peppers, halved • 40 small leaves, divided • 1 (½-inch) piece fresh ginger, minced • Freshly ground black pepper, to taste • ¼ cup water • 1½ (14-ounce) cans coconut milk, divided • 1 teaspoon using apple cider vinegar

Directions:

In a bowl, season the fish with ¼ teaspoon with the turmeric and salt whilst aside. 2. In a sizable skillet, melt coconut oil on medium heat. 3. Add pearl onions, red onions, ginger, Serrano peppers and 20 curry leaves and sauté approximately quarter-hour. 4. Add ginger, remaining turmeric, salt and black pepper and sauté for approximately 2 minutes. 5. Transfer half of the mixture in to a bowl whilst aside. 6. Add remaining curry leaves, fish fillets, water and 1 can of coconut milk and cook for approximately 2 minutes. 7. Now cook, covered approximately 5 minutes. 8. Add apple cider vinegar and remaining half can of coconut milk and cook for around 3-5 minutes or till done completely. 9. Serve hot using the topping of reserved onion mixture.

603. Lemony Shrimp

Yield: 4-6 servings Preparation Time: quarter-hour Cooking Time: 6 minutes

Ingredients:

1 small onion, chopped finely • 1 tablespoon fresh ginger, minced • 3 garlic cloves, minced • 1 tablespoon fresh lemon zest, grated finely • 1 fresh red chili, seeded and minced • 1 teaspoon ground turmeric • ½ cup olive oil • ½ cup freshly squeezed lemon juice • 20-24 raw shrimp, peeled and deveined • 1 tablespoon coconut oil

Directions:

1. In a large bowl, mix together all ingredients except shrimp and coconut oil. 2. Add shrimp and coat with marinade generously. 3. Cover and refrigerate to marinate for overnight. 4. In a big nonstick skillet, melt coconut oil on medium-high heat. 5. Transfer shrimp into skillet, reserving marinade. 6. Stir fry for around 3-4 minutes. 7. Ass reserved marinade and provide to a boil, tossing occasionally.

604. Shrimp with Broccoli

Yield: 2-4 servings Preparation Time: 15 minutes Cooking Time: 12 minutes

Ingredients:

1-2 tablespoons coconut oil, divided • 4 cups broccoli, chopped • 2 pound large shrimp, peeled and deveined • 2 minced garlic cloves • 1 (1-inch) piece fresh ginger, minced • Salt and freshly ground black pepper, to taste

Directions: 1. In a substantial skillet, melt 1 tablespoon of coconut oil on medium-high heat. 2. Add broccoli and sauté for about 1-2 minutes. 3. Cover and cook, stirring occasionally for about 3-4 minutes. 4. With a spoon, push the onion to side from the pan. 5. Add remaining coconut oil and let it melt. 6. Add shrimp and cook, tossing for approximately 2-3 minutes. 7. Add remaining ingredients and sauté approximately 2-3 minutes. 8. Serve hot.

605. Prawns with Veggies

Yield: 4 servings Preparation Time: fifteen minutes Cooking Time: 9 minutes

Ingredients:

2 teaspoons coconut oil • 1½ medium onions, sliced • 1 tablespoon fresh ginger, grated finely • 2 medium green peppers, sliced • 3 medium carrots, peeled and sliced • 1½ pound pawns, peeled and deveined • 3 garlic cloves, minced • 2½ teaspoons curry powder • 1½ tablespoons fish sauce • 1 cup coconut milk • Water, as required • Salt, to taste • 2 tablespoons fresh lime juice

Directions: 1. In a large skillet, melt coconut oil on medium-high heat. 2. Add onion and sauté approximately 1 minute. 3. Add ginger, bell pepper and carrots and stir fry for about 2-3 minutes. 4. Add prawns, garlic, curry powder and fish sauce and stir fry for approximately a few seconds. 5. Add coconut milk plus a little water and stir fry approximately 3-4 minutes.

606. Squid with Veggies

Yield: 2 servings Preparation Time: 20 minutes Cooking Time: 10 min

Ingredients:

1 teaspoon extra virgin olive oil • 2 carrots, peeled and chopped • 2 red bell peppers, seeded and cut into strips • ½ of eggplant, chopped • ¾ pound squids, cleaned • 2 tablespoons fish sauce • 1 teaspoon fresh ginger, minced • ½ teaspoon paprika • 1 cup fresh spinach, chopped • Salt and freshly ground black pepper, to taste • 3 small zucchinis, spiralized with Blade C

Directions: 1. In a sizable skillet, heat oil on medium heat. 2. Add carrots, bell pepper and eggplant and stir fry for around 3-4 minutes. 3. Add remaining ingredients except zucchini and cook for about 1-2 minutes. 4. Stir in spinach and cook for approximately 3-4 minutes. 5. Meanwhile in a very pan of boiling eater, add zucchini noodles and cook for about 1 minute. 6. Drain well. 7. Transfer the zucchini noodles into two serving bowls. 8. Top with squid mixture and gently stir to blend. 9. Serve immediately.

607. Scallops with Broccoli

Yield: 2 servings Preparation Time: fifteen minutes Cooking Time: 6 minutes

Ingredients:

¼ cup fresh ginger, grated • 8 large sea scallops • 1 package frozen broccoli, thawed • 1 tablespoon coconut oil • Freshly ground black pepper, to taste

Directions:

1. Ina pan of water, add ginger on medium heat. 2. Place scallops in the metal steamer basket and arrange inside the pan of water. 3. Cover and steam for approximately 2-5 minutes. 4. Meanwhile in another pan of boiling water, arrange steamer basket. 5. Add broccoli and boil, covered for approximately 5 minutes. 6. Drain well. 7. In a sizable frying pan, melt coconut oil on medium heat. 8. Add scallops and sear for approximately thirty seconds from each party. 9. Serve the scallops over bed of broccoli. 10. Drizzle having a little ginger water and serve.

608. Deep Fried Kingfish

Yield: 4 servings Preparation Time: fifteen minutes Cooking Time: 8 minutes

Ingredients:

½ teaspoon ginger paste • ½ teaspoon garlic paste • 2 tablespoons chickpea flour • 2 teaspoons turmeric powder • 1 teaspoon ground coriander • 1 teaspoon red chili powder • ½ teaspoon garam masala • Salt, to taste • Water, as required • 1 pound kingfisher fillets • Olive oil, as necessary for deep frying

Directions:

1. In a large bowl, add all of the ingredients except the fish and oil and mix till a paste forms. 2. Add the fish fillets and coat using the paste generously. 3. Refrigerate to marinate for approximately 1 hour. 4. In a substantial deep skillet, heat oil on medium-high heat. 5. Add fish fillets and fry for about 3-4 minutes per side or till desired doneness. 6. Transfer onto a paper towel lined plate to drain.

609. Gingered Tilapia

Yield: 5 servings Preparation Time: 15 minutes Cooking Time: 6 minutes

Ingredients:

2 tablespoons coconut oil • 5 tilapia fillets • 3 garlic cloves, minced • 2 tablespoons unswee10ed coconut, shredded • 4-ounce freshly ground ginger • 2 tablespoons coconut aminos • 8 scallions, chopped

Directions:

1. In a large skillet, melt coconut oil on medium heat. 2. Add tilapia fillets and cook for around 2 minutes. 3. Flip the inside and add garlic, coconut and ginger and cook for about 1 minute. 4. Add coconut aminos and cook for around 1 minute. 5. Add scallion and cook for approximately 1-2 minute more. 6. Serve immediately.

610. Crispy Salmon

Yield: 4 servings Preparation Time: fifteen minutes Cooking Time: 12 minutes

Ingredients:

1 teaspoon garlic powder • 1 teaspoon ground coriander • 2 teaspoons red pepper flakes, crushed • 1 teaspoon red chili powder • Salt and freshly ground black pepper, to taste • 2 tablespoons fresh lemon juice • 4 salmon steaks • 1 cup chickpea flour • Olive oil, as essential for deep frying

Directions: 1. In a sizable bowl, mix together all ingredients except salmon, chickpea flour and oil. 2. Add salmon steaks and coat with mixture evenly. 3. Refrigerate to marinate for around 3-4 hours. 4. In a shallow dish, place chickpea flour. 5. In a skillet, heat oil on medium-high heat. 6. Coat the salmon steaks with flour evenly. 7. Fry the salmon fillets approximately 5-6 minutes per side. 8. Transfer onto a paper towel lined plate to drain.

611. Salmon with Vegetables

Yield: 1 serving Preparation Time: twenty minutes Cooking Time: 19 minutes

Ingredients:

5 teaspoons extra virgin olive oil, divided • 1 teaspoon ground turmeric • 1 teaspoon paprika • Salt and freshly ground black pepper, to taste • 1 (4-ounce) salmon fillet • 1 purple baby carrot, cut lengthwise • 1 yellow carrot, cut lengthwise • 1 orange carrot, cut lengthwise • 3 French beans, chopped • 3 button mushrooms, sliced

Directions:

1. In a bowl, mix together 2 teaspoons of oil, turmeric, paprika, salt and black pepper. 2. Add salmon and coat using the oil mixture evenly. Keep aside. 3. In a pan of boiling water, add French beans and carrots and cook for about 3 minutes. 4. Drain well. 5. In a nonstick skillet, heat 2 teaspoons of oil on medium heat. 6. Add mushroom and a pinch of salt and black pepper and stir fry for or about 5-6 minutes. 7. Add the drained vegetables and stir fry approximately 2 minutes. 8. Transfer the vegetables onto a plate and loosely, cover having a foil paper to hold warm. 9. In a similar skillet, heat remaining oil on medium heat. 10. Add salmon filler, skin-side down and cook for approximately 3-5 minutes. 11. Change the inside and cook for approximately 2-3 minutes. 12. Place salmon over vegetables and serve.

612. Haddock with Swiss Chard

Yield: 1 serving Preparation Time: 15 minutes Cooking Time: 10 minutes

Ingredients:

2 tablespoons coconut oil, divided • 2 minced garlic cloves • 2 teaspoons fresh ginger, grated finely • 1 haddock fillet • Salt and freshly ground black pepper, to taste • 2 cups Swiss chard, chopped roughly • 1 teaspoon coconut aminos

Directions:

1. In a skillet, melt 1 tablespoon of coconut oil on medium heat. 2. Add garlic and ginger and sauté approximately 1 minute. 3. Add haddock fillet and sprinkle with salt and black pepper. 4. Cook approximately 3-5 minutes per side or till desired doneness. 5. Meanwhile in another skillet, melt remaining coconut oil on medium heat. 6. Add Swiss chard and coconut aminos and cook for around 5-10 minutes. 7. Serve the salmon fillet over Swiss chard.

613. Citrus Poached Salmon

Yield: 3 servings Preparation Time: fifteen minutes Cooking Time: 12 minutes

Ingredients:

3 garlic cloves, crushed • 1½ teaspoons fresh ginger, grated finely • 1/3 cup fresh orange juice • 3 tablespoons coconut aminos • 3 (6-ounce) salmon fillets

Directions: 1. Ina bowl, mix together all ingredients except salmon. 2. In the bottom of your large pan, squeeze salmon fillet. 3. Place the ginger mixture in the salmon and aside for about quarter-hour. 4. Place the pan on high heat and convey to your boil. 5. Reduce the heat to low and simmer, covered for about 10-12 minutes or till desired doneness.

614. Broiled Spicy Salmon

Yield: 4 servings Preparation Time: fifteen minutes Cooking Time: 14 minutes

Ingredients:

¼ cup low- Fat plain Greek yogurt • ½ teaspoon ground coriander • ½ teaspoon ground turmeric • ½ teaspoon ground ginger • ¼ tsp cayenne pepper • Salt and freshly ground black pepper, to taste • 4 (6-ounce) skinless salmon fillets

Directions:

1. Heat the broiler of the oven. Grease a broiler pan. 2. In a bowl, mix together all ingredients except the salmon. 3. Arrange salmon fillets onto prepared broiler pan inside a single layer. 4. Place the yogurt mixture over each fillet evenly. 5. Broil approximately 12-14 minutes. 6. Serve immediately.

615. Baked Sweet Lemony Salmon

Yield: 2 servings Preparation Time: 15 minutes Cooking Time: 12 minutes

Ingredients:

2 (8-ounce) salmon fillets • ½ teaspoon organic honey and even more for drizzling • 1/3 teaspoon ground turmeric, divided • Freshly ground black pepper, to taste • 2 large lemon slices

Directions:

1. In a zip lock bag, add salmon, ½ teaspoon of honey, ¼ teaspoon of turmeric and black pepper. 2. Seal the bag and shake to coat well. 3. Refrigerate to marinate for around 1 hour. 4. Preheat the oven to 40 degrees F. 5. Transfer the salmon fillets onto a cookie sheet in the single layer. 6. Cover the fillets with marinade. 7. Place the salmon fillets, skin-side up and bake for around 6 minutes. 8. Carefully, customize the side of fillets. 9. Sprinkle with remaining turmeric and black pepper evenly. 10. Place 1 lemon slice over each fillet and drizzle with honey. 11. Bake for approximately 6 minutes.

616. Baked Walnut & Lemon Crusted Salmon

Yield: 4 servings Preparation Time: 15 minutes Cooking Time: twenty minutes

Ingredients:

1 cup walnuts • 1 tablespoon fresh dill, chopped • 2 tablespoons fresh lemon rind, grated • ½ teaspoon garlic salt • Freshly ground black pepper, to taste • 1 tbsp olive oil • 3-4 tablespoons Dijon mustard • 4 (3-ounce) salmon fillets • 4 teaspoons fresh lemon juice

Directions:

1. Preheat the oven to 350 degrees F. Line a substantial baking sheet with parchment paper. 2. In a mixer, add walnuts and pulse till hoped roughly. 3. Add dill, lemon rind, garlic salt, black pepper and oil and pulse till a crumbly mixture forms. 4. Place the salmon fillets, skin-side on to prepared baking sheet in a very single layer. 5. Coat the the surface of each salmon fillet with Dijon mustard evenly. 6. Place the walnut mixture over each fillet evenly and gently, press into the surface of salmon. 7. Bake for about 15-20 min. 8. Serve with the drizzling of fresh lemon juice

617. Baked Cheesy Salmon

Yield: 4 servings Preparation Time: 15 minutes Cooking Time: 25 minutes

Ingredients:

2 garlic cloves, crushed • 1 teaspoon dried dill weed, crushed • Salt and freshly ground black pepper, to taste • 2 pounds salmon fillets • 1 cup cheddar cheese, shredded • 6 scallions, chopped

Directions:

Preheat the oven to 450 degrees F. 2. In a bowl, mix together garlic, dill weed, salt and black pepper. 3. Sprinkle the salmon fillets with garlic mixture evenly. 4. Arrange the salmon fillets over a big foil paper and fold to seal. 5. Place the salmon parcel in a very baking sheet and bake approximately twenty minutes. 6. Now, unfold the parcel and top the salmon fillets with cheese and scallions. 7. Bake for about 5 minutes.

618. Grilled Salmon with Peach & Onion

Yield: 4 servings Preparation Time: fifteen minutes Cooking Time: 12 minutes

Ingredients:

4 salmon steaks • Salt and freshly ground black pepper, to taste • 3 peaches, pitted and cut into wedges • 2 medium red onions, cut into wedges • 1 tablespoon fresh ginger, minced • 1 teaspoon fresh thyme leaves, minced • 3 tablespoons essential olive oil • 1 tablespoon balsamic vinegar

Directions:

1. Preheat the grill to medium heat. Grease the grill grate. 2. Sprinkle the salmon with salt and black pepper evenly. 3. In a bowl, add peach, onion, salt and black pepper and toss to coat well. 4. Grill the salmon steaks for approximately 5-6 minutes. 5. Now, place peaches and onions on grill with salmon steaks. 6. Grill the salmon for about 5-6 minutes per side. 7. Grill the peaches and onion for around 3-4 minutes per side. 8. Meanwhile in a bowl, add remaining ingredients and mix till a smooth paste forms. 9. Place ginger mixture over salmon filets evenly and serve with peaches and onions.

619. Shrimp Curry Delicious

Yield: 4 servings Preparation Time: 15 minutes Cooking Time: 18 minutes

Ingredients:

2 tablespoons peanut oil • ½ sweet onion, minced • 2 minced garlic cloves • 1½ teaspoons ground turmeric • 1 teaspoon ground cumin • 1 teaspoon ground ginger • 1 teaspoon paprika • ½ teaspoon red chili powder • 1 (14-ounce) can coconut milk • 1 (14 ½-ounce) can chopped tomatoes • Salt, to taste • 1 pound cooked shrimp, peeled and deveined • 2 tablespoons fresh cilantro, chopped

Directions:

1. In a big skillet, heat oil on medium heat. 2. Add onion and sauté approximately 5 minutes. 3. Reduce the temperature to low. 4. Add garlic and spices and sauté for around 1 minute. 5. Add coconut milk, tomatoes and salt and simmer for about 10 min, stirring occasionally. 6. Stir in the shrimp and cilantro and simmer approximately 1-2 minutes.

620. Salmon in Spicy Yogurt Gravy

Yield: 5-6 servings Preparation Time: 15 minutes Cooking Time: 35 minutes

Ingredients:

5-6 salmon steaks • 1½ teaspoons ground turmeric, divided • Salt, to taste • 3 tablespoons coconut oil, divided • 1 (1-inch) stick cinnamon, pounded roughly • 3-4 green cardamom, pounded roughly • 4-5 whole cloves, pounded roughly • 2 bay leaves • 1 onion, chopped finely • 1 teaspoon garlic paste • 1½ teaspoons ginger paste • 3-4 green chilies, halved • 1 teaspoon red chili powder • ¾ cup plain Greek yogurt • ¾ cup water • Chopped fresh cilantro, for garnishing

Directions:

1. In a bowl, season the salmon with ½ teaspoon of the turmeric and salt and make aside. 2. In a big skillet, melt 1coconut oil on medium heat. 3. Add salmon and cook approximately 2-3 minutes per side. 4. Transfer the salmon right into a bowl. 5. In the identical skillet, melt remaining oil on medium heat. 6. Add cinnamon, green cardamom, whole cloves and bay leaves and sauté for around 1 minute. 7. Add onion and sauté for about 4-5 minutes. 8. Add garlic paste, ginger paste, green chilies and sauté for about 2 minutes. 9. Reduce the warmth to medium-low. 10. Add remaining turmeric, red chili powder and salt and sauté for about 1 minute. 11. Meanwhile in a very bowl, add yogurt and water and beat till smooth. 12. Now, slow up the heat to low and slowly, add the yogurt mixture, stirring continuously. 13. Simmer, covered for about fifteen minutes. 14. Carefully, add the salmon fillets and simmer for approximately 5 minutes. 15. Serve hot using the topping of cilantro.

POULTRY

621. Chicken with Bell Peppers & Carrot

Yield: 4 servings Preparation Time: fifteen minutes Cooking Time: 24 minutes

Ingredients:

For Chicken Marinade: • 2 minced garlic cloves • 2 teaspoon fresh ginger, minced • 1 egg, bea10 • 2 tablespoons tapioca starch • 2 teaspoon ground turmeric • 1½ teaspoons ground cumin • 1 teaspoon ground coriander • 1 teaspoon red chili powder • 4 skinless, boneless chicken breasts, cut into thin strips For Cooking: • 2 tablespoons olive oil • 1 small red onion, minced • 1 tablespoon ginger paste • 1 tablespoon garlic paste • 2 tablespoons red chili paste • 1 teaspoon red chili powder • ½ teaspoon ground cumin • Salt, to taste • 4 carrots, peeled and sliced • 2 green bell peppers, seeded and cubed • 1-2 green chilies, seeded and sliced

Directions:

1. For marinade inside a bowl, mix together all ingredients except chicken. 2. Add chicken and coat with marinade generously. 3. Refrigerate to marinate for about 120 minutes. 4. In a sizable skillet, heat oil on medium-high heat. 5. Add chicken and stir fry for approximately 3-4 minutes or till golden brown. 6. Transfer chicken right into a plate. 7. In the same skillet, add onion, ginger paste, garlic paste, red chili paste, chili powder, cumin and salt and sauté for approximately 2-3 minutes. 8. Add vegetables and stir fry for about 5 minutes. 9. Add chicken and cook for approximately 5-10 minutes or till desired doneness. 10. Serve hot.

622. Chicken with Veggie Combo

Yield: 2 servings Preparation Time: 25 minutes Cooking Time: fifteen minutes

Ingredients:

1 tbsp olive oil • 1 large skinless, boneless chicken white meat, cubed • 1 cup small cauliflower florets • 1 cup fresh shiitake mushrooms, sliced • 1 cup bokchoy, chopped • 1 cup carrot, peeled and spiralized Blade C • ½ teaspoon ground ginger • ½ teaspoon garlic salt • 1 large zucchini, spiralized Blade C

Directions:

1. In a big skillet, heat oil on medium-high heat. 2. Add chicken and stir fry approximately 2 minutes or till golden brown. 3. Add onion and cabbage and cook for around 4-5 minutes. 4. Add cauliflower whilst without stirring for around 30-45 seconds. 5. Cook, tossing occasionally for about2 minutes. 6. Add mushrooms and cook for approximately 2 minutes. 7. Add bokchoy, carrot, ground ginger and garlic salt and cook, tossing occasionally or about 2-3 minutes. 8. Add zucchini and cook for around 2-3 minutes. 9. Remove from heat and make aside for about 3-5 minutes before serving.

623. Chicken with Mango, Veggies & Cashews

Yield: 4 servings Preparation Time: 25 minutes Cooking Time: 18 minutes

Ingredients:

2 tablespoons coconut oil • 2 skinless, boneless chicken breasts, sliced • 1 red onion, sliced thinly • 2 minced garlic cloves • 2 tablespoons fresh ginger, minced • 1 ripe mango, peeled, pitted and cubed • 1 bunch broccoli, cut into small florets • 1 zucchini, sliced • 1 cup mushrooms, sliced • 1 red bell pepper, seeded and cubed • 2 cups beans sprouts • 3 tablespoons coconut aminos • ¼ teaspoon red chili flakes, crushed • Salt and freshly ground black pepper, to taste • ¼ cup cashews, toasted

Directions: 1. In a big skillet, melt coconut oil on medium-high heat. 2. Add chicken and stir fry for approximately 4-5 minutes or till golden brown. 3. Transfer chicken in a plate. 4. In the same skillet, add onion, garlic and ginger and sauté for about 1-2 minutes. 5. Add mango, broccoli, zucchini and bell pepper and cook for approximately 5-7 minutes. 6. Add chicken, beans sprouts, coconut aminos, red chili flakes, salt and black pepper and cook for approximately 3-4 minutes or till desired doneness. 7. Serve with the topping of cashews.

624. Chicken in Spicy Gravy

Yield: 3-4 servings Preparation Time: 10 min Cooking Time: 38 minutes

Ingredients:

For Marinade: • 1 teaspoon garlic paste • 1 teaspoon ginger paste • 2 teaspoons chili powder • ½ teaspoon ground turmeric • Salt, to taste • 1 teaspoon freshly squeezed lemon juice • Water, as required • 1 pound skinless, boneless chicken breast, cut into medium pieces For Cooking: • 5 tbsp essential olive oil • 2 large onions, sliced thinly • 10 curry leaves • 1½ teaspoons garlic paste • 1½ teaspoons ginger paste • 2 green chilies, chopped • 2 teaspoons ground coriander • 1 teaspoon garam masala • 1 teaspoon chili powder • 1 teaspoon ground turmeric • Salt and freshly ground black pepper, to taste • ½ cup chicken broth • 1 large tomato, chopped finely

Directions:

1. For marinate in a big bowl, mix together all ingredients except water and chicken. 2. Add enough water and mix till a paste forms. 3. Add chicken and coat with marinade generously. 4. Cover and refrigerate to marinate for around 30 minutes. 5. In a big skillet, heat oil on medium-high heat. 6. Add chicken and stir fry approximately 4-5 minutes or till golden brown. 7. Transfer chicken in a plate. 8. In a similar skillet, add onion and curry leaves on medium-low heat 9. Cook, covered for around 15-20 minutes till golden brown, stirring occasionally. 10. Add garlic ginger paste and green chilies and sauté approximately 1-2 minutes. 11. Stir in spices and sauté for approximately 1 minute. 12. Stir in chicken and cook, covered approximately 5-6 minutes. 13. Add broth and cook for approximately 5-6 minutes. 14. Add tomato and cook, stirring occasionally approximately 5 minutes more.

625. Citrus Glazed Chicken

Yield: 6 servings Preparation Time: 10 min Cooking Time: 18 minutes

Ingredients:

3 garlic cloves, minced • ½ cup fresh orange juice • 1 tablespoon apple cider vinegar • 2 tablespoons coconut aminos • ½ teaspoon orange blossom water • ¼ teaspoon ground ginger • ¼ teaspoon ground cinnamon • Salt, to taste • 2 pound skinless, bone-in chicken thighs

Directions:

1. For marinate in a big bowl, mix together all ingredients except chicken. 2. Add chicken and coat with marinade generously. 3. Cover and refrigerate to marinate for around 2 hours. 4. Heat a sizable nonstick skillet, on medium-high heat. 5. Add chicken in skillet, reserving marinade. 6. Cook for about 5-6 minutes or till golden brown. 7. Flip the medial side and cook for about 4 minutes. 8. Add reserved marinade and provide to a boil. 9. Reduce heat to medium-low heat. 10. Cook, covered for about 6-8 minutes or till sauce becomes thick. 11. Serve warm.

626. Chicken with Chickpeas & Veggies

Yield: 4 servings Preparation Time: 15 minutes Cooking Time: 36 minutes

Ingredients:

1 pound skinless, boneless chicken, cubed • Salt, to taste • 2 carrots, peeled and sliced • 1 onion, chopped • 2 celery stalks, chopped • 2 garlic cloves, chopped • 1 tablespoon fresh ginger root, minced • ½ teaspoon dried oregano, crushed • ¾ teaspoon ground cumin • ½ teaspoon paprika • ¼ tsp red pepper cayenne • ¼ teaspoon ground turmeric • 1 cup tomatoes, crushed • 1½ cups chicken broth • 1 zucchini, sliced • 1 cup canned chickpeas, drained • 1 tablespoon freshly squeezed lemon juice

Directions:

1. Heat a big nonstick pan on medium heat. 2. Add chicken and sprinkle with salt and cook for approximately 4-5 minutes. 3. With a slotted spoon, transfer chicken right into a plate. 4. In exactly the same pan, add carrot, onion, celery and garlic and sauté for about 4-5 minutes. 5. Add ginger, oregano and spices and sauté for around 1 minute. 6. Add chicken, tomato and broth and provide to some boil. 7. Reduce the temperature to low and simmer for approximately 10 minutes. 8. Add zucchini and chickpeas and simmer, covered for approximately fifteen minutes. 9. Stir in fresh lemon juice and serve hot.

627. Chicken Chili with Sweet Potato

Yield: 6 servings Preparation Time: 15 minutes Cooking Time: 35 minutes

Ingredients:

2 tablespoons extra-virgin essential olive oil • 1 medium red onion, chopped • 4-6 garlic cloves, minced • 2 medium sweet potatoes, peeled and cubed • 2 teaspoons dried oregano, crushed • 2 teaspoons ground cumin • 2 teaspoons ground ginger • 1 teaspoon red chili powder • ¼ teaspoon red pepper flakes, crushed • Salt, to taste • 4 cups chicken broth • 2 (15-ounce) cans white beans, rinsed and drained • ¾ cup mild roasted green chiles • 4 cups cooked chicken, shredded • 1 tablespoon fresh lime juice • 2 tablespoons fresh cilantro, chopped

Directions:

1. In a substantial pan, heat oil on medium-high heat. 2. Add poblano pepper and onion and sauté for about 2-3 minutes. 3. Add garlic and sauté for approximately 1-2 minutes. 4. Add sweet potato, oregano and spices and stir to combine well. 5. Add broth, beans and green chiles and provide to your boil. 6. Reduce the warmth to low and simmer for about 25-a half-hour. 7. Stir in chicken and lime juice and take off from heat. 8. Serve hot with all the topping of cilantro.

628. Chicken & Tomato Curry

Yield: 4 servings Preparation Time: 15 minutes Cooking Time: 70 minutes

Ingredients:

3 tablespoons organic olive oil • 1 medium onion, chopped • 1 teaspoon ginger paste • 1 teaspoon garlic paste • 4-6 large fresh tomatoes, chopped finely • 1 teaspoon ground cumin • Pinch of ground turmeric • 1½ teaspoons red chili powder • 2 pounds bone-in chicken breasts, cut each breast into 2-3 pieces • 2 cups water, divided • 2 cardamom pods • 2 tablespoons fresh cilantro, chopped

Directions:

1. In a big pan, heat oil on medium heat. 2. Add onion and sauté for about 8-9 minutes. 3. Add ginger and garlic and sauté for about1 minute. 4. Add tomatoes and spices reducing the heat to medium-low. 5. Cook, stirring occasionally for about 15-20 min. 6. Remove from heat whilst aside to chill slightly. 7. In a blender, add tomato mixture and pulse till smooth. 8. Return the mixture to pan with chicken and ½ cup from the water on medium-high heat. 9. Cook, stirring occasionally approximately 15-twenty minutes. 10. Add cardamom pods and remaining water and lower the temperature to low. 11. Simmer for approximately 15-20 min. 12. Serve top with the topping of cilantro.

629. Ground Chicken & Peas Curry

Yield: 3-4 servings Preparation Time: 15 minutes Cooking Time: 6-10 minutes

Ingredients:

For Marinade: • 3 tablespoons essential olive oil • 2 bay leaves • 2 onions, grinded to some paste • ½ tablespoon garlic paste • ½ tablespoon ginger paste • 2 tomatoes, chopped finely • 1 tablespoon ground cumin • 1 tablespoon ground coriander • 1 teaspoon ground turmeric • 1 teaspoon red chili powder • Salt, to taste • 1 pound lean ground chicken • 2 cups frozen peas • 1½ cups water • 1-2 teaspoons garam masala powder

Directions:

In a deep skillet, heat oil on medium heat. 2. Add bay leaves and sauté for approximately half a minute. 3. Add onion paste and sauté for approximately 3-4 minutes. 4. Add garlic and ginger paste and sauté for around 1-1½ minutes. 5. Add tomatoes and spices and cook, stirring occasionally for about 3-4 minutes. 6. Stir in chicken and cook for about 4-5 minutes. 7. Stir in peas and water and bring to a boil on high heat. 8. Reduce the heat to low and simmer approximately 5-8 minutes or till desired doneness. 9. Stir in garam masala and remove from heat. 10. Serve hot.

630. Ground Chicken with Basil

Yield: 8 servings Preparation Time: fifteen minutes Cooking Time: 16 minutes

Ingredients:

2 pounds lean ground chicken • 3 tablespoons coconut oil, divided • 1 zucchini, chopped • 1 red bell pepper, seeded and chopped • ½ of green bell pepper, seeded and chopped • 4 garlic cloves, minced • 1 (1-inch) piece fresh ginger, minced • 1 (1-inch) piece fresh turmeric, minced • 1 fresh red chile, sliced thinly • 1 tablespoon organic honey • 1 tablespoon coconut aminos • 1½ tablespoons fish sauce • ½ cup fresh basil, chopped • Salt and freshly ground black pepper, to taste • 1 tablespoon fresh lime juice

Directions:

1. Heat a large skillet on medium-high heat. 2. Add ground beef and cook for approximately 5 minutes or till browned completely. 3. Transfer the beef in a bowl. 4. In a similar pan, melt 1 tablespoon of coconut oil on medium-high heat. 5. Add zucchini and bell peppers and stir fry for around 3-4 minutes. 6. Transfer the vegetables inside bowl with chicken. 7. In exactly the same pan, melt remaining coconut oil on medium heat. 8. Add garlic, ginger, turmeric and red chile and sauté for approximately 1-2 minutes. 9. Add chicken mixture, honey and coconut aminos and increase the heat to high. 10. Cook, stirring occasionally for approximately 4-5 minutes or till sauce is nearly reduced. 11. Stir in remaining ingredients and take off from heat.

631. Chicken & Cauliflower Rice Casserole

Yield: 8-10 servings Preparation Time: fifteen minutes Cooking Time: an hour fifteen minutes

Ingredients:

2 tablespoons coconut oil, divided • 2-3 pound bone-in chicken thighs and drumsticks • Salt and freshly ground black pepper, to taste • 3 carrots, peeled and sliced • 1 onion, chopped finely • 2 garlic cloves, chopped finely • 2 tablespoons fresh cinnamon, chopped finely • 2 teaspoons ground cumin • 1 teaspoon ground coriander • 12 teaspoon ground cinnamon • ½ teaspoon ground turmeric • 1 teaspoon paprika • ¼ tsp red pepper cayenne • 1 (28-ounce) can diced tomatoes with liquid • 1 red bell pepper, seeded and cut into thin strips • ½ cup fresh parsley leaves, minced • Salt, to taste • 1 head cauliflower, grated to some rice like consis10cy • 1 lemon, sliced thinly

Directions: 1. Preheat the oven to 375 degrees F. 2. In a large pan, melt 1 tablespoon of coconut oil high heat. 3. Add chicken pieces and cook for about 3-5 minutes per side or till golden brown. 4. Transfer the chicken in a plate. 5. In a similar pan, sauté the carrot, onion, garlic and ginger for about 4-5 minutes on medium heat. 6. Stir in spices and remaining coconut oil. 7. Add chicken, tomatoes, bell pepper, parsley and salt and simmer for approximately 3-5 minutes. 8. In the bottom of a 13x9-inch rectangular baking dish, spread the cauliflower rice evenly. 9. Place chicken mixture over cauliflower rice evenly and top with lemon slices. 10. With a foil paper, cover the baking dish and bake for approximately 35 minutes. 11. Uncover the baking dish and bake approximately 25 minutes.

632. Roasted Spatchcock Chicken

Yield: 4-6 servings Preparation Time: twenty or so minutes Cooking Time: 50 minutes

Ingredients:

1 (4-pound) whole chicken • 1 (1-inch) piece fresh ginger, sliced • 4 garlic cloves, chopped • 1 small bunch fresh thyme • Pinch of cayenne • Salt and freshly ground black pepper, to taste • ¼ cup fresh lemon juice • 3 tablespoons extra virgin olive oil

Directions: 1. Arrange chicken, breast side down onto a large cutting board. 2. With a kitchen shear, begin with thigh and cut along 1 side of backbone and turn chicken around. 3. Now, cut along sleep issues and discard the backbone. 4. Change the inside and open it like a book. 5. Flat10 the backbone firmly to flat10. 6. In a food processor, add all ingredients except chicken and pulse till smooth. 7. In a big baking dish, add the marinade mixture. 8. Add chicken and coat with marinade generously. 9. With a plastic wrap, cover the baking dish and refrigerate to marinate for overnight. 10. Preheat the oven to 450 degrees F. Arrange a rack in a very roasting pan. 11. Remove the chicken from refrigerator make onto rack over roasting pan, skin side down. 12. Roast for about 50 minutes, turning once in the middle way.

633. Roasted Chicken Breast

Yield: 4-6 servings Preparation Time: quarter-hour Cooking Time: 40 minutes

Ingredients:

½ of small apple, peeled, cored and chopped • 1 bunch scallion, trimmed and copped roughly • 8 fresh ginger slices, chopped • 2 garlic cloves, chopped • 3 tablespoons essential olive oil • 12 teaspoon sesame oil, toasted • 3 tablespoons using apple cider vinegar • 1 tablespoon fish sauce • 1 tablespoon coconut aminos • Salt and freshly ground black pepper, to taste • 4 pounds chicken thighs

Directions:

1. In a blender, add all ingredients except chicken thighs and pulse till smooth. 2. Transfer a combination and chicken right into a large ziploc bag and seal it. 3. Shake the bag to coat the chicken with marinade well. 4. Refrigerate to marinade for about 12 hours. 5. Preheat the oven to 400 degrees F. Arrange a rack in foil paper lined baking sheet. 6. Place the chicken thighs on rack, skin-side down. 7. Roast for about 40 minutes, flipping once within the middle way.

634. Grilled Chicken

Yield: 8 servings Preparation Time: 15 minutes Cooking Time: 41 minutes

Ingredients:

1 (3-inch) piece fresh ginger, minced • 6 small garlic cloves, minced • 1½ tablespoons tamarind paste • 1 tablespoon organic honey • ¼ cup coconut aminos • 2½ tablespoons extra virgin olive oil • 1½ tablespoons sesame oil, toasted • ½ teaspoon ground cardamom • Salt and freshly ground white pepper, to taste • 1 (4-5-pound)whole chicken, cut into 8 pieces

Directions:

1. In a large glass bowl, mix together all ingredients except chicken pieces. 2. With a fork, pierce the chicken pieces completely. 3. Add chicken pieces in bowl and coat with marinade generously. 4. Cover and refrigerate to marinate for approximately a couple of hours to overnight. 5. Preheat the grill to medium heat. Grease the grill grate. 6. Place the chicken pieces on grill, bone-side down. 7. Grill, covered approximately 20-25 minutes. 8. Change the side and grill, covered approximately 6-8 minutes. 9. Change along side it and grill, covered for about 5-8 minutes.

635. Grilled Chicken with Pineapple & Veggies

Yield: 4 servings Preparation Time: twenty or so minutes Cooking Time: 22 minutes

Ingredients:

For Sauce: • 1 garlic oil, minced • ¾ teaspoon fresh ginger, minced • ½ cup coconut aminos • ¼ cup fresh pineapple juice • 2 tablespoons freshly squeezed lemon juice • 2 tablespoons balsamic vinegar • ¼ teaspoon red pepper flakes, crushed • Salt and freshly ground black pepper, to taste For Grilling: • 4 skinless, boneless chicken breasts • 1 pineapple, peeled and sliced • 1 bell pepper, seeded and cubed • 1 zucchini, sliced • 1red onion, sliced

Directions:

For sauce in a pan, mix together all ingredients on medium-high heat. 2. Bring to a boil reducing the heat to medium-low. 3. Cook approximately 5-6 minutes. 4. Remove from heat and keep aside to cool down the slightly. 5. Coat the chicken breasts about ¼ from the sauce. 6. Keep aside for approximately half an hour. 7. Preheat the grill to medium-high heat. Grease the grill grate. 8. Place the chicken pieces on grill and grill for around 5-8 minutes per side. 9. Now, squeeze pineapple and vegetables on grill grate. 10. Grill the pineapple for around 3 minutes per side. 11. Grill the vegetables for approximately 4-5 minutes, stirring once inside middle way. 12. Cut the chicken breasts into desired size slices. 13. Divide chicken, pineapple and vegetables in serving plates. 14. Serve alongside remaining sauce.

636. Ground Turkey with Asparagus

Yield: 8 servings Preparation Time: 15 minutes Cooking Time: fifteen minutes

Ingredients:

1¾ pound lean ground turkey • 2 tablespoons sesame oil • 1 medium onion, chopped • 1 cup celery, chopped • 6 garlic cloves, minced • 2 cups asparagus, trimmed and cut into 1-inch pieces • 1/3 cup coconut aminos • 2½ teaspoons ginger powder • 2 tablespoons organic coconut crystals • 1 tablespoon arrowroot starch • 1 tablespoon cold water • ¼ teaspoon red pepper flakes, crushed

Directions:

1. Heat a substantial nonstick skillet on medium-high heat. 2. Add turkey and cook for approximately 5-7 minutes or till browned. 3. With a slotted spoon transfer the turkey inside a bowl and discard the grease from skillet. 4. In exactly the same skillet, heat oil on medium heat. 5. Add onion, celery and garlic and sauté for about 5 minutes. 6. Add asparagus and cooked turkey minimizing the temperature to medium-low. 7. Meanwhile inside a pan mix together coconut aminos, ginger powder and coconut crystals n medium heat and convey to some boil. 8. In a smaller bowl, mix together arrowroot starch and water. 9. Slowly, add arrowroot mixture, stirring continuously. 10. Cook approximately 2-3 minutes. 11. Add the sauce in s killed with turkey mixture and stir to blend. 12. Stir in red pepper flakes and cook for approximately 2-3 minutes. 13. Serve hot.

637. Turkey & Pumpkin Chili

Yield: 4-6 servings Preparation Time: quarter-hour Cooking Time: 41 minutes

Ingredients:

2 tablespoons extra-virgin olive oil • 1 green bell pepper, seeded and chopped • 1 small yellow onion, chopped • 2 garlic cloves, chopped finely • 1 pound lean ground turkey • 1 (15-ounce) pumpkin puree • 1 (14 ½-ounce) can diced tomatoes with liquid • 1 teaspoon ground cumin • ½ teaspoon ground turmeric • ½ teaspoon ground cinnamon • 1 cup water • 1 (15-ounce) can chickpeas, rinsed and drained

Directions:

1. In a big pan, heat oil on medium-low heat. 2. Add the bell pepper, onion and garlic and sauté approximately 5 minutes. 3. Add turkey and cook for about 5-6 minutes. 4. Add tomatoes, pumpkin, spices and water and convey to your boil on high heat. 5. Reduce the temperature to medium-low heat and stir in chickpeas. 6. Simmer, covered for approximately a half-hour, stirring occasionally. 7. Serve hot.

638. Ground Turkey with Lentils

Yield: 8 servings Preparation Time: quarter-hour Cooking Time: 35 minutes

Ingredients:

3 tablespoons olive oil, divided • 1 onion, chopped • 1 tablespoon fresh ginger, minced • 4 garlic cloves, minced • 2 Roma tomatoes, seeded and chopped • 3 celery stalks, chopped • 1 large carrot, peeled and chopped • 1 cup dried red lentils, rinsed, soaked for thirty minutes and drained • 2 cups chicken broth • 1 teaspoon black mustard seeds • 1½ teaspoons cumin seeds • 1 teaspoon ground turmeric • ½ teaspoon paprika • 1 pound lean ground turkey • 1 Serrano chile, seeded and chopped • 2 scallions, chopped • Chopped fresh cilantro, for garnishing

Directions:

1. In a Dutch oven, heat 1 tablespoon of oil on medium heat. 2. Add onion, ginger and garlic and sauté for around 5 minutes. 3. Stir in tomatoes, celery, carrot, lentils and broth and convey to your boil 4. Reduce the warmth to medium-low. 5. Simmer, covered for around thirty minutes. 6. Meanwhile in a skillet, heat remaining oil on medium heat. 7. Add mustard seeds and cumin seeds and sauté approximately 30 seconds. 8. Add turmeric and paprika and sauté approximately 25 seconds. 9. Transfer a combination into a small bowl and aside. 10. In exactly the same skillet, add turkey and cook for around 4-5 minutes. 11. Add Serrano chile and scallion and cook for about 3-4 minutes. 12. Add spiced oil mixture and stir to mix well. 13. Transfer the turkey mixture in simmering lentils and simmer for around 5-10 minutes more.

639. Grilled Turkey Breast

Yield: 4 servings Preparation Time: 15 minutes Cooking Time: 6-10 min

Ingredients:

1 large shallot, quartered • (¾-inch) piece fresh ginger, chopped • 2 small garlic cloves, chopped • 1 tablespoon honey • ¼ cup extra virgin olive oil • ¼ cup coconut aminos • 2 tablespoons fresh lime juice • Freshly ground black pepper, to taste • 4 turkey breast 10derloins

Directions:

1. In a food processor, add shallot, ginger and garlic and pulse till minced. 2. Add remaining ingredients except turkey 10derloins and pulse till well combined. 3. Transfer the mixture in a sizable bowl. 4. Add turkey 10derloins and coat with mixture generously. 5. Keep aside, covered for approximately 30 minutes. 6. Preheat the grill to medium heat. Grease the grill grate. 7. Grill for about 6-8 minutes per side.

640. Grilled Duck Breast & Peach

Yield: 2 servings Preparation Time: quarter-hour Cooking Time: 24 minutes

Ingredients:

2 shallots, sliced thinly • 2 tablespoons fresh ginger, minced • 2 tablespoons fresh thyme, chopped • Salt and freshly ground black pepper, to taste • 2 duck breasts • 2 peaches, pitted and quartered • ½ teaspoon ground fennel seeds • ½ tablespoon extra-virgin olive oil

Directions:

1. In a substantial bowl, mix together shallots, ginger, thyme, salt and black pepper. 2. Add duck breasts and coat with marinade evenly. 3. Refrigerate to marinate for about 2-12 hours. 4. Preheat the grill to medium-high heat. Grease the grill grate. 5. In a sizable bowl, add peaches, fennel seeds, salt, black pepper and oil and toss to coat well. 6. Place the duck breast on grill, skin side down and grill for around 6-8 minutes per side. 7. Transfer the duck breast onto a plate. 8. Now, grill the peaches for around 3 minutes per side. 9. Serve the duck breasts with grilled peaches.

641. Creamy Chicken with Broccoli & Spinach

Yield: 4 servings Preparation Time: 15 minutes Cooking Time: 13 minutes

Ingredients:

13-ounce unswee10ed coconut milk • 1 teaspoon fresh ginger, grated • 1½ teaspoons curry powder • 2 tablespoons coconut oil, divided • 1 pound 10der chicken, sliced thinly • 1 large onion, chopped • 2 cups broccoli florets • 1 large bunch fresh spinach, chopped

Directions:

In a bowl, mix together coconut milk, ginger and curry powder. Keep aside. 2. In a big skillet, melt 1 tablespoon of coconut oil on medium-high heat. 3. Add chicken and stir fry for around 3-4 minutes or till golden brown. 4. Transfer chicken right into a plate. 5. In exactly the same skillet, heat remaining oil on medium-high heat. 6. Add onion and sauté for around 2 minutes. 7. Add broccoli and stir fry for about 3 minutes. 8. Add chicken, spinach and coconut mixture and stir fry for approximately 3-4 minute

642. Chicken with Cabbage

Yield: 4-6 servings Preparation Time: 15 minutes Cooking Time: 17 minutes

Ingredients:

½ teaspoon garlic powder • ½ teaspoon fresh ginger powder • Salt and freshly ground black pepper, to taste • ½ teaspoon sesame oil • 3 tablespoons apple cider vinegar treatment • 4 skinless, boneless chicken breasts, sliced thinly • 3 tablespoons coconut oil, divided • 1 onion, sliced thinly • 1 large head cabbage, sliced thinly • ¼ cup organic honey • ¼ cup coconut aminos

Directions:

1. In a big bowl, mix together garlic powder, ginger powder, salt, black pepper, sesame oil and vinegar. 2. Add chicken and coat with mixture generously whilst aside for approximately 5 minutes. 3. In a large skillet, melt 2 tablespoons of coconut oil on medium-high heat. 4. Add chicken and stir fry for about 3-4 minutes or till golden brown. 5. Transfer chicken into a plate. 6. In exactly the same skillet, melt remaining oil on medium heat. 7. Add onion and cabbage and cook for about 4-5 minutes. 8. Add chicken, honey and coconut aminos and cook for around 5-8 minutes or till desired doneness.

643. Chicken with Mixed Veggies & Almonds

Yield: 8-10 servings Preparation Time: 25 minutes Cooking Time: 10 min

Ingredients:

2 tablespoons coconut oil • 2 skinless, boneless chicken breasts, cubed • 2 (8-ounce) cans water chestnuts • 4 cups broccoli florets • 1 cup fresh mushrooms, sliced • ½ cup celery stalk, chopped • 1 head cabbage, shredded • ½ cup green onions, chopped • 4-5 garlic cloves, minced • 2 tablespoons fresh ginger, minced • ½ cup almonds, chopped • 3 tablespoons coconut aminos • White sesame seeds, for garnishing

Directions:

1. In a sizable skillet, melt coconut oil on medium-high heat. 2. Add chicken and stir fry for approximately 3-4 minutes or till golden brown. 3. Add water chestnuts, broccoli, mushrooms and celery and stir fry for around 2 minutes. 4. Add cabbage, green onion, garlic, ginger, almonds and coconut aminos and cook for approximately 2-3 minutes. 5. Serve hot with the garnishing of sesame seeds.

644. Chicken with Strawberries, Rhubarb & Zucchini

Yield: 2 servings Preparation Time: twenty or so minutes Cooking Time: 13 minutes

Ingredients:

2 zucchinis, spiralized with Blade C • Salt, to taste • 1½ teaspoons olive oil • ½ teaspoon fresh ginger, minced • ¾ cup rhubarb, chopped • 1 (8-ounce) skinless, boneless chicken breasts, cubed • 4 teaspoons organic honey • 1 teaspoon fresh lime zest, grated finely • ¼ cup plus 2 teaspoons fresh orange juice, divided • 1 tablespoon fresh lime juice • 2 teaspoons fresh mint leaves, minced • ½ cup fresh strawberries, hulled and sliced • 2 tablespoons almonds, toasted and slivered

Directions:

Arrange a sizable strainer over sink. 2. Place the zucchini noodles in strainer and sprinkle using a pinch of salt. 3. Keep aside release a the moisture. 4. In a sizable skillet, heat oil on medium heat. 5. Add ginger and rhubarb and cook for about 2-3 minutes. 6. Stir in chicken and cook for approximately 4-5 minutes. 7. Add honey, lime zest, ¼ cup of orange juice, lime juice and pinch of salt and cook and raise the heat to high. 8. Bring to your boil reducing heat to medium. 9. Simmer, stirring occasionally approximately 4-5 minutes and take off from heat. 10. Squeeze the moisture from zucchini and pat dry with paper towels. 11. In a smaller bowl, mix together remaining orange juice and mint. 12. Divide zucchini noodles in serving plates and drizzle with mint mixture. 13. Place chicken mixture, strawberries and almonds over zucchini noodles and gently stir to combine. 14. Serve immediately.

645. Lemon Braised Chicken

Yield: 6 servings Preparation Time: fifteen minutes Cooking Time: one hour

Ingredients:

2 tablespoons organic olive oil • 6 bone-in chicken thighs • Salt and freshly ground black pepper, to taste • ½ of onion, sliced • 4 cups chicken broth • 8 sprigs fresh dill • Pinch of cayenne pepper • ½ teaspoon ground turmeric • 2 tablespoons fresh lemon juice • 2 tablespoons arrowroot starch • 1 tablespoon cold water • ½ tablespoon fresh dill, chopped

Directions:

1. In a substantial skillet, heat oil on high heat. 2. Sprinkle the chicken with salt and black pepper. 3. Place inside the skillet, skin side down and cook for about 3-4 minutes. 4. Transfer the thighs in a very plate. 5. In a similar skillet, add onion on medium heat and sauté approximately 4-5 minutes. 6. Return the thighs in skillet, skin side up with broth. 7. Place the dill sprigs over thighs and sprinkle with cayenne, turmeric and salt. 8. Bring to some boil reducing the warmth to medium-low. 9. Simmer, covered for around 40-45 minutes, coating the thighs with cooking liquid. 10. Meanwhile in a small bowl, mix together arrowroot starch and water. 11. Discard the thyme sprigs and transfer the thighs into a bowl. 12. Stir in freshly squeezed lemon juice in sauce. 13. Slowly, add arrowroot starch mixture, stirring continuously. 14. Cook, stirring occasionally for approximately 3-4 minutes or till desired thickness. 15. Serve hot using the topping of chopped dill.

646. Herbed Chicken with Olives

Yield: 4 servings Preparation Time: fifteen minutes Cooking Time: 60 minutes 45 minutes

Ingredients:

4-6 bone-in chicken legs and thighs • Salt and freshly ground black pepper, to taste • 1 tablespoon fresh lemon juice • 1 cup olives, pitted and sliced • ¼ cup essential olive oil • 2 medium yellow onions, sliced thinly • 2 tablespoons fresh lemon zest, grated finely • 3 garlic cloves, crushed • ½ teaspoon ground ginger • ¼ teaspoon saffron threads, crushed • 1½ cups chicken broth • ¼ cup fresh parsley leaves, chopped • ¼ cup fresh cilantro leaves, chopped

Directions:

1. Drizzle the chicken with all the freshly squeezed lemon juice and sprinkle with salt and black pepper. 2. In a substantial Dutch oven, heat oil on medium-high heat. 3. Add chicken and cook for around 4-6 minutes per side. 4. Add remaining ingredients except herbs and bring to a boil. 5. Reduce the heat to medium-low. 6. Simmer for around 75 minutes. 7. Stir in herbs and simmer for quarter-hour more. 8. Serve immediately.

647. Chicken Chili with Zucchini

Yield: 4-5 servings Preparation Time: 15 minutes Cooking Time: 35 minutes

Ingredients:

3 tablespoons organic olive oil • 1 poblano pepper, seeded and chopped • ½ of red onion, chopped • 1 tablespoon garlic, minced • 1 zucchini, halved lengthwise and sliced • 2 (15-ounce) cans cannellini beans, rinsed and drained • 1½ cups rotisserie chicken, shredded • 1 tablespoon fresh oregano, minced • 1 teaspoon ground turmeric • 1 teaspoon ground cumin • Salt and freshly ground black pepper, to taste • 2 cups water • 2 cups chicken broth • 1/3 cup sharp cheddar cheese, shredded • Chopped chives, for garnishing

Directions:

In a substantial pan, heat oil on medium-low heat. 2. Add poblano pepper and onion and sauté for approximately 10 min. 3. Add garlic and zucchini and cook for around 5 minutes. 4. Add remaining ingredients except cheese and chives and produce to your boil. 5. Reduce the heat to low and simmer for around twenty minutes. 6. Add the cheese and stir till well combined. 7. Serve hot with the topping of chives.

648. Chicken Chili with Two Beans & Corn

Yield: 6 servings Preparation Time: quarter-hour Cooking Time: 28 minutes

Ingredients:

1 tbsp essential olive oil • 1 pound skinless, boneless chicken, cubed into 1-inch size • 1 cup onion, chopped • 1 cup green bell pepper, seeded and chopped • 1½ teaspoons dried oregano, crushed • 1 teaspoon garlic powder • 1 teaspoon ground cumin • 1 tablespoon paprika • ¼ teaspoon red pepper flakes, crushed • 1 cup frozen corn • 1 (14½-ounce) can diced tomatoes with liquid • 1 (15-ounce) can great Northern beans, rinsed and drained • 1 (15-ounce) can black beans, rinsed and drained • 1 cup chicken broth

Directions:

1. In a substantial pan, heat oil on medium-high heat. 2. Add chicken, onion and bell pepper and sauté approximately 6-8 minutes. 3. Add oregano and spices and stir to blend well. 4. Add remaining ingredients and provide to your boil. 5. Reduce the temperature to low and simmer for about twenty minutes. 6. Serve hot.

649. Chicken & Sweet Potato Curry

Yield: 4 servings Preparation Time: fifteen minutes Cooking Time: 6-10 minutes

Ingredients:

2 tablespoons organic olive oil, divided • Salt and freshly ground black pepper, to taste • 1 pound skinless, boneless chicken breast, cut into chunks • ½ of onion, chopped • 2 minced garlic cloves • 1 teaspoon ground ginger • 1 teaspoon curry powder • ½ cup chicken broth • 2 large sweet potatoes, peeled and cubed • 1 can coconut milk

Directions:

1. In a sizable skillet, heat 1 tablespoon of oil on medium heat. 2. Add chicken and sprinkle with salt and black pepper. 3. Stir fry approximately 3-4 minutes per side. 4. Transfer chicken right into a plate. 5. In the identical skillet, heat remaining oil on medium heat. 6. Add onion and sauté for about 5-7 minutes. 7. Add garlic, ground ginger and curry powder and sauté for around 1-2 minutes. 8. Add chicken and remaining ingredients and stir to mix well. 9. Simmer, covered for around 15-twenty minutes. 10. Stir in salt and black pepper and serve hot.

650. Chicken Meatballs Curry

Yield: 3-4 servings Preparation Time: 20 min Cooking Time: 25 minutes

Ingredients:

For Meatballs: • 1 pound lean ground chicken • 1 tablespoon onion paste • 1 teaspoons fresh ginger paste • 1 teaspoons garlic paste • 1 green chili, chopped finely • 1 tablespoon fresh cilantro leaves, chopped • 1 teaspoon ground coriander • ½ teaspoon cumin seeds • ½ teaspoon red chili powder • ½ teaspoon ground turmeric • Salt, to taste For Curry: • 3 tablespoons extra-virgin olive oil • ½ teaspoon cumin seeds • 1 (1-inch) cinnamon stick • 3 whole cloves • 3 whole green cardamoms • 1 whole black cardamom • 2 onions, chopped • 1 teaspoons fresh ginger, minced • 1 teaspoons garlic, minced • 4 whole tomatoes, chopped finely • 2 teaspoons ground coriander • 1 teaspoon garam masala powder • ½ teaspoon ground nutmeg • ½ teaspoon red chili powder • ½ teaspoon ground turmeric • Salt, to taste • 1 cup water • Chopped fresh cilantro, for garnishing

Directions:

For meatballs in a substantial bowl, add all ingredients and mix till well combined. 2. Make small equal-sized meatballs from mixture. 3. In a big deep skillet, heat oil on medium heat. 4. Add meatballs and fry approximately 3-5 minutes or till browned from all sides. 5. Transfer the meatballs in a bowl. 6. In the same skillet, add cumin seeds, cinnamon stick, cloves, green cardamom and black cardamom and sauté approximately 1 minute. 7. Add onions and sauté for around 4-5 minutes. 8. Add ginger and garlic paste and sauté approximately 1 minute. 9. Add tomato and spices and cook, crushing with the back of spoon for approximately 2-3 minutes. 10. Add water and meatballs and provide to a boil. 11. Reduce heat to low. 12. Simmer for approximately 10 minutes. 13. Serve hot with all the garnishing of cilantro.

651. Chicken &Veggie Casserole

Yield: 4 servings Preparation Time: quarter-hour Cooking Time: half an hour

Ingredients:

1/3 cup Dijon mustard • 1/3 cup organic honey • 1 teaspoon dried basil • ¼ teaspoon ground turmeric • 1 teaspoon dried basil, crushed • Salt and freshly ground black pepper, to taste • 1¾ pound chicken breasts • 1 cup fresh white mushrooms, sliced • ½ head broccoli, cut into small florets

Directions:

1. Preheat the oven to 350 degrees F. Lightly, grease a baking dish. 2. In a bowl, mix together all ingredients except chicken, mushrooms and broccoli. 3. Arrange chicken in prepared baking dish and top with mushroom slices. 4. Place broccoli florets around chicken evenly. 5. Pour 1 / 2 of honey mixture over chicken and broccoli evenly. 6. Bake for approximately twenty minutes. 7. Now, coat the chicken with remaining sauce and bake for approximately 10 minutes.

652. Chicken Meatloaf with Veggies

Yield: 4 servings Preparation Time: 20 minutes Cooking Time: 1-1¼ hours

Ingredients:

For Meatloaf: • ½ cup cooked chickpeas • 2 egg whites • 2½ teaspoons poultry seasoning • Salt and freshly ground black pepper, to taste • 10-ounce lean ground chicken • 1 cup red bell pepper, seeded and minced • 1 cup celery stalk, minced • 1/3 cup steel-cut oats • 1 cup tomato puree, divided • 2 tablespoons dried onion flakes, crushed • 1 tablespoon prepared mustard For Veggies: • 2 pounds summer squash, sliced • 16-ounce frozen Brussels sprouts • 2 tablespoons extra-virgin extra virgin olive oil • Salt and freshly ground black pepper, to taste

Directions:

1. Preheat the oven to 350 degrees F. Grease a 9x5-inch loaf pan. 2. In a mixer, add chickpeas, egg whites, poultry seasoning, salt and black pepper and pulse till smooth. 3. Transfer a combination in a large bowl. 4. Add chicken, veggies oats, ½ cup of tomato puree and onion flakes and mix till well combined. 5. Transfer the amalgamation into prepared loaf pan evenly. 6. With both hands, press, down the amalgamation slightly. 7. In another bowl mix together mustard and remaining tomato puree. 8. Place the mustard mixture over loaf pan evenly. 9. Bake approximately 1-1¼ hours or till desired doneness. 10. Meanwhile in a big pan of water, arrange a steamer basket. 11. Bring to a boil and set summer time squash I steamer basket. 12. Cover and steam approximately 10-12 minutes. 13. Drain well and aside. 14. Now, prepare the Brussels sprouts according to package's directions. 15. In a big bowl, add veggies, oil, salt and black pepper and toss to coat well. 16. Serve the meatloaf with veggies.

653. Roasted Chicken with Veggies & Orange

Yield: 4 servings Preparation Time: 20 min Cooking Time: 60 minutes

Ingredients:

1 teaspoon ground ginger • ½ teaspoon ground cumin • ½ teaspoon ground coriander • 1 teaspoon paprika • Salt and freshly ground black pepper, to taste • 1 (3 ½-4-pound) whole chicken • 1 unpeeled orange, cut into 8 wedges • 2 medium carrots, peeled and cut 1nto 2-inch pieces • 2 medium sweet potatoes, peeled and cut into ½-inch wedges • ½ cup water

Directions:

Preheat the oven to 450 degrees F. 2. In a little bowl, mix together the spices. 3. Rub the chicken with spice mixture evenly. 4. Arrange the chicken in a substantial Dutch oven and put orange, carrot and sweet potato pieces around it. 5. Add water and cover the pan tightly. 6. Roast for around 30 minutes. 7. Uncover and roast for about half an hour.

654. Roasted Chicken Drumsticks

Yield: 4-6 servings Preparation Time: fifteen minutes Cooking Time: 50 minutes

Ingredients:

1 medium onion, chopped • 1-2 tablespoons fresh turmeric, chopped • 1-2 tablespoons fresh ginger, chopped • 2 lemongrass stalks (bottom third), peeled and chopped • 1-2 jalapeños, seeded and chopped • 1 teaspoon fresh lime zest, grated • 1 tablespoon curry powder • 1¼ cups unswee10ed coconut milk • 3 tablespoons fresh lime juice • 1 tablespoon coconut aminos • 1 tablespoon fish sauce • 3-4 pound chicken kegs • Chopped fresh cilantro, for garnishing

Directions:

1. In a blender, add all ingredients except chicken legs and pulse till smooth. 2. Transfer a combination in a large baking dish. 3. Add chicken and coat with marinade generously. 4. Cover and refrigerate to marinade approximately 12 hours. 5. Remove chicken from refrigerator and in room temperature approximately 25-half an hour before cooking. 6. Preheat the oven to 350 degrees F. 7. Uncover the baking dish and roast or about 50 minutes.

655. Grilled Chicken Breast

Yield: 4 servings Preparation Time: 15 minutes Cooking Time: 20 minutes

Ingredients:

2 scallions, chopped • 1 (1-inch) piece fresh ginger, minced • 2 minced garlic cloves • 1 cup fresh pineapple juice • ¼ cup coconut aminos • ¼ cup extra-virgin organic olive oil • 1 teaspoon ground cinnamon • 1 teaspoon ground cumin • 1 teaspoon ground turmeric • Salt, to taste • 4 skinless, boneless chicken breasts

Directions: 1. In a big ziploc bag add all ingredients and seal it. 2. Shake the bag to coat the chicken with marinade well. 3. Refrigerate to marinade for about twenty or so minutes to an hour. 4. Preheat the grill to medium-high heat. Grease the grill grate. 5. Place the chicken pieces on grill and grill for about 10 min per side.

656. Ground Turkey with Veggies

Yield: 4 servings Preparation Time: quarter-hour Cooking Time: 12 minutes

Ingredients:

1 tablespoon sesame oil • 1 tablespoon coconut oil • 1 pound lean ground turkey • 2 tablespoons fresh ginger, minced • 2 minced garlic cloves • 1 (16-ounce) bag vegetable mix (broccoli, carrot, cabbage, kale and Brussels sprouts) • ¼ cup coconut aminos • 2 tablespoons balsamic vinegar

Directions: 1. In a big skillet heat both oils on medium-high heat. 2. Add turkey, ginger and garlic and cook approximately 5-6 minutes. 3. Add vegetable mix and cook approximately 4-5 minutes. 4. Stir in coconut aminos and vinegar and cook for about 1 minute. 5. Serve hot.

657. Ground Turkey with Peas & Potato

Yield: 4 servings Preparation Time: fifteen minutes Cooking Time: 35 minutes

Ingredients:

3-4 tablespoons coconut oil • 1 pound lean ground turkey • 1-2 fresh red chiles, chopped • 1 onion, chopped • Salt, to taste • 2 minced garlic cloves • 1 (1-inch) piece fresh ginger, grated finely • 1 tablespoon curry powder • 1 teaspoon ground coriander • 1 teaspoon ground cumin • 1 teaspoon ground turmeric • 2 large Yukon gold potatoes, peeled and cubed into 1-inch size • ½ cup water • 1 cup fresh peas, shelled • 2-4 plum tomatoes, chopped • ½ cup fresh cilantro, chopped

Directions: 1. In a substantial pan, heat oil on medium-high heat. 2. Add turkey and cook for about 4-5 minutes. 3. Add chiles and onion and cook for about 4-5 minutes. 4. Add garlic and ginger and cook approximately 1-2 minutes. 5. Stir in spices, potatoes and water and convey to your boil 6. Reduce the warmth to medium-low. 7. Simmer, covered approximately 15-twenty or so minutes. 8. Add peas and tomatoes and cook for about 2-3 minutes. 9. Serve using the garnishing of cilantro.

658. Turkey & Veggies Chili

Yield: 8 servings Preparation Time: quarter-hour Cooking Time: 35 minutes

Ingredients:

3 tablespoons essential olive oil, divided • 1½ pound lean ground turkey • 2 tablespoons tomato paste • 1 teaspoon dried oregano, crushed • 1 teaspoon ground coriander • 1 teaspoon ground cumin • ½ teaspoon ground cinnamon • ½ teaspoon ground turmeric • 1½ cups chicken broth • 3 cups cooked sprouted beans trio • ½ cup mild salsa • 2 carrots, peeled and chopped • 1 (14½-ounce) can crushed tomatoes • 1 medium onion, chopped • 2 garlic cloves, chopped finely • 3 medium zucchinis, chopped • 1 cup cheddar cheese • 4 scallions, chopped

Directions:

1. In a sizable pan, heat 1 tablespoon of oil on medium-high heat. 2. Add turkey and with the spoon, plunge into pieces. 3. Add tomato paste, oregano and spices and cook for about 4-5 minutes. 4. Add broth and provide to a boil, 5. Reduce the temperature to medium and simmer for around 5 minutes. 6. Add beans trio, salsa, carrots and tomatoes and simmer for abbot 10 minutes. 7. Meanwhile in a substantial skillet, heat remaining oil on medium-high heat. 8. Add onion and garlic and sauté for about 5 minutes. 9. Add zucchini and cook for approximately 5 minutes, stirring occasionally. 10. Transfer the zucchini mixture within the chili mixture and transfer the warmth to low. 11. Simmer for around quarter-hour.

659. Roasted Whole Turkey

Yield: 8-10 servings Preparation Time: quarter-hour Cooking Time: 3 hours thirty minutes

Ingredients:

For Turkey Marinade: • 1 (2-inch) piece fresh ginger, grated finely • 3 large garlic cloves, crushed • 1 green chili, chopped finely • 1 teaspoon fresh lemon zest, grated finely • 5-ounce plain Greek yogurt • 3 tablespoons tomato puree • 2 tablespoons fresh lemon juice • 1 tablespoon ground cumin • 1½ tablespoons garam masala • 2 teaspoons ground turmeric For Turkey: • 1 (9-pound) whole turkey, giblets and neck removed • Salt and freshly ground black pepper, to taste • 1 garlic cloves, halved • 1 lime, halved • ½ of lemon

Directions:

1. In a bowl, mix together all marinade ingredients. 2. With a fork, pierce the turkey completely. 3. In a sizable baking dish, put the turkey. 4. Rub the turkey with marinade mixture evenly. 5. Refrigerate to marinate for overnight. 6. Remove from refrigerator and make aside approximately a half-hour before serving. 7. Preheat the oven to 390 degrees F. 8. Sprinkle turkey with salt and black pepper evenly and stuff the cavity with garlic, lime and lemon. 9. Arrange the turkey in a big roasting pan and roast for approximately a half-hour. 10. Now, reduce the temperature of oven to 350 degrees F. 11. Roast for around 3 hours. (if skin becomes brown during roasting, then cover with foil paper)

660. Duck with Bok Choy

Yield: 4-6 servings Preparation Time: 15 minutes Cooking Time: 12 minutes

Ingredients:

2 tablespoons coconut oil • 1 onion, sliced thinly • 2 teaspoons fresh ginger, grated finely • 2 minced garlic cloves • 1 tablespoon fresh orange zest, grated finely • ¼ cup chicken broth • 2/3 cup fresh orange juice • 1 roasted duck, meat picked • 3 pound bokchoy leaves • 1 orange, peeled, seeded and segmented

Directions:

1. In a sizable skillet, melt coconut oil on medium heat. 2. Add onion, ginger and garlic and sauté for around 3 minutes. 3. Add ginger and garlic and sauté for about 1-2 minutes. 4. Stir in orange zest, broth and orange juice. 5. Add duck meat and cook for around 3 minutes. 6. Transfer the meat pieces in a plate. 7. Add bokchoy and cook for about 3-4 minutes. 8. Divide bokchoy mixture in serving plates and top with duck meat. 9. Serve with the garnishing of orange segments.

SIDE DISHES

661. Braised Onion & Cabbage

Yield: 4 servings Preparation Time: 15 minutes Cooking Time: 25 minutes

Ingredients:

1½ teaspoons coconut oil • 2 ½ cups green cabbage, chopped • 1 garlic cloves, chopped • 1 onion, sliced thinly • 1 cup homemade bone broth • Salt, to taste

Directions:

1. In a substantial nonstick skillet, heat oil on high heat. 2. Add cabbage, garlic and onion and sauté approximately 5 minutes. 3. Gradually, stir in water and immediately, lessen the heat to low. 4. Stir in salt and cover the skillet. Cook approximately twenty or so minutes. 5. Serve warm.

662. Lemony Brussels Sprouts

Yield: 4 servings Preparation Time: 10 min Cooking Time: fifteen minutes

Ingredients:

12-ounces Brussels sprouts, trimmed and halved • ½ cup water • Salt and freshly ground black pepper, to taste • 2 tablespoons extra virgin olive oil • 1 tablespoon fresh lemon juice

Directions:

1. In a large skillet, mix together Brussels sprouts, water, salt and black pepper on medium heat. 2. Bring to some gentle boil. Cover and cook approximately 5-8 minutes, stirring occasionally. 3. Stir in oil and improve the heat to medium-high. 4. Cover and cook for approximately 5-7 minutes. 5. Stir in freshly squeezed lemon juice and immediately, remove from heat. Serve warm.

663. Curried Carrot & Leeks

Yield: 3-4 servings Preparation Time: 15 minutes Cooking Time: 26 minutes

Ingredients:

1 tablespoon coconut oil • 2 leeks, halved and sliced • 3 celery ribs, sliced • 3 carrots, peeled and sliced • Salt, to taste • 1 teaspoon curry powder

Directions: 1. In a greater skillet, heat oil on medium heat. 2. Add leeks and cook for approximately 2-4 minutes or till just set out to soft. 3. Stir in celery and carrots and cook for about 5-7 minutes. 4. Stir in salt and curry powder and reduce the heat to low. 5. Cover and cook for about 10-fifteen minutes. 6. Serve warm.

664. Pumpkin & Egg

Yield: 4 servings Preparation Time: 15 minutes Cooking Time: 10 minutes

Ingredients:

8-ounce homemade pumpkin puree • 5 large organic eggs • 1½ cups tapioca flour • ½ teaspoon salt • 2 tablespoons coconut oil

Directions: 1. In a sizable bowl, add all ingredients except oil and mix till well combined. 2. In a frying pan. Heat ½ tablespoon of oil on medium-low heat. 3. Add desired amount of mixture inside pan. Tilt the pan that mixture spreads in the thin consis10cy. 4. Cook approximately 5 minutes. With a flat and big spatula, turn the medial side and cook for 3-5 minutes. 5. Repeat with all the remaining mixture.

665. Kale With Cranberry

Yield: 3-4 servings Preparation Time: 15 minutes Cooking Time: 10 min

Ingredients:

1 tablespoon extra-virgin extra virgin olive oil • 1 small garlic cloves, chopped • 1 large shallot, sliced thinly • 1 teaspoon fresh orange zest, grated finely • 12-16 fresh kale leaves, trimmed and torn • 2 tablespoons water • 2 tablespoons dried cranberries • ½ tablespoon white wine vinegar • 2 tablespoons fresh orange juice • Salt and freshly ground black pepper, to taste • 2 tablespoons pumpkin seeds, toasted

Directions:

1. In a large skillet, heat oil on medium heat. 2. Add garlic and shallots and sauté for approximately 2 minutes. 3. Add orange zest, kale and water and cook for about 2-3 minutes. 4. Stir in cranberries, vinegar and orange juice. 5. Cover and cook approximately 1-2 minutes. 6. Uncover the skillet and cook for 1-2 minute or till all the liquid is absorbed. 7. Remove from heat and stir in salt and black pepper. 8. Serve while using topping of pumpkin seeds.

666. Sweet & Sour Salsa

Yield: 2 servings Preparation Time: fifteen minutes

Ingredients:

1 cup fresh pineapple, chopped • 1 cup fresh mango, chopped • ½ cup avocado, peeled, pitted and chopped • ¼ cup red onion, chopped • ¼ cup red bell pepper, seeded and chopped • 1 jalapeño pepper, seeded and chopped finely • 2-3 tablespoons fresh cilantro leaves, chopped • ¼ cup fresh lime juice

Directions:

1. In a big bowl, add all ingredients and gently, toss to coat well. 2. Serve immediately.

667. Sautéed Garlic Broccolini

Yield: 2 servings Preparation Time: 10 minutes Cooking Time: 8 minutes

Ingredients:

2 tablespoons extra virgin olive oil • ½ pound broccolini • 3 garlic cloves, minced • 1 tablespoon garlic powder • 1 tablespoon fresh lemon juice

Directions:

1. In a substantial skillet, heat oil on medium heat. 2. Add broccolini and sauté for approximately 5 minutes. 3. Stir in garlic, garlic powder and lemon juice and cook for about 2-3 minutes. 4. Serve warm.

668. Gingered Broccoli

Yield: 4 servings Preparation Time: fifteen minutes Cooking Time: 6 minutes

Ingredients:

1 tbsp. olive oil • 4 teaspoons fresh ginger, minced • 2 tablespoons garlic, minced • 6 cups broccoli, chopped • 1 tablespoon fish sauce • 3 tablespoons water • 1 tablespoon apple cider vinegar

Directions:

In a substantial nonstick skillet, heat oil on medium-high heat. 2. Add ginger and garlic and sauté for approximately 1 minute. 3. Add broccoli and stir fry for around 2 minutes. 4. Stir in fish sauce and water and lower the heat to medium. 5. Cook, covered for approximately 3 minutes. 6. Stir in vinegar and take off from heat

669. Broccoli with Coconut

Yield: 4 servings Preparation Time: 15 minutes Cooking Time: 11 minutes

Ingredients:

2 teaspoons coconut oil • ½ teaspoon mustard seeds • 1 medium onion, chopped • 2 green chilies, halved • 3 garlic cloves, crushed • 2-3 curry leaves • 1 head broccoli, cut into florets • ¼ teaspoon ground turmeric • Salt, to taste • 3 tablespoon water • ½ cup coconut, grated

Directions:

1. In a skillet, melt coconut oil on medium heat. 2. Add mustard seeds and sauté for around 1 minute. 3. Add onion, green chilies, garlic and curry leaves and sauté approximately 5 minutes. 4. Add broccoli, turmeric, salt and water and stir to combine. 5. Cook, covered for around 5 minutes. 6. Stir in coconut and serve hot.

670. Gingered Asparagus

Yield: 2-4 servings Preparation Time: 15 minutes Cooking Time: 6 minutes

Ingredients:

2 tablespoons essential olive oil • 1 teaspoon cumin seeds • 1 bunch as asparagus, trimmed and cut into 2-inch pieces diagonally • 1 tablespoon fresh ginger, minced • 2 teaspoons fresh lemon juice • Salt and freshly ground black pepper, to taste

Directions:

1. In a skillet, heat oil on medium heat. 2. Add cumin seeds and sauté for approximately 1 minute. 3. Add remaining ingredients and stir fry for around 4-5 minutes. 4. Serve warm.

671. Spiced Cauliflower

Yield: 4-6 servings Preparation Time: fifteen minutes Cooking Time: 32 minutes

Ingredients:

1 tbsp organic olive oil • ½ of medium onion, sliced thinly • Salt, to taste • 1 dried red chili • 1 teaspoon cumin seeds • 1 teaspoon ground turmeric • 1 head cauliflower, cut into florets • ¼-½ cup vegetable broth • Freshly ground black pepper, to taste

Directions:

1. In a skillet, heat oil on medium-high heat. 2. Add onion and pinch of salt and sauté for around 10 min, 3. Add red chili, cumin seeds and turmeric and sauté for around 2 minutes. 4. Stir in cauliflower after which add broth. 5. Reduce heat to medium and simmer, covered for approximately 20 min. 6. Stir in salt and black pepper and take away from heat. 7. Serve warm.

672. Roasted Cauliflower

Yield: 2-3 servings Preparation Time: fifteen minutes Cooking Time: an hour 15 minutes

Ingredients:

½ of large cauliflower head, cut into florets • 2 tablespoons essential olive oil • 2 teaspoons ground turmeric • Salt, to taste

Directions:

Preheat the oven to 350 degrees F. 2. In a sizable bowl, mix together all ingredients and toss to coat well. 3. Transfer the mix in to a rimmed baking dish. 4. With a foil paper, cover the baking dish and roast for approximately 75 minutes.

673. Roasted Butternut Squash

Yield: 6 servings Preparation Time: quarter-hour Cooking Time: 37 minutes

Ingredients:

3 pounds butternut squash, seeded, peeled and cubed into 1" size • 2 teaspoons smoked paprika • ½ teaspoon garlic powder • ½ teaspoon ground turmeric • Salt, to taste • 2 tablespoons extra-virgin essential olive oil

Directions:

1. Preheat the oven to 375 degrees F. 2. In a substantial bowl, add all ingredients and toss to coat well. 3. Transfer a combination right into a rimmed baking sheet within an even layer. 4. Roast approximately 32-37 minutes, flipping once within the middle way

674. Enoki Mushroom & Spinach

Yield: 2 servings Preparation Time: quarter-hour Cooking Time: 7 minutes

Ingredients:

1 tbsp essential olive oil • ½ tablespoon fresh ginger, grated • 2 bunches enoki mushrooms, trimmed and cleaned • Salt, to taste • ½ bunch fresh spinach chopped • 2 stalks scallions, chopped • 1 tablespoon coconut aminos • Freshly ground black pepper, to taste

Directions:

1. In a nonstick skillet, heat oil on medium-high heat. 2. Add ginger and sauté for around 1 minute. 3. Add mushrooms and salt and sauté approximately 2 minutes. 4. Add spinach and cook for about 2-3 minutes. 5. Stir in scallion, coconut aminos and black pepper and cook for approximately 1 minute. 6. Serve warm.

675. Garlicky Kale

Yield: 2-3 servings Preparation Time: quarter-hour Cooking Time: fifteen minutes

Ingredients:

2 tbsps. extra-virgin extra virgin olive oil • 2 garlic cloves, sliced thinly • 1 bag fresh kale, trimmed and chopped • 1 tablespoon ground turmeric

Directions:

1. In a skillet, heat oil on medium-high heat. 2. Add garlic and sauté for about 1 minute. 3. Add kale and stir fry for around 5-10 minutes or till just wilted. 4. Stir in turmeric and stir fry for approximately 3-4 minutes or till desired doneness of kale.

676. Garlicky Bok Choy

Yield: 2 servings Preparation Time: fifteen minutes Cooking Time: 6 minutes

Ingredients:

1 tablespoon coconut oil • 5 Bok Choy bunches, trimmed and cut into 1-inch chunks • 1 teaspoon fresh ginger, grated finely • 2 minced garlic cloves • Salt, to taste

Directions:

In a skillet, melt coconut oil on medium heat. 2. Add Bok Choy and stir fry approximately 3-4 minutes. 3. Add ginger, garlic and salt and stir fry for approximately 2 minutes more. 4. Serve warm.

677. Citrus Carrot

Yield: 4 servings Preparation Time: fifteen minutes Cooking Time: 5 minutes

Ingredients:

2 teaspoons extra virgin olive oil • 2 teaspoons fresh ginger, minced • 3 cups carrots, peeled and grated • ½ cup fresh orange juice • Salt and freshly ground black pepper, to taste

Directions:

1. In a large nonstick skillet, heat oil on medium-high heat. 2. Add ginger and carrot and cook, stirring occasionally for approximately 2 minutes. 3. Reduce heat and stir in orange juice, salt and black pepper. 4. Simmer for approximately 1-2 minutes or till desired doneness of carrots.

678. Roasted Spicy Baby Carrot

Yield: 2-4 servings Preparation Time: 15 minutes Cooking Time: 20 minutes

Ingredients:

1 pound baby carrots, trimmed • 1 teaspoon fresh lime zest, grated finely • ½ teaspoon ground cumin • ¼ teaspoon smoked paprika • ¼ teaspoon ground coriander • Salt, to taste • 1 teaspoon organic honey • 2 tablespoons fresh lime juice • 1 tbsp organic olive oil • 2 scallion, sliced thinly • 2 tablespoons fresh mint leaves, chopped

Directions:

1. Preheat the oven to 400 degrees F. 2. In a baking dish, arrange the carrots. 3. In a bowl, mix together remaining ingredients except scallion and mint. 4. Place the honey mixture over carrots evenly. 5. Roast for approximately 20 min. 6. Serve with the garnishing of scallion and mint.

679. Spicy Cabbage

Yield: 2-4 servings Preparation Time: quarter-hour Cooking Time: 13 minutes

Ingredients:

1 teaspoon extra-virgin extra virgin olive oil • 1 onion, sliced thinly • 2 teaspoons curry powder • 1 teaspoon ground cumin • 1 teaspoon ground turmeric • 8 cups cabbage, sliced thinly • Salt and freshly ground black pepper, to taste • 2 tablespoons fresh lemon juice • ¼ cup water

Directions:

1. In a skillet, heat oil on medium heat. 2. Add onion and sauté for approximately 4-5 minutes. 3. Add curry powder and spices and sauté for about 1 minute. 4. Add cabbage and cook approximately 2-3 minutes. 5. Stir in water and cook, covered for around 4-5 minutes or till desired doneness.

680. Roasted Sweet Potato

Yield: 2-3 servings Preparation Time: 15 minutes Cooking Time: twenty minutes

Ingredients:

1 teaspoon coconut oil • 1 onion, chopped • 2 medium sweet potatoes, peeled and cubed • ½ tablespoon ground turmeric • 1-2 fresh parsley sprigs • Salt and freshly ground black pepper, to taste • Water, as required

Directions:

In a skillet, melt coconut oil on low heat. 2. Add onion and sauté approximately 810 minutes. 3. Stir in sweet potato turmeric, parsley, salt and black pepper. 4. Add enough water that covers the sweet potato midway. 5. Cook for around 68 minutes or till desired doneness.

681. Roasted Summer Squash & Fennel Bulb

Yield: 4 servings Preparation Time: quarter-hour Cooking Time: fifteen minutes

Ingredients:

2 small summer squash, cubed into 1-inch size • 1½ cups fennel bulb, sliced • 1 tablespoon fresh thyme, chopped • 1 tablespoon extra-virgin organic olive oil • Salt and freshly ground black pepper, to taste • ¼ cup garlic, sliced thinly • 1 tablespoon fennel fronds, chopped

Directions:

1. Preheat the oven to 450 degrees F. 2. In a substantial bowl, add all ingredients except garlic and fennel fronds and toss to coat well. 3. Transfer a combination right into a large rimmed baking sheet. 4. Roast for approximately 10 min. 5. Remove from oven and stir in sliced garlic. 6. Roast for 5 minutes more. 7. Remove from oven and stir inside the fennel fronds. 8. Serve immediately

682. Potato Mash

Yield: 32 servings Preparation Time: fifteen minutes Cooking Time: 20 minutes

Ingredients:

10 large baking potatoes, peeled and cubed • 3 tablespoons organic olive oil, divided • 1 onion, chopped • 1 tablespoon ground turmeric • ½ teaspoon ground cumin • Salt and freshly ground black pepper, to taste

Directions:

1. In a large pan of water, add potatoes and produce with a boil on medium-high heat. 2. Cook approximately twenty or so minutes. 3. Drain well and transfer in to a large bowl. 4. With a potato masher, mash the potatoes. 5. Meanwhile in a very skillet, heat 1 tablespoon of oil on medium-high heat. 6. Add onion and sauté for about 6 minutes. 7. Add onion mixture in the bowl with mashed potatoes. 8. Add turmeric, cumin, salt and black pepper and mash till well combined. 9. Stir in remaining oil and serve.

683. Gingered Cauliflower Rice

Yield: 3-4 servings Preparation Time: quarter-hour Cooking Time: 10 minutes

Ingredients:

3 tablespoons coconut oil • 4 (1/8-inch thick) fresh ginger slices • 1 small head cauliflower, trimmed and processed into rice consis10cy • 3 garlic cloves, crushed • 1 tablespoon chives, chopped • 1 tablespoon coconut vinegar • Salt, to taste

Directions:

1. In a skillet, melt coconut oil on medium-high heat. 2. Add ginger and sauté for about 2-3 minutes. 3. Discard the ginger slices and stir in cauliflower and garlic. 4. Cook, stirring occasionally approximately 7-8 minutes. 5. Stir in remaining ingredients and take off from heat. 6. Serve immediately

684. Simple Brown Rice

Yield: 4 servings Preparation Time: 10 min Cooking Time: 50 minutes

Ingredients:

1 cup brown rice • 2 cups chicken broth • 1 tablespoon ground turmeric • 1 tbsp extra virgin olive oil

Directions:

In a pan, add rice, broth and turmeric and provide with a boil. 2. Reduce the warmth to low. 3. Simmer, covered for about 50 minutes. 4. Add the organic olive oil and fluff using a fork. 5. Keep aside, covered approximately 10 minutes before serving.

685. Quinoa With Apricots

Yield: 4 servings Preparation Time: 15 minutes Cooking Time: 12 minutes

Ingredients:

2 cups water • 1 cup quinoa • ½ teaspoon fresh ginger, grated finely • ½ cup dried apricots, chopped roughly • Salt and freshly ground black pepper, to taste

Directions:

1. In a pan, add water on high heat and bring to your boil. 2. Add quinoa and reduce the heat to medium. 3. Cover and reduce the heat to low. 4. Simmer for about 12 minutes. 5. Remove from heat and immediately, stir in ginger and apricots. 6. Keep aside, covered for approximately fifteen minutes before serving.

686. Sautéed Spinach & Tomatoes

Yield: 2 servings Preparation Time: fifteen minutes Cooking Time: 10 minutes

Ingredients:

1 tablespoon coconut oil • ½ of medium onion, chopped • 2 medium tomatoes, chopped • ½ cup fresh basil, chopped • 4 cups fresh spinach, chopped

Directions:

1. In a skillet, heat oil on medium-high heat. 2. Add onion and sauté for about 5 minutes. 3. Add tomatoes and cook for approximately 1-2 minutes. 4. Stir in basil and spinach and cook for around 2-3 minutes. 5. Serve warm.

687. Steamed Simple Asparagus

Yield: 4 servings Preparation Time: 10 min Cooking Time: 6-8 minutes

Ingredients:

1 bunch fresh asparagus, trimmed, peeled and cut into desired size • Salt and freshly ground black pepper, to taste

Directions: 1. Arrange a steamer basket in a substantial pan of boiling water. 2. Place the asparagus in steamer basket. 3. Cover and steam for about 6-8 minutes or till crisp 10der. 4. Remove from steamer basket and transfer into a serving plate. 5. Sprinkle with salt and black pepper and serve.

688. Stir Fried Eggplant

Yield: 2-3 servings Preparation Time: 10 minutes Cooking Time: 2-3 minutes

Ingredients:

3-4 tablespoons lard • 1 large eggplant, sliced

Directions: 1. In a greater skillet, heat lard on medium heat. 2. Add eggplant and stir fry for approximately 2-3 minutes or till desired doneness.

689. Garlicky Cauliflower Mash

Yield: 2 servings Preparation Time: quarter-hour Cooking Time: 26 minutes

Ingredients:

1 head cauliflower, chopped finely • 2-3 garlic cloves, chopped • ¼ cup grass-fed salted butter • Salt, to taste

Directions: 1. Arrange a steamer basket in a sizable pan of boiling water. 2. Place the chopped cauliflower in steamer basket. 3. Cover and steam for around 15-20 min or till 10der. 4. Remove from steamer basket and transfer in a bowl and allow it to go cool slightly. 5. Now, squeeze cauliflower in a blender and pulse till chopped very finely. 6. Add remaining ingredients and pulse till smooth. 7. Transfer into a serving bowl and serve.

690. Pesto Coated Carrot Sticks

Yield: 6 servings Preparation Time: 15 minutes Cooking Time: 25 minutes

Ingredients:

12 large carrots, peeled and cut into 2-inch long sticks • ¼ cup plus 1 tablespoon olive oil • ½ of jalapeño pepper, chopped roughly • 1 cup fresh cilantro, chopped • 1 tablespoon fresh lime juice • 2 garlic cloves, chopped • 1 teaspoon ground cumin • Pinch of salt and black pepper

Directions:

1. Preheat the oven to 400 degrees F. Lightly, grease a big baking sheet. 2. Place carrot sticks into prepared baking sheet inside a single layer. 3. Drizzle with 1 tablespoon of oil. Roast approximately twenty or so minutes. 4. Meanwhile in a blender, add remaining all ingredients except ¼ cup of oil and pulse till smooth. 5. While motor is running, gradually, add remaining oil and pulse till smooth. 6. Remove the carrots from oven and toss with pesto. 7. Roast for 5 minutes more.

691. Zucchini With Mint

Yield: 2 servings Preparation Time: 10 min Cooking Time: 7 minutes

Ingredients:

1 tablespoon extra-virgin essential olive oil • 2 large zucchinis, sliced thickly • 1 tablespoon freshly squeezed lemon juice • 1 garlic clove, minced • Salt and freshly ground black pepper, to taste • 4 fresh mint leaves, minced

Directions:

1. In a sizable skillet, heat oil on medium-high heat. 2. Add zucchini and stir fry for about 2-3 minutes 3. Add freshly squeezed lemon juice, garlic, salt and black pepper and stir fry approximately 2 minutes. 4. Stir in mint and cook approximately 1-2 minutes. 5. Serve hot.

692. Fried Avocado Slices

Yield: 2 servings Preparation Time: 10 min Cooking Time: 5 minutes

Ingredients:

1 tablespoon coconut oil • 1 ripe avocado, peeled, pitted and sliced • 1 tablespoon freshly squeezed lemon juice • Sat, to taste

Directions:

1. In a sizable skillet, heat oil on medium-high heat. 2. Add avocado slices and stir fry for around 3-5 minutes or till golden brown coming from all sides. 3. Stir in lemon juice and salt and remove from heat. 4. Serve warm.

693. Stir Fried Cauliflower Rice

Yield: 2-3 servings Preparation Time: 10 minutes Cooking Time: 10 minutes

Ingredients:

1 tablespoon coconut oil • ½ of Vidalia onion, chopped • 3 garlic cloves, minced • 1 head cauliflower, stemmed and grated as being a rice consis10cy • Salt and freshly ground black pepper, to taste

Directions:

In a large skillet, heat oil on medium heat. 2. Add onion and garlic and sauté approximately 5 minutes. 3. Add cauliflower, salt and black pepper and cook approximately 3-5 minutes. 4. Serve warm.

694. Spiced Broccoli

Yield: 2 servings Preparation Time: 15 minutes Cooking Time: 11 minutes

Ingredients:

8-ounce broccoli, chopped • 1 tablespoon coconut oil • 1 teaspoon mustard seeds • 1 onion, chopped • 2 tomatoes, chopped • 1 teaspoon garam masala • 1 teaspoon ground turmeric • ½ teaspoon ground coriander • 1 tablespoon coconut, shredded • 2 tablespoons coconut milk • 1 tablespoon fresh lemon juice • ¼ cup water

Directions:

1. In a pan of boiling water, arrange a steamer basket. 2. Place the broccoli in steamer basket and steam, covered for around 5 minutes. 3. Drain well. 4. In a skillet, melt coconut oil on medium heat. 5. Add mustard seeds and sauté approximately 1 minute. 6. Add onion and sauté for approximately 5 minutes. 7. Add remaining ingredients and bring to a gentle simmer. 8. Stir in broccoli and simmer for about 5 minutes.

695. Broccoli with Asparagus

Yield: 4 servings Preparation Time: fifteen minutes Cooking Time: 8 minutes

Ingredients:

½ tablespoon fresh ginger paste • ½ tablespoon garlic paste • ½ teaspoon garam masala • Salt and freshly ground black pepper, to taste • 2 tablespoons extra virgin olive oil, divided • 1 pound asparagus, trimmed and cut into 1-inch pieces • ½ cup broccoli florets • 2 tablespoons fresh lemon juice

Directions:

1. In a bowl, mix together, ginger, garlic paste, garam masala, salt, black pepper and 1 teaspoon oil. 2. Add asparagus and broccoli and toss to coat well. 3. In a sizable skillet, heat remaining oil on medium heat. 4. Add onion and sauté for around 2 minutes. 5. Add asparagus mixture and stir fry for around 5 minutes. 6. Stir in freshly squeezed lemon juice and take off from heat.

696. Spiced Brussels Sprout

Yield: 4 servings Preparation Time: quarter-hour Cooking Time: 12 minutes

Ingredients:

2 tablespoons extra virgin olive oil • 1 tablespoon fresh ginger, minced • 1 tablespoon garlic, minced • 1 tablespoon dried fenugreek leaves • 1 tablespoon cumin seeds • 1 teaspoon smoked paprika • Salt and freshly ground black pepper, to taste • 1 pound Brussels sprouts, trimmed and halved • ½ cup water

Directions:

1. In a skillet, heat oil on medium heat. 2. Add ginger and garlic and sauté for about 2 minutes. 3. Add fenugreek leaves, cumin seeds, paprika, salt and black pepper and sauté for around 2 minutes. 4. Add Brussels sprouts and water and stir to blend. 5. Cook, covered approximately 6-8 minutes.

697. Cauliflower with Capers

Yield: 2 servings Preparation Time: fifteen minutes Cooking Time: 12 minutes

Ingredients:

½ cup water • 2 cups cauliflower, cut into 1-inch florets • Salt, to taste • ¼ cup coconut oil • 1 (½-inch) fresh turmeric root, sliced thinly • 5-7 fresh thyme stalks • 2 tablespoon capers • Chopped fresh thyme leaves, for garnishing

Directions: 1. In a pan, add water, cauliflower and salt and provide with a boil on medium heat. 2. Cover and cook for approximately 10-12 minutes. 3. Drain well and transfer right into a serving platter. 4. Meanwhile in a small skillet, melt the coconut oil on medium-low heat. 5. Add ginger and thyme stalks and swirl the pan occasionally for around 2-3 minutes. 6. Discard the turmeric and thyme stalks. 7. Pour the oil over cauliflower and top while using capers and thyme.

698. Roasted Spicy Cauliflower

Yield: 8 servings Preparation Time: fifteen minutes Cooking Time: 60 minutes

Ingredients:

2 teaspoons ground turmeric • 1 tablespoon ground cumin • 2 teaspoons red pepper flakes, crushed • Salt, to taste • 1 cup olive oil • 4 heads cauliflower, cut into 1-inch florets • 2 tablespoons fresh mint leaves, chopped • 1 tablespoon fresh cilantro, chopped • ¼ cup pine nuts, toasted and chopped

Directions:

1. Preheat the oven to 425 degrees F. 2. In a big bowl, mix together turmeric, cumin, red pepper flakes, salt and oil. 3. Add cauliflower and toss to coat well. 4. Transfer a combination into 2 rimmed baking sheets in the even layer. 5. Roast for about 60 minutes, flipping once inside the middle way. 6. Top with mint, cilantro and pine nuts and serve

699. Spicy Button Mushrooms

Yield: 2 servings Preparation Time: quarter-hour Cooking Time: 7 minutes

Ingredients:

2 tablespoons olive oil • ½ teaspoon cumin seeds, crushed lightly • 2 medium onions, sliced thinly • ½ pound white button mushrooms, chopped • 1 green chili, chopped • 1 teaspoon ground coriander • ½ teaspoon garam masala • ½ teaspoon red chili powder • 1/8 teaspoon ground turmeric • Salt, to taste • 2 tablespoons fresh cilantro leaves, chopped

Directions:

1. In a skillet, heat oil on medium heat. 2. Add cumin seeds and sauté for about 1 minute. 3. Add onion and sauté for around 4-5 minutes. 4. Add mushrooms and sauté approximately 5-7minutes. 5. Add green chili and spices and sauté for around 1-2 minutes. 6. Stir in cilantro and sauté for approximately 1 minute more.

700. Spicy Spinach

Yield: 4 servings Preparation Time: 10 min Cooking Time: 21 minutes

Ingredients:

1 tablespoon coconut oil • 1 red onion, chopped finely • 6 garlic cloves, minced • 1 (1-inch) piece fresh ginger, minced • 1 teaspoon garam masala • 1 teaspoon ground coriander • ½ teaspoon ground cumin • ¼ teaspoon ground turmeric • 6 cups fresh spinach, chopped • Salt and freshly ground black pepper, to taste • 1-2 tablespoons water

Directions: 1. In a substantial skillet, melt coconut oil on medium heat. 2. Add onion and sauté for about 8 minutes. 3. Add garlic, ginger and spices and sauté for approximately 1 minute. 4. Add spinach, salt and black pepper and cook, stirring occasionally for around 2 minutes. 5. Add water and cook for approximately 3 minutes. 6. Cook, covered for approximately fifteen minutes. 7. Uncover and stir fry for about 2 minutes. 8. Serve warm.

701. Spinach with Kale

Yield: 2 servings Preparation Time: 15 minutes Cooking Time: 22 minutes

Ingredients:

3 tablespoons extra-virgin olive oil, divided • 8 garlic cloves, minced • ½ of red onion, chopped finely • 1 bunch fresh kale, trimmed and chopped • Water, as required • 1 bag fresh baby spinach • Salt and freshly ground black pepper, to taste

Directions: 1. In a big nonstick skillet, heat 2 tablespoons of oil on medium heat. 2. Add garlic and sauté for approximately 1 minute. 3. Reduce the heat to medium-lo. 4. Add onion and a pinch of salt sauté for about 4-5 minutes. 5. Stir fry kale along with a few teaspoons of water and improve the heat to medium. 6. Cook, covered for approximately 2-3 minutes. 7. Stir in spinach and 1-2 teaspoons of water. 8. Cook, covered approximately 5-8 minutes. 9. Stir in remaining oil and improve the heat to medium-high. 10. Stir fry for about 3-4 minutes. 11. Stir in sat and black pepper and take away from heat. 12. Serve warm.

702. Turmeric Potato

Yield: 1 serving Preparation Time: fifteen minutes Cooking Time: 10 min

Ingredients:

2 tablespoons olive oil • 1 medium potato, scrubbed and sliced thinly • 1 garlic oil, minced • ½ teaspoon ground turmeric • 1 small onion, sliced thinly

Directions:

1. In a frying pan, heat oil on medium heat. 2. Add potato slices, garlic and turmeric and cook for about 10 min. 3. Add onion and cook, stirring occasionally for about 4 minutes.

703. Roasted Honey Carrot

Yield: 4 servings Preparation Time: fifteen minutes Cooking Time: 40 minutes

Ingredients:

1 pound carrots, peeled and halved lengthwise • 1 (1-inch) piece fresh ginger, grated • ¼ cup honey • ¼ cup essential olive oil • 3 tablespoons coconut aminos • Salt, to taste • 1 tablespoon sesame seeds

Directions:

1. Preheat the oven to 400 degrees F. 2. In a baking dish, arrange the carrot halves. 3. In a bowl, mix together remaining ingredients except sesame seeds. 4. Place the honey mixture over carrots evenly. 5. Roast for about 30-40 minutes. 6. Serve with all the sprinkling of sesame seeds.

704. Sweet & Citrus Glazed Carrot

Yield: 4 servings Preparation Time: quarter-hour Cooking Time: 8 minutes

Ingredients:

1 cup water • 1 pound carrots, peeled and cut into ½-inch slices • Salt, to taste • 1 tablespoon coconut oil • 2 teaspoons fresh orange zest, grated finely • 2 tablespoons organic honey • 2 tablespoons fresh orange juice • ½ teaspoon ground ginger • Freshly ground black pepper, to taste

Directions:

1. In a pan, add water, carrots as well as a pinch of salt and provide with a boil on high heat. 2. Reduce the temperature to medium and simmer approximately 5 minutes. 3. Drain the river well. 4. In the same pan, add remaining ingredients with carrot on medium heat. 5. Sauté for about 2-3 minutes or till glaze becomes slightly thick.

705. Cabbage with Apple

Yield: 2-4 servings Preparation Time: 15 minutes Cooking Time: 9 minutes

Ingredients:

2 teaspoons coconut oil • 1 large apple, cored and sliced thinly • 1 onion, sliced thinly • 1½ pound cabbage, chopped finely • 1 tablespoon fresh thyme, chopped • 1 red chili, chopped • 1 tablespoon using apple cider vinegar • 2/3 cup almonds, chopped

Directions:

In a nonstick skillet, melt 1 teaspoon of coconut oil on medium heat. 2. Add apple and stir fry for around 2-3 minutes. 3. Transfer the apple right into a bowl. 4. In a similar skillet, melt 1 teaspoon of coconut oil on medium heat. 5. Add onion and sauté for about 1-2 minutes. 6. Add cabbage and stir fry for about 3 minutes. 7. Add apple, thyme and vinegar and cook, covered for approximately 1 minute. 8. Serve warm with all the garnishing of almonds.

706. Beetroot with Coconut

Yield: 2 servings Preparation Time: fifteen minutes Cooking Time: twenty minutes

Ingredients:

4 beetroots, peeled and cubed • 1 small onion, cubed • ¼ cup extra virgin olive oil • 1 small cinnamon stick • 2 whole cardamoms • 2 whole cloves • 1 teaspoon garlic paste • 1 teaspoon ginger paste • Pinch of ground turmeric • 1 tablespoon red chili powder • Salt, to taste • 2-3 tablespoons fresh coconut powder • 1 tablespoon garam masala powder

Directions:

1. In a mixer grinder, add beetroot and onion and grind till chopped very finely. (Mixture needs to be just a little chunky). Keep aside. 2. In a skillet, heat oil on medium heat. 3. Add cinnamon stick, cardamoms and cloves and sauté for about 1 minute. 4. Add garlic paste, ginger paste, turmeric, chili powder and salt and sauté approximately 1 minute. 5. Add beetroot mixture and stir fry for about fifteen minutes. 6. Add coconut powder and garam masala powder and cook for about 2-3 minutes. 7. Serve hot.

707. Roasted Brussels Sprouts & Sweet Potato

Yield: 6-8 servings Preparation Time: 15 minutes Cooking Time: 45 minutes

Ingredients:

1 large sweet potato, peeled and cut into 1-2-nch pieces • 1 pound Brussels sprouts, trimmed and halved • 2 minced garlic cloves • 1 teaspoon ground cumin • ½ teaspoon garlic salt • Salt and freshly ground black pepper, to taste • 1/3 cup olive oil • 1 tablespoon apple cider vinegar • Chopped fresh thyme, for garnishing

Directions:

1. Preheat the oven to 400 degrees F. Grease a sheet pan. 2. In a large bowl, add all ingredients except vinegar and thyme and toss to coat well. 3. Transfer the mix into prepared baking pan. 4. Roast for 40-45 minutes more. 5. Transfer the vegetable mixture in a serving plate and drizzle with vinegar. 6. Garnish with thyme and serve.

708. Creamy Sweet Potato Mash

Yield: 4 servings Preparation Time: fifteen minutes Cooking Time: 21 minutes

Ingredients:

1 tbsp extra virgin olive oil • 2 large sweet potatoes, peeled and chopped • 2 teaspoons ground turmeric • 1 garlic herb, minced • 2 cups vegetable broth • 2 tablespoons unswee10ed coconut milk • Salt and freshly ground black pepper, to taste • Chopped pistachios, for garnishing

Directions:

In a big skillet, heat oil on medium-high heat. 2. Add sweet potato and stir fry for bout 2-3 minutes. 3. Add turmeric and stir fry for approximately 1 minute. 4. Add garlic and stir fry approximately 2 minutes. 5. Add broth and provide to a boil. 6. Reduce the heat to low and cook for approximately 10-15 minutes or till every one of the liquid is absorbed. 7. Transfer the sweet potato mixture in to a bowl. 8. Add coconut milk, salt and black pepper and mash it completely. 9. Garnish with pistachio and serve.

709. Spicy Cauliflower Rice

Yield: 4 servings Preparation Time: 15 minutes Cooking Time: 10 min

Ingredients:

3 tablespoons coconut oil • 1 small white onion, chopped • 3 garlic cloves, minced • 1 large head cauliflower, trimmed and processed into rice consis10cy • ½ teaspoon ground cumin • ½ teaspoon paprika • Salt and freshly ground black pepper, to taste • 1large tomato, chopped • ¼ cup tomato paste • ¼ cup fresh cilantro, chopped • Chopped fresh cilantro, for garnishing • 2 limes, quarters

Directions:

1. In a sizable skillet, melt coconut oil on medium-high heat. 2. Add onion and sauté for approximately 2 minutes. 3. Add garlic and sauté approximately 1 minute. 4. Stir in cauliflower rice. 5. Add cumin, paprika, salt and black pepper and cook, stirring occasionally approximately 2-3 minutes. 6. Stir in tomato, tomato paste and cilantro and cook approximately 2-3 minutes. 7. Garnish with cilantro and serve alongside lime.

710. Spicy Quinoa

Yield: 4 servings Preparation Time: 10 minutes Cooking Time: 25 minutes

Ingredients:

2 tablespoons extra-virgin essential olive oil • 1 teaspoon curry powder • 1 teaspoon ground turmeric • 12 teaspoon ground cumin • 1 cup quinoa, rinsed and drained • 2 cups chicken broth • ¾ cup almonds, toasted • ½ cup raisins • ¾ cup fresh parsley, chopped

Directions:

1. In a medium pan, heat oil on medium-low heat. 2. Add curry powder, turmeric and cumin and sauté for approximately 1-2 minutes. 3. Add quinoa and sauté approximately 2-3 minutes. 4. Add broth and stir to blend. 5. Cover reducing the warmth to low. 6. Simmer for around twenty minutes. 7. Remove from heat whilst aside, covered approximately 5 minutes. 8. Just before serving, add almonds and raisins and toss to coat. 9. Drizzle with lemon juice and serve.

SALAD VEGETARIAN And SNACK

711. Roasted Veggies

Yield: 12 servings Preparation Time: 25 minutes Cooking Time: 55 minutes

Ingredients:

1½ cups pecans • 1 small butternut squash, peeled, seeded and cut into ¼-thick slices • 1 medium head cauliflower, cut into florets • 1 pound Brussels sprouts, trimmed and halved • 2 large parsnips, peeled and cut into ¼-thick slices • 4 medium carrots, peeled and cut into ¼-thick slices • ¼ teaspoon nutmeg, grated freshly • Salt and freshly ground black pepper, to taste • ½ cup extra-virgin organic olive oil • 2 tablespoons fresh ginger, minced • 1/3 cup raw honey

Directions:

1. Preheat the oven to 425 degrees F. 2. In a pie plate, put the pecans. 3. Roast approximately 6 minutes or till toasted. 4. Remove from heat and keep aside to cool down the. 5. In a big bowl, add all vegetables, nutmeg, salt, black pepper and oil and toss to coat well. 6. In 2 large rimmed baking sheets, spread the vegetable mixture evenly. 7. Roast for about thirty minutes. 8. Remove the baking sheets from oven. 9. Sprinkle the vegetables with ginger and pecans e and drizzle with honey evenly. 10. Roast approximately 25 minutes. 11. Serve warm.

712. Grilled Veggie Skewers

Yield: 5 servings Preparation Time: 20 minutes Cooking Time: fifteen minutes

Ingredients:

For Marinade Mixture: • 3 garlic cloves, chopped • 1 (1-inch) pieces fresh ginger, chopped • 1 teaspoon ground cumin • 1 teaspoon ground coriander • 1teaspoon sweet paprika • 1/8 teaspoon red chili powder • Salt and freshly ground black pepper, to taste • ¼ cup fresh lemon juice • ¼ cup organic olive oil • ½ lot of fresh cilantro • ½ couple of fresh parsley For Vegetables: • 2 medium red bell pepper, seeded and cut into 1-inch pieces • 2 medium zucchinis, cut into 1/3-inch thick round slices • 1 pound small mushrooms • 1 large yellow onion, sliced into 1-inch pieces • 1 large eggplant, quartered lengthwise and cut into ½-inch thick slices diagonally

Directions:

1. For marinade mixture in the blender, add all ingredients except herbs and pulse till well combined. 2. Add fresh herbs and pulse till smooth. 3. In a sizable bowl, add vegetables and marinade and toss to coat well. 4. Refrigerate, covered approximately 4 hours. 5. Preheat the grill to medium-low heat. Grease the grill grate. 6. Thread the skewers for around 15 minutes, flipping occasionally. Mushrooms with

713. Three Mushrooms Medley

Yield: 3 servings Preparation Time: 15 minutes Cooking Time: 17 minutes

Ingredients:

3 tablespoons extra-virgin extra virgin olive oil • 3 portabella mushrooms, sliced • 6-ounce shiitake mushrooms, stemmed and sliced • 7½-ounce baby beech mushrooms • 1 tablespoon fresh ginger, minced • 5 garlic cloves, minced • 1 dried red chili, crushed • 2 teaspoons coconut aminos • 1 teaspoon sesame oil

Directions: 1. In a skillet, heat 1 tablespoon of essential olive oil on medium heat. 2. Add portabella mushrooms and cook stirring occasionally for approximately 4-5 minutes. 3. Transfer the mushrooms in a large bowl. 4. In a similar skillet, heat 1 tablespoon of extra virgin olive oil on medium heat. 5. Add shiitake mushrooms and cook for approximately 4-5 minutes. 6. Transfer the mushrooms in to the large bowl with portabella mushrooms. 7. In a similar skillet, heat ½ tablespoon from the organic olive oil on medium heat. 8. Add baby beech mushrooms and cook approximately 3-4 minutes. 9. Transfer the mushrooms to the large bowl with portabella mushrooms. 10. In exactly the same skillet, heat remaining extra virgin olive oil on medium heat. 11. Add ginger, garlic and red chili and sauté for around 1 minute. 12. Add the mushroom mixture, coconut aminos and sesame oil and stir till well combined. 13. Cook for around 1-2 minutes. 14. Serve hot.

714. Nutty Spinach

Yield: 4 servings Preparation Time: fifteen minutes Cooking Time: 23 minutes

Ingredients:

3 tablespoons coconut oil • 1½ tablespoons coconut sugar • ½ teaspoon cumin seeds • 1 tablespoon black mustard seeds • ¼ teaspoon fenugreek seeds • 2 pounds fresh spinach, trimmed • 1 tablespoon green chili, minced • ½ tablespoon fresh ginger, grated • 2/3 cup almonds, soaked in warm water for 4 hours and drained • 1/3 cup coconut, shredded • Salt and freshly ground black pepper, to taste • 2 tablespoons water • 1/8 teaspoon ground nutmeg

Directions:

1. In a big skillet, melt coconut oil on medium heat. 2. Add brown sugar, cumin seeds, mustard seeds and fenugreek seeds and sauté for around 1 minute. 3. Stir in spinach, green chili, ginger, almonds, coconut, salt and black pepper. 4. Reduce the heat to low and simmer, covered approximately 10 minutes. 5. Uncover and stir in water and simmer approximately 10 min. 6. Stir within the nutmeg and simmer for about 1-2 minutes more.

715. Mixed Vegetables Stew

Yield: 4 servings Preparation Time: 20 min Cooking Time: 52 minutes

Ingredients:

2 tablespoons organic olive oil • 1¼ cups yellow onion, chopped • 1 tablespoon garlic, minced • 1 tablespoon chile paste • 1½ tablespoons fresh turmeric, grated • 1½ teaspoons ground cumin • 1 teaspoon ground cinnamon • 1 cup carrots, peeled and chopped roughly • 1 cup cauliflower, chopped roughly • 2 cups broccoli, chopped roughly • 4 cups green cabbage, chopped roughly • 1 cup coconut water • 2 cups canned crushed tomatoes • ¾ cup frozen peas, thawed • Salt and freshly ground black pepper, to taste

Directions:

1. In a sizable pan, heat poi on medium heat. 2. Add onion and garlic and sauté approximately 10 min. 3. Add chile paste, turmeric, cumin and cinnamon and sate for around 1 minute. 4. Stir in carrots and cook for around 3-4 minutes. 5. Stir in cauliflower and broccoli and cook for about 2-3 minutes. 6. Stir in cabbage reducing heat to low. 7. Simmer for about 4 minutes. 8. Add coconut water and tomatoes and produce to some boil on medium-high heat. 9. Reduce heat to low and simmer, covered for approximately thirty minutes. 10. Stir in peas, salt and black pepper and remove from heat. 11. Serve hot.

716. Veggies Curry in Pumpkin Puree

Yield: 4 servings Preparation Time: fifteen minutes Cooking Time: a half-hour

Ingredients:

1 tablespoon coconut oil • 1 green bell pepper, seeded and chopped • 1 onion, chopped • 1 cup homemade pumpkin puree • 1 tablespoon curry powder • 1 teaspoon ground cinnamon • ¼ teaspoon ground ginger • Salt, to taste • 1 (14-ounce) can coconut milk • 1 cup water • 1 sweet potato, peeled and cut into 1-inch cubes • 1 head broccoli, cut into florets

Directions:

In a big pan, melt coconut oil on medium heat. 2. Add onion and sauté for about 8 minutes. 3. Add pumpkin puree, curry powder, cinnamon, ginger, salt, coconut milk and water and stir to blend well. 4. Stir in pumpkin and broccoli and bring with a gentle simmer. 5. Simmer, covered approximately 15-twenty minutes. 6. Serve hot.

717. Stuffed Zucchini

Yield: 6 servings Preparation Time: twenty minutes Cooking Time: half an hour

Ingredients

6 medium zucchinis, halved lengthwise • Salt, to taste • 1½ baking potatoes, peeled and cubed • 4 teaspoons olive oil • 2½ cups onion, chopped • 1 Serrano chile, mined • 2 minced garlic cloves • 1½ tablespoons fresh ginger, minced • 2 tablespoons chickpea flour • 1 teaspoon ground coriander • ¼ teaspoon ground cumin • ¼ teaspoon ground turmeric • Freshly ground black pepper, to taste • 1½ cups frozen green peas, thawed • 2 tablespoons fresh cilantro, chopped

Directions:

1. Preheat the oven to 375 degrees F. 2. With a scooper, scoop your pulp from zucchini halves, leaving about ¼-inch thick shell. 3. In a shallow roasting pan, arrange the zucchini halves, cut side up. 4. Sprinkle the zucchini halves which has a little salt. 5. In a pan of boiling water, cook the potatoes for around 2 minutes. 6. Drain well whilst aside. 7. In a nonstick skillet, heat oil on medium-high heat. 8. Add onion, Serrano, garlic and dinger and sauté for around 3 minutes. 9. Reduce the heat to medium-low. 10. Stir in chickpea flour and spices and cook for about 5 minutes. 11. Sir in cooked potato, green peas and cilantro and take off from heat. 12. With a paper towel, pat dry the zucchini halves. 13. Stuff the zucchini halves with all the veggie mixture evenly, 14. Bake, covered for about twenty or so minutes.

718. Veggies with Red Lentils

Yield: 6 servings Preparation Time: twenty or so minutes Cooking Time: 35 minutes

Ingredients:

2 tablespoons coconut oil • 12 fresh curry leaves • 1 teaspoon cumin seeds • 1 teaspoon brown mustard seeds • 1 medium onion, chopped finely • 4 garlic cloves, chopped finely • 3 tablespoons fresh ginger, minced • 1 Serrano chile, chopped finely • 1½ cups red lentils • 1 teaspoon ground turmeric • Salt, to taste • (1 (14-ounce) can coconut milk • 4½ cups water • 2 cups cauliflower, cut into 1-inch florets • 2½ cups butternut squash, peeled and cubed • 1 large Yukon gold potato, peeled and cut into ½-inch cubes • 2 tablespoons fresh lime juice • 1 tablespoon garam masala

Directions: 1. In a sizable pan, melt coconut oil on medium-high heat. 2. Add curry leaves, cumin seeds and mustard seeds and sauté for around a few seconds. 3. Add onion and sauté approximately 5 minutes. 4. Add garlic, ginger and Serrano chile and sauté for approximately half a minute. 5. Add lentils, turmeric, salt, coconut milk and water and produce to your boil, stirring occasionally. 6. Stir inside the vegetables and again bring to your boil. 7. Reduce heat to low and simmer, covered for around 20-25 minutes or till desired doneness. 8. Stir in lime juice and garam masala and immediately, remove from heat. 9. Serve hot.

719. Veggies with Chickpeas

Yield: 2 servings Preparation Time: 20 min Cooking Time: 25 minutes

Ingredients:

¼ cup onion, chopped • 1 (1-inch) fresh piece ginger, chopped • 4 garlic cloves, chopped • 2-3 tablespoons water • 1 teaspoon organic olive oil • ½ teaspoon ground coriander • ½ teaspoon ground cumin • ½ teaspoon ground turmeric • ¼ teaspoon ground cardamom • ¼ teaspoon ground cinnamon • 1/3 teaspoon red pepper cayenne • ½ cup coconut milk • 3 tablespoons almond butter • ¾ cup vegetable broth • 1 (15-ounce) can chickpeas, rinsed and drained • ½ cup zucchini, sliced • ½ cup carrot, peeled and sliced • ½ of red bell pepper, seeded and sliced • Crushed red pepper flakes, to taste • Salt and freshly ground black pepper, to taste • 1 teaspoon fresh lime juice • ¼ cup fresh cilantro, chopped

Directions: 1. In blender, add onion, ginger, garlic and water and pulse till smooth. 2. In a pan, heat oil on medium heat. 3. Add spices and sauté for about 30 seconds. 4. Reduce the temperature to medium-low. 5. Add onion mixture and sauté for about 7-9 minutes. 6. Add coconut milk and almond butter and stir to blend well. 7. Increase heat to medium-high. 8. Stir in broth, chickpeas, vegetables, red pepper flakes, salt and black pepper and bring to your boil for about 4 minutes. 9. Reduce the warmth to medium-low and simmer for approximately 5 minutes. 10. Stir in lime juice and cilantro and simmer for approximately 3-4 minutes.

720. Red Kidney Beans with Tomato

Yield: 6 servings Preparation Time: quarter-hour Cooking Time: twenty or so minutes

Ingredients:

1/3 cup extra-virgin organic olive oil • 1 medium onion, chopped finely • 3 garlic cloves, minced • 2 tablespoons fresh ginger, minced • 1 (8-ounce) can no-added sugar tomato sauce • 1 teaspoon ground coriander • 1 teaspoon ground cumin • 12 teaspoon ground turmeric • ¼ tsp cayenne • Salt and freshly ground black pepper, to taste • 1 (30-ounce) can red kidney beans with liquid • 1 plum tomato, chopped finely • 1 cup water • ½ cup fresh parsley, chopped

Directions:

1. In a large pan, heat oil on medium heat. 2. Add onion, garlic and ginger and sauté for approximately 2-3 minutes. 3. Stir in tomato sauce and spices cook for around 5 minutes. 4. Stir in kidney beans with liquid, tomato and water and bring with a boil on high heat. 5. Reduce the heat to medium and simmer for about 10 min. 6. Serve hot with the garnishing of parsley.

721. Spicy Three Beans Chili

Yield: 6 servings Preparation Time: fifteen minutes Cooking Time: 60 minutes

Ingredients:

For spice Mixture: • 1 teaspoon dried oregano, crushed • 1 tablespoon red chili powder • 1 tablespoon red pepper flakes, crushed • 2 teaspoons ground cumin • 1 teaspoon ground turmeric • 1 teaspoon onion powder • 1 teaspoon garlic powder • 1 teaspoon paprika • Salt and freshly ground black pepper, to taste For Chili: • 2 tablespoons extra virgin olive oil • 1 red bell pepper, seeded and chopped • 1 green bell pepper, seeded and chopped • 3 large celery stalks, chopped • 1 scallion, chopped • 3 garlic cloves, minced • 1 (28-ounce) can salt-free diced tomatoes • 4 cups water • 1 (16-ounce) can kidney beans, rinsed and drained • 1 (16-ounce) can cannellini beans, rinsed and drained • 1 (8-ounce) can black beans, rinsed and drained • 1 jalapeño pepper, seeded and chopped

Directions:

1. For spice mixture in a bowl, mix together all ingredients. Keep aside. 2. In a big pan, heat oil on medium heat. 3. Add bell peppers, celery, scallion and garlic and sauté approximately 8-10 min. 4. Add spice mixture, tomatoes and water and provide to your boil. 5. Simmer for about 20 min. 6. Stir in beans and jalapeño pepper and simmer approximately 30 minutes. 7. Serve hot.

722. Lentils Chili

Yield: 8 servings Preparation Time: fifteen minutes Cooking Time: couple of hours 6 minutes

Ingredients:

2 teaspoons extra virgin olive oil • 1 large onion, chopped • 3 medium carrot, peeled and chopped • 4 celery stalks, chopped • 2 minced garlic cloves • 2 tablespoons tomato paste • 1½ tablespoons ground coriander • 1½ tablespoons ground cumin • 1½ teaspoons ground turmeric • 1 teaspoon chipotle chili powder • Salt and freshly ground black pepper, to taste • 1 pound lentils, rinsed • 8 cups vegetable broth • 1 cup fresh spinach, chopped • ¼ cup fresh mint leaves, chopped • ¼ cup fresh cilantro, chopped

Directions:

In a big pan, heat oil on medium heat. 2. Add onion, carrot and celery and sauté for around 5 minutes. 3. Add garlic, tomato paste and spices and sauté for approximately 1 minute. 4. Add lentils and broth and bring to some boil. 5. Reduce the heat to low and simmer approximately 120 minutes. 6. Stir in spinach and take off from heat. 7. Serve hot using the garnishing of mint and cilantro.

723. Red Lentils Curry

Yield: 8 servings Preparation Time: fifteen minutes Cooking Time: 23 minutes

Ingredients:

2 cups red lentils, rinsed • 1 tbsp extra virgin olive oil • 1 large onion, chopped • 1 teaspoon fresh ginger, minced • 1 teaspoon garlic, minced • 2 tablespoons curry paste • 1 tablespoon curry powder • 1 teaspoon ground cumin • 1 teaspoon ground turmeric • 1 teaspoon red chili powder • Salt and freshly ground black pepper, to taste • 1 (14¼-ounce) can tomato puree

Directions:

1. In a substantial pan of water, add lentils and produce with a boil on high heat. 2. Reduce the heat to medium-low and simmer, covered for about 15-twenty or so minutes. 3. Drain well. 4. Meanwhile in a large skillet, heat oil on medium heat. 5. Add onion and sauté for approximately twenty minutes. 6. Meanwhile in a very bowl, mix together all remaining ingredients except tomato puree. 7. Add spice mixture in the skillet with onions on medium-high heat. 8. Sauté for around 1-2 minutes. 9. Stir in tomato puree and cook for around 1 minute. 10. Transfer a combination to the pan with the lentils and stir to mix. 11. Serve hot.

724. Vegetarian Balls in Gravy

Yield: 4-6 servings Preparation Time: twenty minutes Cooking Time: 25 minutes

Ingredients:

For Balls: • 1 cup cooked chickpeas • 1 cup cooked red kidney beans • ½ cup cooked quinoa • Salt and freshly ground black pepper, to taste • 2 tablespoons black beans flour • 1 medium onion, chopped • 2 garlic cloves, chopped • ¼ cup fresh cilantro, chopped • 1 teaspoon cumin seeds • Pinch of baking soda • 1 tablespoon fresh lemon juice • 2 teaspoons essential olive oil For Gravy: • 1 teaspoon extra virgin olive oil • 1 teaspoon cumin seeds • 1 medium onion, chopped finely • 1 (1-inch) piece fresh ginger, grated finely • 2 tomatoes, chopped finely • 2 green chilies, chopped finely • ½ teaspoon garam masala • ½ teaspoon ground turmeric • ½ teaspoon red chili powder • Salt, to taste • 2 cups water • ¼ cup fresh cilantro, chopped

Directions:

1. For balls in a very blender, add all ingredients except oil and pulse till a coarse meal forms. 2. Transfer the amalgamation right into a bowl. 3. Cover the bowl which has a foil paper and refrigerate not less than one hour. 4. Remove the mixture from refrigerator making equal sized balls. 5. In a nonstick skillet, heat oil on medium heat. 6. Cook the balls for around 2-3 minutes or till golden brown all sides. 7. For gravy inside a nonstick pan, heat oil on medium heat. 8. Add cumin seeds and sauté approximately 1 minute. 9. Add onion and sauté approximately 6-7 minutes. 10. Stir in ginger, tomatoes, green chilies and spices and cook for approximately 1-2 minutes. 11. Add water and produce with a boil. 12. Reduce the warmth to low and simmer, covered for around 10 min. 13. Carefully, place the balls within the gravy and cook for approximately 1-2 minutes. 14. Sprinkle with cilantro and serve.

725. Quinoa with Asparagus

Yield: 4 servings Preparation Time: quarter-hour Cooking Time: 18 minutes

Ingredients:

1 pound fresh asparagus, trimmed • 2 teaspoons coconut oil • ½ of onion, chopped • 2 minced garlic cloves • 1 cup cooked red quinoa • 1 tablespoon ground turmeric • ½ cup reduced-sodium vegetable broth • ½ cup nutritional yeast • 1 tablespoon fresh lemon juice

Directions:

In a large pan of boiling water, cook the asparagus approximately 2-3 minutes. 2. Drain well and rinse under cold water. 3. In a big skillet, melt coconut oil on medium heat. 4. Add onion and garlic and sauté for around 5 minutes. 5. Stir in quinoa, turmeric and broth and cook for around 5-6 minutes. 6. Stir in nutritional yeast, fresh lemon juice and asparagus and cook for approximately 3-4 minutes.

726. Coconut Brown Rice

Yield: 14 servings Preparation Time: fifteen minutes Cooking Time: an hour

Ingredients:

12 cups water • 1 tablespoon dried turmeric • 2 pound brown rice • 2 (13½-ounce) cans lite coconut milk • 2 (13½-ounce) cans coconut milk • 1 tablespoon fresh ginger, minced • 1½ teaspoons fresh lemon zest, grated finely • 4 dried bay leaves • Salt and freshly ground black pepper, to taste • Chopped cashews, for garnishing • Chopped fresh cilantro, for garnishing

Directions:

1. In a small bowl, add water and turmeric and beat till well combined. 2. In a big pan, add turmeric water and remaining ingredients except cashews and stir well. 3. Bring with a boil on high heat. 4. Reduce heat to medium and simmer, stirring occasionally for about 30-35 minutes. 5. Reduce the temperature to low and simmer, covered for about 20-25 minutes. 6. Remove bay leaf before serving. 7. Garnish with cashews and cilantro and serve.

727. Brown Rice Casserole

Yield: 2 servings Preparation Time: quarter-hour Cooking Time: 60 minutes

Ingredients:

1 teaspoon extra-virgin olive oil • 1 red onion, sliced thinly • 1½ teaspoons ground turmeric • 9-ounce brown mushrooms, sliced • 1 teaspoon raisins • ½ cup brown rice, rinsed • 1¼ cups vegetable broth • ¼ cup fresh cilantro, chopped • ½ tablespoons pine nuts, toasted • 1 tablespoon fresh lemon juice • Salt and freshly ground black pepper, to taste

Directions:

1. Preheat the oven to 400 degrees F. 2. In an ovenproof casserole, heat oil on medium heat. 3. Add onion and turmeric and sauté for about 3 minutes. 4. Add mushrooms and stir fry approximately 2 minutes. 5. Stir in raisins, rice and broth and transfer into oven. 6. Bake for around 45-55 minutes or till desired doneness. 7. Just before serving, stir in remaining ingredients.

728. Herbed Bulgur Pilaf

Yield: 6 servings Preparation Time: 20 minutes Cooking Time: 35 minutes

Ingredients:

2 tablespoons extra-virgin organic olive oil • 2 cups onion, chopped • 1 garlic clove, minced • 1½ cups medium bulgur • ½ teaspoon ground cumin • ½ teaspoon ground turmeric • 1½ cups carrot, peeled and chopped • 2 teaspoons fresh ginger, grated finely • Salt, to taste • 2 cups vegetable broth • 3 tablespoons freshly squeezed lemon juice • ¼ cup fresh parsley, chopped • ¼ cup fresh mint leaves, chopped • ¼ cup fresh dill, chopped • ½ cup walnuts, toasted and chopped

Directions:

In a big deep skillet, heat oil on medium-low heat. 2. Add onion and cook, stirring occasionally for around 12-18 minutes. 3. Add garlic and sauté fir about 1 minute. 4. Add bulgur, cumin and turmeric and stir fry for approximately 1 minute. 5. Add carrot, ginger, salt and broth and provide to a boil, stirring occasionally. 6. Simmer, covered for around quarter-hour. 7. Remove from heat and keep aside, covered for about 5 minutes. 8. Stir in fresh lemon juice and fresh herbs and serve while using garnishing of walnuts.

729. Mango Salad

Yield: 6 servings Preparation Time: fifteen minutes

Ingredients:

For Dressing: • 1 fresh Serrano chile, chopped • 1 tablespoon fresh cilantro, chopped • 1 teaspoon fresh ginger, chopped • ¼ cup golden raisins, soaked in boiling water approximately half an hour and drained • 3 tablespoons extra-virgin organic olive oil • 2 tablespoons balsamic vinegar • Salt, to taste For Salad: • 8 cups fresh mixed baby greens • 1 medium red bell pepper, seeded and sliced thinly • 1 large mango, peeled, pitted and cubed

Directions:

1. For dressing in a very blender, add all ingredients and pulse till smooth. 2. Reserve 1 tablespoon of the dressing. 3. In a large bowl, squeeze greens and remaining dressing and toss to coat well. 4. In another bowl, add bell pepper, mango and reserved dressing and toss to coat. 5. Divide the greens and mango mixture in serving bowls. 6. Serve immediately

730. Lemony Fruit Salad

Yield: 16 servings Preparation Time: 25 minutes

Ingredients:

1 fresh pineapple, peeled, cored and chopped • 2 large mangoes, peeled, pitted and chopped • 2 large Fuji apples, cored and chopped • 2 large red Bartlett pears, cored and chopped • 2 large navel oranges, peeled, seeded and sectioned • 2 teaspoons fresh ginger, grated finely • 2 tablespoons organic honey • ¼ cup fresh lemon juice

Directions:

1. In a big bowl, mix together all fruits. 2. In a little bowl, add remaining ingredients and beat well. 3. Place honey mixture over fruit mixture and toss to coat well. 4. Refrigerate, covered till chilled completely.

731. Wheat Berries & Mango Salad

Yield: 4 servings Preparation Time: 20 minutes Cooking Time: 35 minutes

Ingredients:

For Salad: • 2 cups water • 1 cup wheat berries • 1 mango, peeled, pitted and cubed • ½ of red bell pepper, seeded and chopped • 2 scallions, chopped • ½ cup fresh mint leaves, chopped • ½ cup cranberries • ½ cup walnuts, toasted and chopped For Dressing: • 1 tablespoon fresh ginger, minced • cup plain Greek yogurt • 3 tablespoons raw honey • ½ teaspoon balsamic vinegar • Salt and freshly ground black pepper, to taste

Directions:

1. In a pan, add water and warmth berries and bring to your boil. 2. Cover and cook approximately 35 minutes. 3. Remove from heat whilst aside for cooling. 4. In a large bowl, add wheat berries and remaining ingredients and mix. 5. In a little bowl, add dressing ingredients and beat well. 6. Place dressing over fruit mixture and toss to coat well. 7. Serve immediately.

732. Berries & Watermelon Salad

Yield: 8-10 servings Preparation Time: 20 min

Ingredients:

2½ pound seedless watermelon, cubed • 2 cartons fresh strawberries, hulled and sliced • 2 cups fresh blueberries • 1 tablespoon fresh gingerroot, grated • ¼-ounce fresh mint leaves, chopped • 1 tablespoon raw honey • ¼ cup fresh lime juice

Directions: 1. In a sizable bowl, mix together all ingredients. 2. Serve immediately.

733. Pear & Jicama Salad

Yield: 4 servings Preparation Time: quarter-hour

Ingredients:

For Salad: • 2 small pears, cored and sliced thinly • 1 pound jicama, sliced into matchsticks • 1 sprig fresh mint • 1 sprig fresh parsley For Dressing: • 2 tablespoons extra virgin olive oil • 3 tablespoons fresh orange juice • 1 tablespoon using apple cider vinegar • ¼ teaspoon ginger powder • Salt, to taste

Directions:

1. In a big bowl, mix together all salad ingredients. 2. In a smaller bowl, add dressing ingredients and beat well. 3. Place dressing over salad mixture and toss to coat well. 4. Serve immediately.

734. Carrot & Almond Salad

Yield: 4 servings Preparation Time: 15 minutes

Ingredients:

1 garlic clove, minced • 2 teaspoons fresh ginger, grated finely • ¼ cup coconut milk • 2 tablespoons almond butter • 2 tablespoons coconut aminos • 1 tablespoon fresh lemon juice • Pinch of cayenne • Salt, to taste • 5 large carrots, peeled and grated • Chopped almonds, to taste

Directions:

1. In a large bowl, add all ingredients except carrots and almonds and mix till well combined. 2. Add carrots and stir to mix. 3. Serve with the garnishing of almonds.

735. Beet, Carrot & Parsley Salad

Yield: 5 servings Preparation Time: 15 minutes

Ingredients:

For Salad: • 1 cup Daikon radishes, trimmed, peeled and julienned • 3 cups carrots, peeled and julienned • ½ cup fresh parsley, chopped For Dressing: • 1 teaspoon fresh ginger, grated finely • 2 tablespoons balsamic vinegar • 1 tablespoon extra-virgin extra virgin olive oil • 2 teaspoons coconut aminos • 2 teaspoons raw honey • ¼ teaspoon granulated garlic • Salt, to taste

Directions: 1. In a big bowl, mix together all salad ingredients. 2. In a tiny bowl, add dressing ingredients and beat well. 3. Place dressing over fruit mixture and toss to coat well. 4. Serve immediately.

736. Greens & Seeds Salad

Yield: 4 servings Preparation Time: 20 minutes Cooking Time: 6 minutes

Ingredients:

1½ teaspoons fresh ginger, grated finely • 2 tablespoons apple cider vinegar treatment • 3 tablespoons olive oil • 1 teaspoon sesame oil, toasted • 3 teaspoons raw honey, divided • ½ teaspoon red pepper flakes, crushed and divided • Salt, to taste • 1 tablespoon water • 2 tablespoons raw sunflower seeds • 1 tablespoon raw sesame seeds • 1 tablespoon raw pumpkin seeds • 10-ounce collard greens, stems and ribs removed and thinly sliced leaves

Directions: 1. For dressing inside a bowl, add ginger, vinegar, both oils, 1 teaspoon of honey, ¼ teaspoon red pepper flakes and salt and bat till well combined. Keep aside. 2. In another bowl, add remaining honey, remaining red pepper flakes and water and mix till well combined. 3. Heat a medium nonstick skillet on medium heat. 4. Add all seeds and cook, stirring for approximately 3 minutes. 5. Stir in honey mixture and cook, stirring continuously for about 3 minutes. 6. Transfer the seeds mixture onto a parchment paper and make aside to cool down the completely. 7. Break the seeds mixture into small pieces. 8. In a large bowl, add the greens, 2 teaspoons with the dressing plus a little salt and toss to coat well. 9. With both your hands, rub the greens for around a few seconds. 10. Add remaining dressing and toss to coat well. 11. Serve with a garnishing of seeds pieces.

737. Cucumber Salad

Yield: 4 servings Preparation Time: 10 min

Ingredients:

For Salad: • 2 cucumbers, spiralized with blade C • 1 avocado, peeled, pitted and sliced • 2-3 green onions, sliced • Toasted sesame seeds, as required For Dressing: • 1 teaspoon fresh ginger, grated finely • 1 garlic clove, minced • 1 teaspoon raw honey • 1 tablespoon coconut aminos • 1 tablespoon sesame oil, toasted • 1 tbsp olive oil

Directions:

1. In a large bowl, squeeze cucumber pasta. 2. In another small bowl, add all dressing ingredients and beat till well combined. 3. Place dressing over cucumber and toss to coat well. 4. Serve with all the topping of remaining ingredients.

738. Kale, Carrot & Radish Salad

Yield: 4 servings Preparation Time: 10 min

Ingredients:

1 bunch fresh kale, trimmed and sliced thinly • 1 large garlic herb, minced • 2 tablespoons coconut aminos • 2 tablespoons fresh lemon juice • 1 tablespoon extra-virgin organic olive oil • 2 tablespoons extra-virgin coconut oil • 2 medium carrots, peeled and sliced thinly • 6 radishes, trimmed and sliced thinly • 2 tablespoons apple cider vinegar treatment • Salt, to taste • 1/3 cup coconut flakes, toasted • 1 avocado, peeled, pitted and chopped

Directions:

1. In a large bowl, add kale, garlic, coconut aminos, freshly squeezed lemon juice and olive oil and toss to coat well. 2. With the hands, rub the kale generously. 3. Add coconut oil and toss to coat well. 4. Keep aside for about quarter-hour, stringing occasionally. 5. In another bowl, mix together the carrots, radishes and vinegar and keep aside for around quarter-hour, stirring occasionally. 6. Add the carrot mixture inside bowl with kale mixture and toss to combine. 7. Serve using a garnishing of coconut flakes and avocado.

739. Citrus Mixed Veggie Salad

Yield: 4 servings Preparation Time: 20 minutes

Ingredients:

For Salad: • ½ of the cabbage head, sliced thinly • 2 carrots, peeled and cut into matchsticks • 1 zucchini, peeled and cut into matchsticks • 1 raw beetroot, peeled and cut into matchsticks • 1 red bell pepper, seeded and sliced thinly • 2 scallions, sliced thinly • 3 tablespoons cashews, toasted • 2 tablespoons sunflower seeds, toasted • Lime wedges, for serving For Dressing: • 3 tablespoons cashews, toasted • 2 tablespoons sunflower seeds, toasted • 1 large thumb size piece fresh ginger, chopped • ½ cup fresh cilantro • ¼ cup fresh mint leaves • 2 tablespoons fresh lime juice • 2 tablespoons fresh lemon juice • 1 tbsp essential olive oil

Directions:

In a big bowl, mix together all salad ingredients except cashews, sunflower seeds and lime wedges. 2. In a smaller bowl, add dressing ingredients and beat well. 3. Place dressing over salad mixture and toss to coat well. 4. Serve immediately with the garnishing of cashews, sunflower seeds alongside the lime wedges.

740. Warm Chickpeas Salad

Yield: 4 servings Preparation Time: 10 min Cooking Time: 10 min

Ingredients:

5 tablespoons virgin olive oil • 1 large red onion, chopped finely • 2 minced garlic cloves • 2 (15-ounce) cans chickpeas, rinsed and drained • Pinch of red pepper flakes, crushed • ½ teaspoon ground ginger • 1 tablespoon freshly squeezed lemon juice • Salt and freshly ground black pepper, to taste • ¼ teaspoon paprika • ½ teaspoon ground cumin • 2 tablespoons fresh cilantro, chopped

Directions:

1. In a skillet, heat 1 tablespoon of oil on medium-low heat. 2. Add onion and garlic and sauté for approximately 5-7 minutes. 3. Add chickpeas, red pepper flakes and ground ginger and cook approximately 1 minute. 4. Add fresh lemon juice and cook for around 1-2 minutes or till each of the liquid is absorbed. 5. Transfer the chickpea mixture in the serving bowl. 6. Add remaining oil, paprika and cumin and gently, stir to blend. 7. Serve warm using the garnishing of cilantro.

741. Black Beans & Mango Salad

Yield: 6 servings Preparation Time: 15 minutes

Ingredients:

For salad: • 2 (15½-ounce) cans black beans, rinsed and drained • 2 mangoes, peeled, pitted and chopped • ½ cup red onion, chopped • 2 tablespoons fresh cilantro, chopped For Dressing: • 1 (½-inch) pieces fresh ginger, grated • 2 teaspoons fresh orange zest, grated finely • 3-4 tablespoons fresh orange juice • 1 tablespoon using apple cider vinegar • 2 teaspoons extra-virgin olive oil • ¼ teaspoon red pepper flakes, crushed

Directions: 1. In a large bowl, mix together all salad ingredients. 2. In another bowl, add all dressing ingredients and beat till well combined. 3. Place dressing over beans mixture and mix till well combined. 4. Serve immediately.

742. Lentil & Beet Salad

Yield: 2-3 servings Preparation Time: quarter-hour Cooking Time: twenty or so minutes

Ingredients:

For Salad: • 2¾ cups water • 1 cup puy lentils, rinsed • Salt, to taste • 3 cooked beetroots, peeled and cubed • 2 scallions, chopped • 2 tablespoons fresh parsley, chopped • 2 tablespoons fresh mint leaves, chopped • 2 tablespoons hazelnuts, chopped For Dressing: • 1 (¾-inch) piece fresh ginger, chopped • 1 teaspoon Dijon mustard • 1/3 cup extra-virgin essential olive oil • 1 tablespoon using apple cider vinegar • Salt and freshly ground black pepper, to taste

Directions: 1. In a sizable pan, add water, lentils and salt on high heat and bring with a boil. 2. Reduce the heat to low and simmer for about 15-twenty minutes or till each of the liquid is absorbed. 3. Transfer the lentils right into a large bowl and make aside to cool down the. 4. Add remaining salad ingredients and mix. 5. In another bowl, add all dressing ingredients and beat till well combined. 6. Place dressing over lentils mixture and mix till well combined. 7. Serve immediately.

743. Nutty Chicken Salad

Yield: 6-8 servings Preparation Time: twenty minutes

Ingredients:

For dressing: • 2-3 tablespoons plain Greek yogurt • 3 tablespoons Dijon mustard • 2 tablespoons sunflower seeds • 1 teaspoon kelp powder • ½-1 teaspoon ground turmeric • ¼ teaspoon garlic powder • ¼ teaspoon onion powder • Salt and freshly ground black pepper, to taste For Salad: • 4 cooked chicken breasts, shredded • 2-3 celery stalks, chopped • 7-10 sprigs fresh parsley • 2 tablespoons dried cherries • 2 tablespoons pecan • 2 tablespoons slivered almonds

Directions: 1. For dressing inside a bowl, add all dressing ingredients and mix till well combined. 2. In another large bowl, mix together salad ingredients. 3. Pour dressing over salad and toss to coat well. 4. Serve immediately.

744. Chicken, Bok Choy & Jicama Salad

Yield: 4 servings Preparation Time: twenty or so minutes

Ingredients:

For Dressing: • 1 tablespoon fresh ginger, chopped • 2 tablespoons coconut cream • 2 tablespoons fresh lime juice • 1 tablespoon sesame oil • 1 tablespoon coconut aminos • 1 tablespoon fish sauce • 1 teaspoon stevia powder For Salad: • 2 cups grilled chicken, chopped • 6 baby bokchoy, grilled and chopped • 2 scallions, chopped • ½ cup jicama, chopped • ¼ cup fresh cilantro, chopped • 1 tablespoon sesame seeds

Directions:

1. For dressing in the blender, add all dressing ingredients and mix till well combined. 2. In another large bowl, mix together salad ingredients. 3. Pour dressing over salad and toss to coat well. 4. Serve immediately

745. Chicken &Broccolini Salad

Yield: 2 servings Preparation Time: 25 minutes Cooking Time: 12 minutes

Ingredients:

For Chicken: • 1 tablespoon coconut oil • ½ medium onion, chopped • 9-ounce boneless chicken thigh, chopped finely • 1 large garlic herb, minced • 1 teaspoon fresh lime zest, grated finely • 1 teaspoon ground turmeric • 1 teaspoon fresh lime juice • Salt and freshly ground black pepper, to taste For Salad: • 6 broccolini stalks • 3 large kale leaves, trimmed and chopped • ½ of avocado, peeled, pitted and chopped • 2 tablespoons fresh parsley leaves, chopped • 2 tablespoons fresh cilantro, chopped • 2 tablespoons pumpkin seeds, toasted For Dressing: • 1 small garlic cloves, grated finely • ½ teaspoon Dijon mustard • 3 tablespoons extra-virgin olive oil • 3 tablespoons fresh lime juice • 1 teaspoon raw honey • Salt and freshly ground black pepper, to taste

Directions:

1. In a small skillet, melt coconut oil on medium-high heat. 2. Add onion and sauté for approximately 4-5 minutes. 3. Add chicken and garlic and stir fry for about 2-3 minutes. 4. Add remaining ingredients and cook, stirring occasionally approximately 3-4 minutes. 5. Meanwhile in the pan of boiling water, add broccolini and cook for around 2 minutes. 6. Drain well and rinse under cold water and after that cut each stalk in 3-4 pieces. 7. In a bowl, add all dressing ingredients and mix till well combined. 8. Add kale and along with your hands rub till coated with dressing generously. 9. Add chicken, broccolini, avocado, herbs and pumpkin seeds and toss to coat well. 10. Serve immediately.

746. Smoked Salmon & Veggie Salad

Yield: 2 servings Preparation Time: 20 minutes

Ingredients:

4 radishes, trimmed and sliced thinly • 2 tomatoes, chopped • ½ of cucumber, peeled and chopped • 1 carrot, peeled and sliced diagonally • 1 small head romaine lettuce • 5-ounce smoked salmon, sliced thinly For Dressing: • 1 teaspoon fresh ginger, minced • 1 tablespoon fresh lemon juice • 1 tbsp olive oil

Directions:

In a bowl, mix together radishes, tomatoes, cucumber and carrot. 2. In another bowl, add all dressing ingredients and beat till well combined. 3. Divide lettuce in serving plates and top with carrot mixture, then salmon evenly. 4. Pour dressing over salad and serve immediately.

747. Salmon, Spinach & Kale Salad

Yield: 1 serving Preparation Time: 10 min

Ingredients:

For Salad: • ¼ cup fresh orange juice • 1 (4-ounce) salmon fillet • 1 teaspoon raw honey • 1½ cups fresh baby spinach • 1 teaspoon coconut oil • 1½ cups fresh baby kale • ½ of avocado, peeled, pitted and sliced • 1 orange, peeled, seeded and sectioned • 3 tablespoons pomegranate seeds For Dressing: • ½ tablespoon coconut oil • 1 teaspoon raw honey • 2½ tablespoons fresh orange juice • Salt, to taste

Directions:

1. In a bowl, mix together ¼ cup of orange juice and salmon. 2. Refrigerate, covered for approximately a couple of hours. 3. Preheat the oven to 400 degrees F. Grease a tiny baking dish. 4. Coat the each side of salmon fillet with honey evenly. 5. In a smaller frying pan, melt coconut oil on medium heat. 6. Add salmon fillet and cook for around 1-2 minutes per side. 7. Transfer the salmon fillet into prepared baking dish and bake for approximately 8-10 minutes. 8. Meanwhile in a substantial bowl, mix together all salad ingredients. 9. For dressing inside a microwave safe bowl, add coconut oil and homey and microwave for approximately 20 seconds or till melted. 10. Add orange juice and salt and beat well. 11. Pour dressing over salad and toss to coat well. 12. Top with salmon fillet and serve.

748. Salmon & Beans Salad

Yield: 4 servings Preparation Time: 15 minutes Cooking Time: 7 minutes

Ingredients:

For Salmon: • 4 (6-ounce) salmon fillets • Ground cumin, to taste • Salt and freshly ground black pepper, to taste • 2 tablespoons olive oil For Salad: • 1 (15-ounce) can pinto beans, rinsed and drained • 1 (15-ounce) can kidney beans, rinsed and drained • 1 (15-ounce) can navy beans, rinsed and drained • 1 medium bunch scallion, chopped • 1 small bunch fresh parsley, chopped • 1/3 cup extra-virgin essential olive oil • ¼ cup freshly squeezed lemon juice • Salt and freshly ground black pepper, to taste

Directions: 1. Sprinkle the salmon fillets with cumin, salt and black pepper evenly. 2. In a sizable nonstick skillet, heat oil on medium heat. 3. Ass salmon, skin-side down and cook for about 3-4 minutes. 4. Carefully flip the side and cook for about 3 minutes. 5. Meanwhile in the bowl, mix together all salad ingredients. 6. Top with salmon fillets and serve.

749. Parsnip Fries

Yield: 4 servings Preparation Time: fifteen minutes Cooking Time: 40 minutes

Ingredients:

2 tablespoons extra-virgin organic olive oil · 1¼ pound small parsnips, peeled and quartered · 1½ tablespoons fresh ginger, minced · Salt and freshly ground black pepper, to taste

Directions: 1. Preheat the oven to 325 degrees F. 2. In a 13x9-inch baking dish, place the oil evenly. 3. Add remaining ingredients and toss to coat well. 4. With a foil paper, cover the baking dish and bake for about 40 minutes. 5. Serve immediately.

750. Sweet Potato Fries

Yield: 2 servings Preparation Time: 10 minutes Cooking Time: 25 minutes

Ingredients:

1 large sweet potato, peeled and cut into wedges • 1 teaspoon ground turmeric • 1 teaspoon ground cinnamon • Salt and freshly ground black pepper, to taste • 2 tablespoons extra-virgin olive oil

Directions: 1. Preheat the oven to 425 degrees F. Line a baking sheet having a foil paper. 2. In a sizable bowl, add all ingredients and toss to coat well. 3. Transfer the mixture into prepared baking sheet. 4. Bake for around 25 minutes, flipping once after 15 minutes. 5. Serve immediately.

751. Jicama Fries

Yield: 3 servings Preparation Time: 15 minutes Cooking Time: 51 minutes

Ingredients:

1 medium jicama, peeled and cut into fries • 3 tablespoons water • ½ teaspoon ground turmeric • ½ teaspoon ground cumin • ½ teaspoon garlic powder • ¼ teaspoon onion powder • ¼ teaspoon smoked paprika • Pinch of cayenne pepper • Salt and freshly ground black pepper, to taste

Directions:

1. Preheat the oven to 400 degrees F. Line a baking sheet having a foil paper. 2. In a substantial microwave safe bowl, add jicama fries and water. 3. Cover and microwave for about 6 minutes. 4. Drain the water if you have any left within the bowl. 5. Add the spices and oil and toss to coat well. 6. Transfer the mixture into prepared baking sheet. 7. Bake for approximately 35-45 minutes, flipping once in the middle way. 8. Serve immediately.

752. Zucchini Chips

Yield: 2 servings Preparation Time: fifteen minutes Cooking Time: 15 minutes

Ingredients:

1 medium zucchini, cut into thin slices • 1/8 teaspoon ground turmeric • 1/8 teaspoon ground cumin • Salt, to taste • 2 teaspoons essential olive oil

Directions:

1. Preheat the oven to 400 degrees F. Line 2 baking sheets with parchment papers. 2. In a substantial bowl, add all ingredients and toss to coat well. 3. Transfer a combination into prepared baking sheets in a single layer. 4. Bake approximately 10-fifteen minutes. 5. Serve immediately.

753. Beet Greens Chips

Yield: 2 servings Preparation Time: fifteen minutes Cooking Time: 25 minutes

Ingredients:

1 large bunch beet greens, tough ribs removed • Salt and freshly ground black pepper, to taste • Olive oil, as required

Directions:

1. Preheat the oven to 350 degrees F. Line a baking sheet having a parchment paper. 2. In a sizable bowl, add all ingredients and toss to coat well. 3. Transfer the leaves into prepared baking sheet inside a single layer. 4. Bake for approximately 25 minutes, flipping once after fifteen minutes. 5. Serve immediately.

754. Plantain Chips

Yield: 1 serving Preparation Time: quarter-hour Cooking Time: 10 min

Ingredients:

1 plantain, peeled and sliced • ½ teaspoon ground turmeric • Salt, to taste • 1 teaspoon coconut oil, melted

Directions:

In a large bowl, add all ingredients and toss to coat well. 2. Transfer the half in the mixture in a large greased microwave safe bowl. 3. Microwave on high for around 3 minutes. 4. Now, decrease the capacity to 50% and microwave approximately 2 minutes. 5. Repeat with the remaining plantain mixture.

755. Sweet & Tangy Seeds Crackers

Yield: 10 servings Preparation Time: 15 minutes Cooking Time: 12 hours

Ingredients:

2 cups water • 1 cup sunflower seeds • 1 cup flaxseeds • 1 tablespoon fresh ginger, chopped • 1 teaspoon raw honey • ¼ cup freshly squeezed lemon juice • 1 teaspoon ground turmeric • Salt, to taste

Directions

1. In a bowl, add water, sunflower seeds and flaxseeds and soak for around overnight. 2. Drain the seeds. 3. In a food processor, add soaked seeds and remaining ingredients and pulse till well combined. 4. Set dehydrator at 115 degrees F. Line a dehydrator tray with unbleached parchment paper. 5. Place the mix onto prepared dehydrator tray evenly. 6. With a knife, score how big crackers. 7. Dehydrate for about 12 hours.

756. Beet Crackers

Yield: 15 servings Preparation Time: twenty or so minutes Cooking Time: 50 minutes

Ingredients:

1 cup raw beets, chopped • 3 tablespoons arrowroot flour • 3 tablespoons coconut flour • 2 egg whites • 1 tablespoon coconut oil • ¼ teaspoon ground turmeric • 1/8 teaspoon cayenne • Salt and freshly ground black pepper, to taste

Directions:

1. Preheat the oven to 350 degrees F. Grease a sizable baking sheet. 2. In a mixer, add beets and pulse till merely a puree forms. 3. Add remaining ingredients and pulse till well combined. 4. Place a parchment paper onto an easy surface. 5. Place the dough onto parchment paper and top with another paper. 6. With a rolling pin, roll the dough to at least one/8-inch thickness. 7. Remove the parchment papers. 8. Place the rolled dough onto prepared baking sheet. 9. Bake for around 40-50 minutes.

757. Apple Leather

Yield: 4 servings Preparation Time: 15 minutes Cooking Time: 12 hours 25 minutes

Ingredients: •

1 cup water • 8 cups apples, peeled, cored and chopped • 1 tablespoon ground cinnamon • 2 tablespoons freshly squeezed lemon juice

Directions: 1. In a big pan, add water and apples on medium-low heat. 2. Simmer, stirring occasionally for around 10-quarter-hour. 3. Remove from heat and make aside to cool slightly. 4. In a blender, add apple mixture and pulse till smooth. 5. Return the mixture into pan on medium-low heat. 6. Stir in cinnamon and fresh lemon juice and simmer approximately 10 minutes. 7. Transfer the mix onto dehydrator trays and with the back of spoon smooth the very best. 8. Set the dehydrator at 135 degrees F. 9. Dehydrate for around 10-12 hours. 10. Cut the apple leather into equal sized rectangles. 11. Now, roll each rectangle to make fruit rolls.

758. Roasted Almonds

Yield: 32 servings Preparation Time: 5 minutes Cooking Time: 10 min

Ingredients:

2 cups whole almonds • 1 tablespoon chili powder • ½ teaspoon ground cinnamon • ½ teaspoon ground cumin • ½ teaspoon ground coriander • Salt and freshly ground black pepper, to taste • 1 tablespoon extra-virgin organic olive oil

Directions: 1. Preheat the oven to 350 degrees F. Line a baking dish with a parchment paper. 2. In a bowl, add all ingredients and toss to coat well. 3. Transfer the almond mixture into prepared baking dish in a single layer. 4. Roast for around 10 minutes, flipping twice inside the middle way. 5. Remove from oven and make aside to cool down the completely before serving. 6. You can preserve these roasted almonds in airtight jar.

759. Roasted Chickpeas

Yield: 8-10 servings Preparation Time: 10 min Cooking Time: one hour

Ingredients:

3 cups canned chickpeas, rinsed and dried • 2 tablespoons nutritional yeast • 1 tablespoon ground turmeric • ½ teaspoon garlic powder • Pinch of cayenne pepper. • Salt and freshly ground black pepper, to taste • 2 tablespoons extra-virgin organic olive oil

Directions:

1. Preheat the oven to 400 degrees F. 2. In a bowl, add all ingredients except freshly squeezed lemon juice and toss to coat well. 3. Transfer the almond mixture right into a baking sheet. 4. Roast for around 1 hour, flipping after every quarter-hour. 5. Remove from oven and keep aside for cooling completely before serving. 6. Drizzle with freshly squeezed lemon juice and serve.

760. Cucumber Bites

Yield: 4 servings Preparation Time: quarter-hour

Ingredients:

½ cup prepared hummus • 2 teaspoons nutritional yeast • ¼-½ teaspoon ground turmeric • Pinch of red pepper cayenne • Pinch of salt • 1 cucumber, cut diagonally into ¼-½-inch thick slices • 1 teaspoon black sesame seeds • Fresh mint leaves, for garnishing

Directions:

1. In a bowl, mix together hummus, turmeric, cayenne and salt. 2. Transfer the hummus mixture in the pastry bag and pipe on each cucumber slice. 3. Serve while using garnishing of sesame seeds and mint leaves.

761. Crispy Chicken Fingers

Yield: 4-6 servings Preparation Time: fifteen minutes Cooking Time: 18 minutes

Ingredients:

2/3 cup almond meal • ½ teaspoon ground turmeric • ½ teaspoon red pepper cayenne • ½ teaspoon paprika • ½ teaspoon garlic powder • Salt and freshly ground black pepper, to taste • 1 egg • 1 pound skinless, boneless chicken breasts, cut into strips

Directions:

Preheat the oven to 375 degrees F. Line a substantial baking sheet with parchment paper. 2. In a shallow dish, beat the egg. 3. In another shallow dish, mix together almond meal and spices. 4. Coat each chicken strip with egg after which roll into spice mixture evenly. 5. Arrange the chicken strips onto prepared baking sheet in the single layer. 6. Bake for approximately 16-18 minutes.

762. Tuna & Sweet Potato Croquettes

Yield: 8 servings Preparation Time: fifteen minutes Cooking Time: 12 minutes

Ingredients:

1 tablespoon coconut oil • ½ of large onion, chopped • 1 (1-inch) piece fresh ginger, minced • 3 garlic cloves, minced • 1 Serrano pepper, seeded and minced • ½ teaspoon ground coriander • ¼ teaspoon ground turmeric • ¼ teaspoon red chili powder • ¼ teaspoon garam masala • Salt and freshly ground black pepper, to taste • 2 (5-ounce) cans tuna • 1 cup cooked sweet potato, peeled and mashed • 1 egg • ¼ cup tapioca flour • ¼ cup almond flour • Olive oil, as required

Directions:

1. In a frying pan, melt coconut oil on medium heat. 2. Add onion, ginger, garlic and Serrano pepper and sauté for approximately 5-6 minutes. 3. Stir in spices and sauté approximately 1 minute more. 4. Transfer the onion mixture in a bowl. 5. Add tuna and sweet potato and mix till well combined. 6. Make equal sized oblong shaped patties in the mixture. 7. Arrange the croquettes inside a baking sheet in a very single layer and refrigerate for overnight. 8. In a shallow dish, beat the egg. 9. In another shallow dish mix together both flours. 10. In a big skillet, heat the enough oil. 11. Add croquettes in batches and shallow fry for around 2-3 minutes per side.

763. Turkey Burgers

Yield: 5 servings Preparation Time: quarter-hour Cooking Time: 8 minutes

Ingredients:

1 ripe pear, peeled, cored and chopped roughly • 1 pound lean ground turkey • 1 teaspoon fresh ginger, grated finely • 2 minced garlic cloves • 1 teaspoon fresh rosemary, minced • 1 teaspoon fresh sage, minced • Salt and freshly ground black pepper, to taste • 1-2 tablespoons coconut oil

Directions:

1. In a blender, add pear and pulse till smooth. 2. Transfer the pear mixture in a large bowl with remaining ingredients except oil and mix till well combined. 3. Make small equal sized 10 patties from mixture. 4. In a heavy-bottomed frying pan, heat oil on medium heat. 5. Add the patties and cook for around 4-5 minutes. 6. Flip the inside and cook for approximately 2-3 minutes.

764. Salmon Burgers

Yield: 3 servings Preparation Time: fifteen minutes Cooking Time: 8 minutes

Ingredients:

1 (6-ounce) can skinless, boneless salon, drained • 1 celery rib, chopped • ½ of medium onion, chopped • 2 large eggs • 1 tablespoon plus 1 teaspoon coconut flour • 1 tablespoon dried dill, crushed • 1 teaspoon lemon pepper • Salt and freshly ground black pepper, to taste • 3 tablespoons coconut oil

Directions:

In a substantial bowl, add salmon and which has a fork, break it into small pieces. 2. Add remaining ingredients except oil and mix till well combined. 3. Make 6 equal sized small patties from mixture. 4. In a substantial skillet, melt coconut oil on medium-high heat. 5. Cook the patties for around 3-4 minutes per side.

765. Veggie Balls

Yield: 5-6 servings Preparation Time: 15 minutes Cooking Time: 25 minutes

Ingredients:

2 medium sweet potatoes, peeled and cubed into ½-inch size • 2 tablespoons coconut milk • 1 cup fresh kale leaves, trimmed and chopped • 1 medium shallot, chopped finely • 1 teaspoon ground cumin • ½ teaspoon granulated garlic • ¼ teaspoon ground turmeric • Salt and freshly ground black pepper, to taste • Ground flax seeds, as required

Directions:

1. Preheat the oven to 400 degrees F. Line a baking sheet with parchment paper. 2. In a pan of water, arrange a steamer basket. 3. Place the sweet potato in steamer basket and steam approximately 10-15 minutes. 4. In a sizable bowl, put the sweet potato. 5. Add coconut milk and mash well. 6. Add remaining ingredients except flax seeds and mix till well combined. 7. Make about 1½-2-inch balls from your mixture. 8. Arrange the balls onto prepared baking sheet inside a single layer. 9. Sprinkle with flax seeds. 10. Bake for around 20-25 minutes.

766. Fennel Seeds Cookies

Yield: 5 servings Preparation Time: 10 minutes Cooking Time: 20 minutes

Ingredients:

1/3 cup coconut flour • ¼ teaspoon whole fennel seeds • ½ teaspoon fresh ginger, grated finely • ¼ cup coconut oil, sof10ed • 2 tablespoons raw honey • 1 teaspoon vanilla extract • Pinch of ground cinnamon • Pinch of salt and freshly ground black pepper

Directions:

1. Preheat the oven to 360 degrees F. Line a cookie sheet which has a parchment paper. 2. In a substantial bowl, add all ingredients and mix till an even dough forms. 3. Make small balls in the mixture make onto prepared cookie sheet inside a single layer. 4. With your fingers, gently press along the balls in order to create the cookies. 5. Bake approximately 9 minutes or till golden brown.

767. Mango & Avocado Salad

Yield: 16 servings Preparation Time: 25 minutes

Ingredients:

For Dressing: • 2 teaspoons coconut oil • 1 cup fresh raspberries • 1 (¼-inch) piece fresh ginger, chopped • 2 teaspoons raw honey • 1 tablespoon extra-virgin olive oil • 2 tablespoons fresh lemon juice • Salt and freshly ground black pepper, to taste For Salad: • 3 large mangoes, peeled, pitted and cubed • 1 avocado, peeled, pitted and sliced • 8 radishes, trimmed and sliced thinly • 2 cups fresh baby spinach • 1 cup watercress leaves • 3 scallions, sliced thinly • 3tablespoons fresh cilantro, chopped • 2 tablespoons fresh mint leaves, chopped • 2 tablespoons fresh parsley, chopped • ½ cup sunflower seeds, shelled and toasted

Directions:

For dressing inside a small pan, melt coconut oil on medium heat. 2. Add raspberries and cook, stirring occasionally approximately 3 minutes. 3. Remove from heat and keep aside to chill slightly. 4. In a blender, add coked raspberries and remaining ingredients and pulse till smooth. 5. In a sizable bowl, add all salad ingredients except sunflower seeds and mix. 6. Pour dressing and toss to coat well. 7. Serve immediately with the garnishing of sunflower seeds.

768. Berries & Fruit Salad

Yield: 15-20 servings Preparation Time: 10 minutes

Ingredients:

For Salad: • 1 whole fresh cantaloupe, peeled, seeded and cubed • 1 whole pineapple, peeled, cored and cut into 1-inch pieces • 6 kiwi fruit, peeled and sliced • 4-5 fresh nectarine, peeled and sliced • 1 pound fresh strawberries, hulled and quartered • 1 cup fresh blueberries • 1 cup fresh black berries For Dressing: • 1-2 tablespoons fresh ginger, grated finely • 1 teaspoon fresh lime zest, grated finely • 1-2 teaspoons poppy seeds • 2 tablespoons fresh lime juice • ½ cup raw honey

Directions:

1. In a big bowl, mix together every one of the fruit. 2. In a little bowl, add dressing ingredients and beat well. 3. Place dressing over fruit mixture and toss to coat well. 4. Serve immediately.

769. Berries & Pineapple Salad

Yield: 8-10 servings Preparation Time: 20 minutes

Ingredients:

1 pineapple peeled, cored and chopped • 32-ounce fresh strawberries, hulled and sliced • 12-ounce fresh blackberries • 12-ounce fresh blueberries • 4 cups fresh baby spinach • 2-ounce gorgonzola cheese, crumbled For Dressing: • ¼ cup white onion, minced • 1½ teaspoons fresh ginger, grated • 5½ tablespoons raw honey • 1/3 cup apple cider vinegar • ¼ cup plain Greek yogurt • ¼ cup extra-virgin extra virgin olive oil • 1 teaspoon Dijon mustard • 1½ teaspoons poppy seeds • Salt, to taste

Directions:

1. In a substantial bowl, mix together all salad ingredients. 2. In a smaller bowl, add dressing ingredients and beat well. 3. Place dressing over fruit mixture and toss to coat well. 4. Serve immediately.

770. Berries & Papaya Salad

Yield: 6 servings Preparation Time: twenty or so minutes

Ingredients:

1 papaya, peeled and cubed • ½ cup fresh blackberries • ½ cup fresh blueberries • 2 tablespoons fresh ginger, minced • 2 teaspoons raw honey • 3 tablespoons fresh lime juice

Directions:

1. In a big bowl, mix together all ingredients. 2. Refrigerate before serving.

771. Kiwi & Orange Salad

Yield: 2-4 servings Preparation Time: 15 minutes

Ingredients:

For Salad: • 3 kiwi fruit, peeled and cut into chunks • 2 oranges, peeled, seeded and cut into chunks • 2 tablespoons fresh mint leaves, chopped • ¼ cup almonds, toasted and chopped For Dressing: • 1½ teaspoons fresh ginger, grated finely • 1 tablespoon raw honey • 1 tablespoon extra-virgin extra virgin olive oil • 1 tablespoon fresh lime juice

Directions:

In a substantial bowl, mix together all salad ingredients except almonds. 2. In a little bowl, add dressing ingredients and beat well. 3. Place dressing over salad mixture and toss to coat well. 4. Serve immediately while using garnishing of almonds.

772. Apple, Carrot & Beet Salad

. Yield: 8 servings Preparation Time: fifteen minutes

Ingredients:

For Salad: • 1¾ cups Brae burn apple, peeled, cored and grated • 1¾ cups beetroot, peeled and grated • 1¾ cups carrots, peeled and grated For Dressing: • 1 tablespoon fresh gingerroot, grated finely • 1 tablespoon raw honey • 3-4 tablespoons fresh lime juice • 1-3 tablespoons extra-virgin organic olive oil

Directions:

1. In a big bowl, mix together all salad ingredients. 2. In a little bowl, add dressing ingredients and beat well. 3. Place dressing over salad mixture and toss to coat well. 4. Refrigerate before serving.

773. Bok Choy & Carrot Salad

Yield: 2 servings Preparation Time: 20 min

Ingredients:

½ head bokchoy, leaves torn and white, sliced diagonally • 1 carrot, peeled and shaved with vegetable peeler • 1 small red bell pepper, seeded and sliced • 5 scallions, chopped • ¼ cup unsalted peanuts, roasted For Dressing: • 2 medium garlic cloves, chopped • 1 (1-inch) piece fresh ginger, chopped • 1 tablespoon Dijon mustard • ¼ cup olive oil • 2 tablespoons balsamic vinegar • 1 tablespoon freshly squeezed lemon juice • 1 teaspoon coconut aminos • Pinch of red pepper flakes, crushed

Directions:

1. In a substantial bowl, mix together all salad ingredients except peanuts. 2. In a mixer, add dressing ingredients and pulse till smooth. 3. Place dressing over fruit mixture and toss to coat well. 4. Serve immediately using the garnishing of peanuts.

774. Beet & Carrot Salad

Yield: 1 serving Preparation Time: 10 minutes

Ingredients:

½ cup carrot, peeled and grated • ½ cup beets, peeled and grated • ½ teaspoon fresh ginger, minced • 2 tablespoons fresh apple juice • 1 tablespoon extra-virgin olive oil • Salt, to taste

Directions:

1. In a bowl, add all ingredients and toss to coat well. 2. Serve immediately.

775. Kale Salad

Yield: 4 servings Preparation Time: 10 min Cooking Time: 30 seconds

Ingredients:

1 bunch fresh kale, chopped into 2-inch pieces • 1 tablespoon fresh ginger, minced • 2 tablespoons sesame seeds, toasted • 2 tablespoons using apple cider vinegar • 2 tablespoons sesame oil, tasted • Salt and freshly ground black pepper, to taste

Directions:

In a large pan of boiling water, cook the kale approximately half a minute. 2. Immediately, transfer the kale in a bowl of ice water. 3. Keep aside to cool completely. 4. Meanwhile in a very bowl, add all remaining ingredients and beat till well combined. 5. Drain the kale completely and transfer in to a bowl. 6. Add dressing and toss to coat well.

776. Green Beans Salad

Yield: 2 servings Preparation Time: fifteen minutes Cooking Time: 4 minutes

Ingredients:

4-5 tablespoons water • 4 cups green beans, trimmed • Salt, to taste • 1 tablespoon sesame seeds, toasted For Dressing: • 1 tablespoon fresh ginger, grated finely • 1- 1½ teaspoons raw honey • 2 tablespoons sesame oil, toasted • 1 tablespoon apple cider vinegar • Salt, to taste

Directions:

1. In a medium pan, add water and bring to a boil. 2. Add beans and sprinkle with some salt on medium-low heat. 3. Cook, covered approximately 4-5 minutes. 4. Immediately, transfer the beans right into a bowl of ice water. 5. Keep aside to cool down the completely. 6. Meanwhile in the bowl, add all dressing ingredients and beat till well combined. 7. Drain the beans completely and cut into thirds. 8. Transfer the beans into a bowl. 9. Add dressing and toss to coat well. 10. Serve which has a garnishing of sesame seeds.

777. Roasted Veggie Salad

Yield: 4 servings Preparation Time: fifteen minutes Cooking Time: twenty minutes

Ingredients:

For Dressing: • 1 cup pomegranate arils • 1 teaspoon fresh ginger, grated finely • 1 teaspoon Dijon mustard • 2 tablespoons extra-virgin essential olive oil • 1 tablespoon freshly squeezed lemon juice • ¼ teaspoon ground cinnamon • Salt and freshly ground black pepper, to taste For Salad: • 1 cup sweet potatoes, peeled and cubed • 1 cup beet, peeled and cubed • 1 cup butternut squash, peeled and cubed • 1 cup parsnips, peeled and cubed • 1 cup carrot, peeled and cubed • 1 cup Brussels sprouts, quartered • 2 tablespoons olive oil, divided • 6 cups arugula • ¼ cup pecan halves, toasted • ¼ cup pomegranate seeds

Directions:

1. Preheat the oven to 400 degrees F. Line 2 large baking sheets with parchment paper. 2. For dressing in a very mixer, add pomegranate arils and pulse till juiced. 3. In a bowl, add pomegranate juice and remaining ingredients and pulse till well combined 4. In first prepared baking sheet, add sweet potato, butternut squash, beet and 1 tablespoon of oil and toss to coat well. 5. Spread the veggie mixture in a single layer. 6. In second prepared baking sheet, add parsnip, carrot and Brussels sprouts and remaining oil and toss to coat well. 7. Spread the veggie mixture in a single layer. 8. Bake the carrot mixture for around quarter-hour, stirring once inside the midway. 9. Bake the beet mixture for about 20 min, stirring once within the midway. 10. In a big bowl, add roasted vegetables, arugula, pecans, pomegranate seeds and dressing and toss to coat well.

778. Quinoa & Veggie Salad A

Yield: 4 servings Preparation Time: twenty minutes Cooking Time: quarter-hour

Ingredients:

For Salad: • 2 cups water • 1 cup quinoa • Salt, to taste • 3 medium carrots, peeled and chopped • 1½ cups frozen edamame, shelled • 1 cup red cabbage, chopped • ½ of yellow bell pepper, seeded and chopped • ½ of red bell pepper, seeded and chopped For Dressing: • 3 tablespoons fresh ginger, minced finely • 1 tablespoon sesame seeds • 2 tablespoons sesame oil • 2 tablespoons apple cider vinegar treatment

Directions:

In a pan, add water, quinoa and salt and convey to some boil on high heat. 2. Reduce the heat to low and simmer, covered for around 15 minutes or till the liquid is absorbed. 3. Transfer the quinoa right into a large bowl. 4. Add remaining salad ingredients and stir to mix. 5. In another bowl, add all dressing ingredients and mix till well combined. 6. Place dressing over quinoa mixture and mix till well combined. 7. Serve immediately.

779. Couscous & Chickpeas Salad

Yield: 6 servings Preparation Time: twenty or so minutes Cooking Time: 4 minutes

Ingredients:

For Dressing: • 2 teaspoons fresh ginger, grated finely • 1 garlic clove, minced • ½ teaspoon raw honey • 1/3 cup fresh lime juice • 1½ tablespoons fresh lime juice • ¾ teaspoon ground cumin • Salt and freshly ground black pepper, to taste For Salad: • 2 cups water • 1½ cups uncooked couscous • ½ cup raisins • ½ teaspoon ground turmeric • 1 (15-ounce) can chickpeas, rinsed and drained • 1 cup cucumber, peeled and chopped • 1 cup tomato, chopped • ¼ cup scallion, sliced thinly • 2 tablespoons fresh mint leaves, chopped • 4-ounce feta cheese, crumbled

Directions:

1. In a bowl, add all dressing ingredients and beat till well combined. 2. In a pan, add water and provide to your boil. 3. Slowly, add couscous, raisins and turmeric and stir to blend. 4. Remove from heat and make aside, covered approximately 5 minutes. 5. With a fork, fluff the couscous and transfer into a bowl. 6. Add remaining salad ingredients and dressing and gently mix to blend.

780. Lentil & Apple Salad

Yield: 10 servings Preparation Time: quarter-hour Cooking Time: 25 minutes

Ingredients:

For Salad: • 2 cups French green lentils • 1 Granny Smith apple, cored and chopped finely • ½ cup unsalted sunflower seeds, toasted • ½ cup fresh cilantro, chopped For Dressing: • 2 teaspoons fresh ginger, grated • 2 teaspoons raw honey • ½ cup fresh lime juice • ½ cup extra-virgin olive oil • Salt and freshly ground black pepper, to taste

Directions: 1. In a substantial pan of water, add lentils on high heat and produce to some boil. 2. Reduce the heat to low and simmer, covered for around 22-25 minutes. 3. Drain completely and transfer in to a large bowl and make aside to chill. 4. Add remaining salad ingredients and mix. 5. In another bowl, add all dressing ingredients and beat till well combined. 6. Place dressing over lentils mixture and mix till well combined. 7. Serve immediately.

781. Creamy Chicken Salad

Yield: 4-6 servings Preparation Time: quarter-hour

Ingredients:

1 large ripe avocado, peeled, pitted and chopped • ½ cup coconut cream • 1 tablespoon fresh lemon juice • 2 teaspoons ground turmeric • ½ teaspoon onion powder • ½ teaspoon garlic powder • Salt, to taste • 1 pound cooked skinless, boneless chicken breasts, shredded • ¼ cup fresh parsley, chopped • 2 scallions, chopped

Directions: 1. In a food processor, add avocado, coconut cream, lemon juice, turmeric, onion powder, garlic powder and salt and pulse till smooth. 2. Transfer a combination in to a bowl. 3. Add chicken, parsley and scallion and stir to mix.

782. Chicken Salad

Yield: 4 servings Preparation Time: 20 minutes

Ingredients:

For Dressing: • 1 cup raw cashews • ½ cup water • 1 (1-inch) pieces fresh turmeric, grated finely • 2 tablespoons fresh parsley, chopped • ¾ teaspoon Dijon mustard • 1 tablespoon extra-virgin olive oil • 2 teaspoons fresh lemon juice • 2 teaspoons coconut aminos • 1 teaspoon apple cider vinegar • Salt and freshly ground black pepper, to taste For salad: • 3 cups cooked chicken, chopped • 1 shallot, chopped finely • 2 celery ribs, chopped finely

Directions: 1. For cashew cream in a very blender, add cashews and water and pulse till a whipped cream like consis10cy forms. 2. For dressing in a bowl, add cashew cream and remaining dressing ingredients and mix till well combined. 3. In another large bowl, mix together salad ingredients. 4. Pour dressing over salad and toss to coat well. 5. Serve immediately.

783. Chicken & Cabbage Salad

Yield: 4 servings Preparation Time: 25 minutes Cooking Time: 12 minutes

Ingredients:

For Chicken Marinade: • ¼ cup scallion, chopped • 2 tablespoons fresh ginger, minced • ¼ cup coconut aminos • ¼ cup olive oil • 1 tablespoon honey • Salt and freshly ground black pepper, to taste • 2 skinless, boneless chicken breasts For Salad: • ¼ cup balsamic vinegar • 2 cups red cabbage, shredded • 1 cup green cabbage, shredded • 2 cups carrots, peeled and shredded • 4 cups fresh kale, trimmed and chopped • 3 scallions, chopped

Directions:

1. For chicken in a very bowl, mix together all ingredients except chicken. 2. In another bowl, coat chicken with 3 tablespoons of marinade. 3. Refrigerate to marinate approximately 30-60 minutes. 4. For dressing in a very bowl, mix together remaining marinade and vinegar. 5. Preheat the grill to medium-high heat. Grease the grill grate. 6. Remove chicken from refrigerator and discard any excess marinade. 7. Grill for about 5-6 minutes per side. 8. Remove from grill whilst aside to cool down the slightly. 9. Cut the chicken breasts in thin slices. 10. In a large serving bowl, mix together salad ingredients. 11. Add dressing and toss to coat well. 12. Top with chicken slices and serve.

784. Beef & Broccoli Salad

Yield: 4 servings Preparation Time: 15 minutes Cooking Time: 7 minutes

Ingredients:

For Dressing: • 2 tablespoons shallots, minced • 1 tablespoon fresh ginger, minced • ½ cup extra-virgin essential olive oil • 2 tablespoons fresh lime juice • 1 tablespoon balsamic vinegar • Salt and freshly ground black pepper, to taste For Salad: • 3 cups broccoli florets • 1 pound beef sirloin steak, trimmed and cut into thin strips • 1 red bell pepper, seeded and sliced thinly • 1 red onion, sliced thinly • 8 cups fresh baby salad greens

Directions:

1. In a bowl, add all dressing ingredients and beat till well combined. 2. Ina skillet, add 2 tablespoons of dressing as well as heat on medium-high heat. 3. Add broccoli and cook for about 3 minutes. 4. Add beef and stir fry approximately 3-4 minutes. 5. Remove from heat whilst aside to cool slightly. 6. In a big serving bowl, mix together beef mixture and remaining salad ingredients. 7. Add dressing and toss to coat well.

785. Salmon, Orange & Beet Salad

Yield: 1-2 servings Preparation Time: fifteen minutes

Ingredients:

For Salad: • 6-ounce cooked salmon, chopped • 1 large orange, peeled, seeded and chopped roughly • ½ cup cooked beets, peeled and chopped • ¼ of avocado, peeled, pitted and chopped • 1 small red onion, chopped • 3 cups lettuce, torn • 10 pistachios, chopped For Dressing: • ½ teaspoon fresh orange zest, grated finely • 2 tablespoons fresh orange juice • 1 tablespoon extra-virgin olive oil • 2 teaspoons balsamic vinegar • ½ teaspoon Dijon mustard • ¼-½ teaspoon red chili powder • Salt and freshly ground black pepper, to taste

Directions:

In a big bowl, mix together all salad ingredients. 2. In another bowl, add all dressing ingredients and mix till well combined. 3. Place dressing over quinoa mixture and mix till well combined. 4. Serve immediately.

786. Salmon & Tomato Salad

Yield: 2 servings Preparation Time: 10 minutes

Ingredients:

1 (14-ounce) can salmon, flaked • 1 large tomato, chopped • 1 bunch fresh parsley. Chopped • 1 tablespoon fresh lime juice • Freshly ground black pepper, to taste

Directions:

1. In a substantial bowl, add all ingredients and toss to coat well. 2. Refrigerate to chill before serving.

787. Grilled Veggies

Yield: 6 servings Preparation Time: twenty or so minutes Cooking Time: 12 minutes

Ingredients:

¼ cup essential olive oil • 4 teaspoons balsamic vinegar • 2tablespoons raw honey • 1 teaspoon dried oregano, crushed • 1 teaspoon ground cumin • 12 teaspoon garlic powder • Salt and freshly ground black pepper, to taste • 3 small carrots, peeled and halved lengthwise • 1 medium yellow squash, cut into ½-inch slices • 1 large red bell pepper, seeded and cut into1-inch strips • 1 pound fresh as asparagus, trimmed • 1 medium red onion, cut into wedges

Directions:

1. In a tiny bowl, mix together all ingredients except vegetables. 2. In a substantial bowl, add 3 tablespoons of marinade, reserving the residual. 3. Add vegetables and toss to coat well. 4. Keep aside, covered approximately 1½ hours. 5. Preheat the grill to medium heat. Grease the grill grate. 6. Place the vegetables over grill grate inside a single layer and arrange in the grill rack. 7. Grill, covered approximately 8-12 minutes, flipping occasionally.

788. Broccolini& Bell Pepper

Yield: 2-3 servings Preparation Time: 15 minutes Cooking Time: 12 minutes

Ingredients:

For Mushroom Marinade: • 2 teaspoons fresh ginger, minced • 2 minced garlic cloves • 3-4 tablespoons organic honey • 3-4 tablespoons coconut aminos • 3 tablespoons fresh lime juice • 1 tablespoon sesame oil • 1 tablespoon water • 2 Portobello mushrooms, sliced into thin strips For Vegetables: • 1 tablespoon sesame seeds • 1 cup broccolini, chopped • 1 red bell pepper, seeded and sliced thinly • 1 cup scallion, chopped

Directions:

For mushrooms in a big bowl, add all ingredients except mushrooms and mix till well combined. 2. Add mushrooms and coat with marinade generously. 3. Keep aside for about 10-12 minutes. 4. In a big nonstick skillet, heat sesame oil on medium heat. 5. Remove the mushrooms from marinade and add inside skillet in 2 batches and sauté for approximately 2-4 minutes per side. 6. Transfer the mushrooms in a very bowl and cover which has a foil paper to maintain warm. 7. In exactly the same skillet, add broccolini and bell pepper and sauté for about 2-3 minutes. 8. Add scallion and then for any remaining marinade from the bowl and sauté approximately 1 minute. 9. Remove from heat and immediately mix with mushrooms. 10. Serve immediately.

789. Mushroom with Spinach

Yield: 2 servings Preparation Time: quarter-hour Cooking Time: 13 minutes

Ingredients:

1 teaspoon coconut oil • 5-6 button mushrooms, sliced • 2 tablespoons olive oil • ½ of red onion, sliced • 1 garlic oil, minced • ½ teaspoon fresh lemon rind, grated finely • ¼ cup cherry tomatoes, halved • Salt and freshly ground black pepper, to taste • Pinch of ground nutmeg • 3 cups fresh spinach, torn • ½ tablespoon fresh lemon juice

Directions:

1. I a skillet, melt coconut oil on medium heat. 2. Add mushrooms and sauté for around 3-4 minutes. 3. Transfer the mushrooms in a bowl and make aside. 4. In a similar skillet, heat olive oil on medium heat. 5. Add onion and sauté for about 2-3 minutes. 6. Add garlic, lemon rind and tomatoes, salt and black pepper and cook approximately 2-3 minutes, revealing the tomatoes slightly which has a spatula. 7. Stir inside spinach and cook for approximately 2-3 minutes. 8. Stir in mushrooms and freshly squeezed lemon juice and take off from heat. 9. Serve hot.

790. Mixed Root Vegetables & Kale

Yield: 6-8 servings Preparation Time: fifteen minutes Cooking Time: 20 minutes

Ingredients:

2 tablespoons essential olive oil • 1 large sweet onion, chopped • 1 medium parsnip, peeled and chopped • 2 minced garlic cloves • 3 tablespoons tomato paste • 1 teaspoon ground cumin • ½ teaspoon ground cinnamon • ½ teaspoon ground ginger • ¼ tsp cayenne • Salt and freshly ground black pepper, to taste • 2 medium carrots, peeled and chopped • 2 medium purple potatoes, peeled and chopped • 2 medium sweet potatoes, peeled and chopped • 4 cups vegetable broth • 2 cups fresh kale, trimmed and chopped roughly • 2 tablespoons fresh lemon juice • ¼ cup fresh cilantro, chopped

Directions:

1. In a sizable soup pan, heat oil on medium-high heat. 2. Add onion and sauté approximately 5 minutes. 3. Add parsnip and cook approximately 3 minutes. 4. Add garlic, tomato paste and spices and sauté for approximately 2 minutes. 5. Add carrots, potatoes, sweet potatoes and broth and bring with a boil. 6. Reduce the warmth to medium-low and simmer for about 20 min, stirring occasionally. 7. Stir in kale and freshly squeezed lemon juice and simmer approximately 2-3 minutes. 8. Garnish with cilantro and serve.

791. Veggie Curry

Yield: 2-4 servings Preparation Time: quarter-hour Cooking Time: 22 minutes

Ingredients:

2 teaspoons coconut oil • 1 small white onion, chopped • 2 garlic cloves, chopped finely • 1 tablespoon fresh ginger, chopped finely • Salt, to taste • 3 carrots, peeled and cut into ¾-inch round slices • 2 cups asparagus, trimmed and cut into 2-inch pieces • 2 tablespoons green curry paste • 1½ teaspoons coconut sugar • 1 (14-ounce) can coconut milk • ½ cup water • 2 cups fresh baby spinach, chopped roughly • 1½ teaspoons coconut aminos • 1½ teaspoons balsamic vinegar • Crushed red pepper flakes, to taste

Directions:

In a substantial deep skillet, melt coconut oil on medium heat. 2. Add onion, garlic, ginger as well as a pinch of salt and sauté for around 5 minutes. 3. Add carrots and asparagus and cook, stirring occasionally for around 3 minutes. 4. Stir inside the curry paste and cook, stirring occasionally for approximately 2 minutes. 5. Add coconut sugar, coconut milk and water and provide to a gentle simmer. 6. Cook for about 5-10 minutes or till desired doneness of vegetables. 7. Stir within the spinach and cook for approximately 1 minute. 8. Stir in coconut aminos, vinegar, salt and red pepper flakes and take away from heat. 9. Serve hot.

792. Spicy Mixed Veggies

Yield: 6 servings Preparation Time: 25 minutes Cooking Time: 35 minutes

Ingredients:

2 tablespoons extra virgin olive oil • 1 teaspoon mustard seeds • 2 onions, chopped finely • 2 fresh green chilies, seeded and chopped • 1 bunch curry leaves • ½ teaspoon garam masala • ½ teaspoon ground cumin • ½ teaspoon ground coriander • ¼ teaspoon ground turmeric • ¼ teaspoon red chili powder • 6 tomatoes, chopped • 1 eggplant, cubed • 2 potatoes, peeled and cubed • 2 sweet potatoes, peeled and cubed • ½ cup coconut milk • ½ cup okra, trimmed and chopped • ½ cup French beans • ½ cup fresh peas, shelled • Salt and freshly ground black pepper, to taste

Directions:

1. In a sizable pan, heat oil on medium heat. 2. Add mustard seeds and sauté for about 1 minute. 3. Add onion, green chilies, curry leaves and spices and sauté for approximately 4-5 minutes. 4. Add tomatoes and cook approximately 2-3 minutes. 5. Stir in eggplant, potatoes, sweet potatoes and coconut milk and provide to some gentle simmer. 6. Reduce the warmth to medium-low. 7. Simmer, covered for about 15-twenty minutes or till desired doneness. 8. Stir in the remaining ingredients and cook for around 5 minutes. 9. Serve hot.

793. Stuffed Bell Peppers

Yield: 4 servings Preparation Time: 15 minutes Cooking Time: 23 minutes (plus time of brown rice)

Ingredients:

1 cup brown rice, rinsed and drained • 2 cups vegetable broth • 1 tablespoon coconut oil • 1 small can unswee10ed sweet corn • 1 (15-ounce) can kidney beans, rinsed and drained • 2 teaspoons ground cumin • 1 teaspoon ground turmeric • 1 teaspoon garlic powder • 1 teaspoon red chili powder • Salt and freshly ground black pepper, to taste • 2 tablespoons fresh parsley, chopped • 4 large peppers, tops and seeds removed

Directions:

1. Preheat the oven to 375 degrees F. Grease a large baking sheet. 2. Prepare the brown rice as outlined by package's directions in vegetable broth. 3. In a substantial nonstick skillet, melt coconut oil on medium heat. 4. Add cooked rice, corns, beans and spices and cook for around 2-3 minutes. 5. Stir in parsley and take off from heat. 6. Stuff the sweet peppers with rice mixture evenly. 7. Arrange the bell peppers in prepared baking sheet. 8. Bake for around 15-20 minutes.

794. Veggies with Green Lentils

Yield: 4 servings Preparation Time: 20 minutes Cooking Time: 37 minutes

Ingredients:

1 tbsp extra virgin olive oil • 1 onion, chopped • 2 minced garlic cloves • 1 teaspoon fresh ginger, minced • 1 russet potato, peeled and chopped • 1 large carrot, peeled and chopped • 2celery stalks, chopped • 1 zucchini, chopped • 1½ cups green lentils, soaked for about quarter-hour and drained • 3 cups canned tomatoes • 1 teaspoon ground cumin • 1 teaspoon ground coriander • 1 teaspoon ground turmeric • ½ teaspoon cayenne • Salt and freshly ground black pepper, to taste • 2½ cups water • ½ cup fresh parsley, chopped

Directions:

In a large pan, heat oil on medium heat. 2. Add onion, garlic and ginger and sauté for about 4-5 minutes. 3. Add vegetables and cook for about 5-7 minutes. 4. Stir in lentils, tomatoes, spices and water and bring to some boil. 5. Boil for around 5 minutes, stirring occasionally. 6. Reduce heat to low and simmer, covered for about twenty or so minutes. 7. Stir in parsley and remove from heat.

795. Spicy Black Beans

Yield: 6 servings Preparation Time: quarter-hour Cooking Time: 1 hour 25 minutes

Ingredients:

4 cups water • 1½ cups dried black beans, soaked for 8 hours and drained • ½ teaspoon ground turmeric • 3 tablespoons organic olive oil • 1 teaspoon cumin seeds • 1 teaspoon black mustard seeds • 1 small onion, chopped finely • 2 green chilies, chopped • 1 (1-inch) piece fresh ginger, minced • 1 garlic oil minced • 1 tablespoon dried curry leaves • 1 tablespoon dried fenugreek leaves • 1½ tablespoons ground coriander • 1 teaspoon garam masala • 1 teaspoon ground cumin • ½ teaspoon mustard powder • ½ teaspoon ground turmeric • ½ teaspoon cayenne pepper • Salt, to taste • 2 medium tomatoes, chopped finely • ½ cup fresh cilantro, chopped

Directions:

1. In a substantial pan, add water, black beans and turmeric and produce to some boil on high heat. 2. Reduce the warmth to low and simmer, covered for around 1 hour or till desired doneness of beans. 3. Meanwhile in the skillet, heat oil on medium heat. 4. Add cumin seeds and mustard seeds and sauté for about 1 minute. 5. Add onion and sauté for about 4-5 minutes. 6. Add green chilies, ginger and garlic and sauté for approximately 1-2 minutes. 7. Add dried leaves and spices and sauté for around 1 minute. 8. Stir in tomatoes and cook, stirring occasionally for about 10 min. 9. Transfer the tomato mixture in the pan with black beans and stir to blend on medium-low heat. 10. Simmer approximately 15-20 minutes. 11. Stir in cilantro and simmer approximately 5 minutes. 12. Serve hot.

796. Vegetables Chili

Yield: 10 servings Preparation Time: 20 min Cooking Time: an hour 10 min

Ingredients:

For Spice Mixture: • 1 teaspoon ground cinnamon • ½ teaspoon ground nutmeg • 1/8 teaspoon ground cloves • 1 tablespoon red chili powder • ¼ tsp red pepper cayenne • Salt, to taste For Chili: • 2 teaspoons organic olive oil • 1 medium onion, chopped • 1 jalapeño pepper, seeded and chopped • 2 tablespoons fresh ginger, minced • 2 large garlic cloves, minced • 4 large Portobello mushrooms, stemmed and cubed • 2 medium carrots, peeled and cubed • 1 (15-ounce) can black beans, rinsed and drained • 2 cups frozen corns • 1 (28-ounce) can fire roasted tomatoes • 1 (15-ounce) can pumpkin puree • 2 cups vegetable broth

Directions:

1. For spice mixture in the bowl, mix together all ingredients. Keep aside. 2. In a sizable pan, heat oil on medium heat. 3. Add onion, jalapeño pepper, ginger and garlic and sauté for approximately 3-4 minutes. 4. Add mushrooms and carrots and cook, stirring occasionally for about 6 minutes. 5. Stir in spice mixture and remaining ingredients and bring to some boil. 6. Reduce the heat to medium-low and simmer, covered for about 20 min. 7. Stir in beans and jalapeño pepper and simmer for approximately 40-45 minutes. 8. Serve hot.

797. Chickpeas Chili

Yield: 4 servings Preparation Time: quarter-hour Cooking Time: 25 minutes

Ingredients:

2 teaspoons olive oil • 1 cup onion, chopped • ½ cup carrot, peeled and chopped • ¾ cup celery, chopped • 1 teaspoon garlic, minced • 2 teaspoons ground cumin • 1 teaspoon ground ginger • ½ teaspoon ground turmeric • 1/8 teaspoon ground cinnamon • 2 teaspoons paprika • 1/8 teaspoon red chili powder • Salt and freshly ground black pepper, to taste • 2 (15½-ounce) cans chickpeas, rinsed and drained • 1 (14½-ounce) can salt-free diced tomatoes • 2 tablespoons salt-free tomato paste • 1½ cups water • 1 tablespoon fresh lemon juice • 2 tablespoons fresh cilantro, chopped

Directions: 1. In a large pan, heat oil on medium heat. 2. Add onion, carrot, celery and garlic and sauté for around 5 minutes. 3. Add spices and sauté for around 1 minute. 4. Add chickpeas, tomatoes, tomato paste and water and produce to a boil. 5. Reduce heat to low and simmer, covered for about twenty minutes. 6. Stir in freshly squeezed lemon juice and cilantro and remove from heat. 7. Serve hot.

798. Grains Chili

. Yield: 12 servings Preparation Time: fifteen minutes Cooking Time: 51 minutes

Ingredients:

2 tablespoons organic olive oil • 2 shallots, chopped • 1 large yellow onion, chopped • 1 tablespoon fresh ginger, grated finely • 8 garlic cloves, minced • 1 teaspoon ground cumin • 3 tablespoons red chili powder • Salt and freshly ground black pepper, to taste • 1 (28-ounce) can crushed tomatoes • 1 canned chipotle pepper, minced • 1 Serrano pepper, seeded and chopped finely • 2/3 cup bulgur wheat • 2/3 cup pearl barley • 2¼ cups mixed lentils (green, black, brown), rinsed • 1½ cups canned chickpeas • 3 scallions, chopped

Directions:

1. In a big pan heat oil on medium heat. 2. Add shallot and onion and sauté for around 4-5 minutes. 3. Add ginger, garlic, cumin and chili powder and sauté for about 1 minute. 4. Stir in tomatoes, both peppers and broth. 5. Stir inside remaining ingredients except the scallion and produce to a boil. 6. Reduce the temperature to low and simmer for about 35-45 minutes or till desired thickness with the chili. 7. Serve hot using the topping of scallion.

799. Red Lentils with Spinach

Yield: 4 servings Preparation Time: quarter-hour Cooking Time: 30 minutes

Ingredients:

3½ cups water • 1½ cups red lentils, soaked for 20 min and drained • ½ teaspoon red chili powder • ½ teaspoon ground turmeric • Salt, to taste • 1 pound fresh spinach, chopped • 2 tablespoons coconut oil • 1 onion, chopped • 1 teaspoon mustard seeds • 1 teaspoon ground cumin • ½ cup coconut milk • 1 teaspoon garam masala

Directions:

1. In a large pan, add water, lentils, red chili powder, turmeric and salt and produce to your boil on high heat. 2. Reduce the warmth to low and simmer, covered for about 15 minutes. 3. Stir in spinach and simmer for approximately 5 minutes. 4. In a frying pan, melt coconut oil on medium heat. 5. Add onion, mustard seeds and cumin and sauté approximately 4-5 minutes. 6. Transfer the onion mixture in the pan using the lentils and stir to combine. 7. Stir in coconut milk and garam masala and simmer for about 3-4 minutes. 8. Serve hot.

800. Quinoa with Veggies

Yield: 3 servings Preparation Time: fifteen minutes Cooking Time: 35 minutes

Ingredients:

2 tablespoons essential olive oil • 1 small onion, minced • 2 carrots, peeled and sliced • 1 celery stalk, chopped • 1 garlic clove, minced • ½ cup uncooked quinoa, rinsed • 1 teaspoon ground turmeric • ¼ teaspoon dried basil, crushed • Salt, to taste • 1 cup vegetable broth • 1 teaspoon fresh lime juice

Directions:

In a pan, heat oil on medium heat. 2. Add onion, carrot, celery and garlic and sauté for around t minutes. 3. Stir in remaining ingredients except lime juice and bring with a gentle simmer. 4. Reduce heat to low and simmer, covered for about 25-30 minutes or till all of the liquid is absorbed. 5. Stir in lime juice and serve.

801. Quinoa & Beans with Veggies

Yield: 6 servings Preparation Time: 20 minutes Cooking Time: 26 minutes

Ingredients:

2 cups water • 1 cup dry quinoa • 2 tablespoons coconut oil • 1 medium onion, chopped • 4 garlic cloves, chopped finely • 2 tablespoons curry powder • ½ teaspoon ground turmeric • Cayenne pepper, to taste • Salt, to taste • 2 cups broccoli, chopped • 1 cup fresh kale, trimmed and chopped • 1 cup green peas, shelled • 1 red bell pepper, seeded and chopped • 2 cups canned kidney beans, rinsed and drained • 2 tablespoons fresh lime juice

Directions:

1. In a pan, add water and convey to a boil on high heat. 2. Add quinoa minimizing heat to low. 3. Simmer for around 10-15 minutes or till every one of the liquid is absorbed. 4. In a sizable skillet, melt coconut oil on medium heart. 5. Add onion, garlic, curry powder, turmeric and salt and sauté approximately 4-5 minutes. 6. Add the vegetables and cook approximately 5-6 minutes. 7. Stir in quinoa and beans, 8. Drizzle with lime juice and serve.

802. Brown Rice & Cherries Pilaf

Yield: 8 servings Preparation Time: 20 min Cooking Time: 35 minutes

Ingredients:

1 (14-ounce) can low-sodium vegetable broth • 1/3 cup water • 1 cup brown basmati rice • 1 tablespoon curry powder • ½ teaspoon ground turmeric • Pinch of saffron threads, crumbled • 1/3 cup fresh lemon juice • 3 tablespoons organic olive oil • 3 tablespoons raw honey • 1 tablespoon fresh ginger, minced • 1 tablespoon fresh orange zest, grated finely • Salt, to taste • ¾ cup celery stalk, chopped • ½ cup scallion, chopped, divided • ¾ cup dried cherries, chopped roughly • 1 cup fresh dark sweet cherries, pitted and chopped • ¾ cup unsalted mixed nuts

Directions:

1. In a pan, mix together broth, water, rice, curry powder, turmeric and saffron and produce with a boil on medium-high heat. 2. Reduce the warmth to low and simmer, covered for around 35 minutes. 3. Remove from heat and keep aside, covered approximately 5 minutes. 4. With a fork, fluff the rice. 5. In a large glass bowl, mix together lemon juice, oil, honey, ginger, orange zest and salt. 6. Stir in cooked rice, celery, ¼ cup of scallion and dried cherries. 7. Serve immediately using the topping of fresh cherries, nuts and remaining scallion.

803. Rice, Lentils & Veggie Casserole

Yield: 10 servings Preparation Time: twenty or so minutes Cooking Time: 60 minutes 36 minutes

Ingredients:

3¾ cups water, divided • ½ cup brown lentils, rinsed • ½ cup wild rice, rinsed • 1 tbsp organic olive oil • ½ of medium onion, chopped • 1 cup button mushrooms, sliced • 1 cup tomato sauce • 1 (10-ounce) package frozen spinach, thawed and squeezed • 1 (16-ounce) package frozen peas, thawed • 2 minced garlic cloves • 1 tablespoon dried oregano, crushed • 1 teaspoon smoked paprika • ½ teaspoon ground turmeric • ¼ cup nutritional yeast For Sauce • 1¼ cups unswee1oed almond milk • 1 cup unsalted cashews, soaked for half an hour and drained • 1 teaspoon coconut aminos • ½ teaspoon dried garlic

Directions:

1. In a pan, add 3 ½ servings of water, lentils and rice and convey to a boil. 2. Reduce the temperature to low and simmer, covered for about 35 minutes. 3. Remove from heat whilst aside to cool. 4. Preheat the oven to 350 degrees F. Grease a 13x9-inch casserole dish. 5. In a substantial skillet, heat 2 tablespoons of water on high heat. 6. Add onion and sauté for around 2-3 minutes. 7. Add mushrooms and cook for approximately 2 minutes. 8. Add remaining 2 tablespoons of water and remaining ingredients except nutritional yeast and cook approximately 1 minute. 9. Remove from heat and mix with rice mixture. 10. Transfer the amalgamation into prepared casserole dish evenly. 11. In a blender, add all sauce ingredients and pulse till smooth. 12. Spread the sauce in the rice mixture evenly and stir to mix well. 13. Top with nutritional yeast evenly. 14. Bake for approximately 45 minutes.

804. Okra Fries

. Yield: 4 servings Preparation Time: quarter-hour Cooking Time: 35 minutes

Ingredients:

2 tablespoons olive oil, divided • 3 tablespoons creole seasoning • ½ teaspoon ground turmeric • 1 teaspoon water • 1 pound okra, trimmed and slit in middle

Directions:

1. Preheat the oven to 450 degrees F. Line a baking sheet which has a foil paper and grease with 1 tablespoon of oil. 2. In a bowl, mix together creole seasoning, turmeric and water. 3. Fill the slits of okra with turmeric mixture. 4. Place the okra onto prepared baking sheet in a very single layer. 5. Bake for around 30-35 minutes, flipping once inside middle way.

805. Potato Sticks

Yield: 2 servings Preparation Time: quarter-hour Cooking Time: 10 min

Ingredients:

1 large russet potato, peeled and cut into 1/8-inch thick sticks lengthwise • 10 curry leaves • ¼ teaspoon ground turmeric • ¼ teaspoon red chili powder • Salt, to taste • 1 tbsp essential olive oil

Directions:

1. Preheat the oven to 400 degrees F. Line 2 baking sheets with parchment papers. 2. In a sizable bowl, add all ingredients and toss to coat well. 3. Transfer the amalgamation into prepared baking sheets in the single layer. 4. Bake for around 10 minutes. 5. Serve immediately.

806. Beet Chips

Yield: 2 servings Preparation Time: quarter-hour Cooking Time: 20 minutes

Ingredients:

1 beetroot, trimmed, peeled and sliced thinly • 1 teaspoon garlic, minced • 1 tablespoon nutritional yeast • ½ teaspoon red chili powder • 2 teaspoons coconut oil, melted

Directions:

1. Preheat the oven to 375 degrees F. Line a baking sheet using a parchment paper. 2. In a large bowl, add all ingredients and toss to coat well. 3. Transfer the mixture into prepared baking sheet in a very single layer. 4. Bake approximately twenty minutes, flipping once inside the middle way. 5. Serve immediately.

807. Spinach Chips

Yield: 1 serving Preparation Time: 10 minutes Cooking Time: 8 minutes

Ingredients:

2 cups fresh spinach leaves • Few drops of extra-virgin olive oil • Salt, to taste • Italian seasoning, to taste

Directions:

Preheat the oven to 325 degrees F. Line a baking sheet with a parchment paper. 2. In a substantial bowl, add spinach leaves and drizzle with oil. 3. With the hands, rub the spinach leaves till al the leaves are coated with oil. 4. Transfer the leaves into prepared baking sheet in a very single layer. 5. Bake for about 8 minutes. 6. Serve immediately.

808. Apple Chips

Yield: 8 servings Preparation Time: quarter-hour Cooking Time: couple of hours

Ingredients:

Salt and freshly ground black pepper, to taste • 2 tablespoons ground cinnamon • 1 tablespoon ground ginger • 1½ teaspoons ground cloves • 1½ teaspoons ground nutmeg • 3 Fuji apples, sliced thinly in rounds

Directions:

1. Preheat the oven to 200 degrees F. Line a baking sheet with a parchment paper. 2. In a bowl, mix together all spices. 3. Arrange the apple slices into prepared baking sheet in the single layer. 4. Sprinkle the apple slices with spice mixture generously. 5. Roast for around an hour. 6. Flip the medial side and sprinkle with spice mixture. 7. Serve immediately. 8. Bake approximately one hour.

809. Fruit Crackers

Yield: 15 servings Preparation Time: 20 minutes Cooking Time: 12 hours

Ingredients:

8 carrots • 1 orange, peeled • 1 apple • 1 (1-inch) piece fresh ginger • 1 onion • 1 cup chia seeds • ½ cup sesame seeds • 1 tablespoon ground turmeric • Salt and freshly ground black pepper, to taste

Directions:

1. In a juicer, add carrots and extract juice based on manufacturer's directions. 2. In a bowl, transfer the carrot juice and pulp. 3. Now, in juicer, add orange, apple and ginger and extract the juice. 4. Transfer the juice inside the bowl with carrot juice and pulp. 5. In a food processor, add juice mixture and remaining ingredients and pulse till a puree forms. 6. Spread a combination into 3 dehydrator trays evenly. 7. With a knife, score how big crackers. 8. Set dehydrator at 115 degrees F. 9. Dehydrate for about 12 hours.

810. Quinoa & Seeds Crackers

Yield: 6 servings Preparation Time: 15 minutes Cooking Time: twenty or so minutes

Ingredients:

3 tablespoons water • 1 tablespoon chia seeds • 3 tablespoons sunflower seeds • 1 tablespoon quinoa flour • 1 teaspoon ground turmeric • Pinch of ground cinnamon • Salt, to taste

Directions:

1. Preheat the oven to 345 degrees F. Line a baking sheet with parchment paper. 2. In a bowl, add water and chia seeds and soak for approximately quarter-hour. 3. After fifteen minutes, add remaining ingredients and mix well. 4. Spread the mix onto prepared baking sheet. 5. Bake approximately 20 min.

811. Roasted Cashews O

Yield: 16 servings Preparation Time: 5 minutes Cooking Time: twenty or so minutes

Ingredients:

2 cups cashews • 2 teaspoons raw honey • 1½ teaspoons smoked paprika • ½ teaspoon chili flakes • Salt, to taste • 1 tablespoon freshly squeezed lemon juice • 1 teaspoon organic olive oil

Directions:

1. Preheat the oven to 350 degrees F. Line a baking dish with a parchment paper. 2. In a bowl, add all ingredients and toss to coat well. 3. Transfer the cashew mixture into prepared baking dish inside a single layer. 4. Roast for approximately 20 min, flipping once inside middle way. 5. Remove from oven and make aside to cool completely before serving. 6. You can preserve these roasted cashews in airtight jar.

812. Roasted Pumpkin Seeds

Yield: 4 servings Preparation Time: 10 minutes Cooking Time: 20 min

Ingredients:

1 cup pumpkin seeds, washed and dried • 2 teaspoons garam masala • 1/3 teaspoon red chili powder • ¼ teaspoon ground turmeric • Salt, to taste • 3 tablespoons coconut oil, meted • ½ tablespoon fresh lemon juice

Directions:

1. Preheat the oven to 350 degrees F. 2. In a bowl, add all ingredients except lemon juice and toss to coat well. 3. Transfer the almond mixture right into a baking sheet. 4. Roast approximately twenty or so minutes, flipping occasionally. 5. Remove from oven and make aside to cool completely before serving. 6. Drizzle with freshly squeezed lemon juice and serve.

813. Spiced Popcorn

Yield: 2-3 servings Preparation Time: 5 minutes Cooking Time: 2 minutes

Ingredients:

3 tablespoons coconut oil • ½ cup popping corn • 1 tbsp olive oil • 1 teaspoon ground turmeric • ¼ teaspoon garlic powder • Salt, to taste

Directions:

1. In a pan, melt coconut oil on medium-high heat. 2. Add popping corn and cover the pan tightly. 3. Cook, shaking the pan occasionally for around 1-2 minutes or till corn kernels begin to pop. 4. Remove from heat and transfer right into a large heatproof bowl. 5. Add essential olive oil and spices and mix well. 6. Serve immediately

814. Spinach Fritters

Yield: 2-3 servings Preparation Time: 15 minutes Cooking Time: 5 minutes

Ingredients:

2 cups chickpea flour • ¾ teaspoons white sesame seeds • ½ teaspoon garam masala powder • ½ teaspoon red chili powder • ¼ teaspoon ground cumin • 2 pinches of baking soda • Salt, to taste • 1 cup water • 12-14 fresh spinach leaves • Olive oil, for frying

Directions:

1. In a sizable bowl, add all ingredients except spinach and oil and mix till an easy mixture forms. 2. In a sizable skillet, heat oil on medium heat. 3. Dip each spinach leaf in chickpea flour mixture evenly and place in the hot oil in batches. 4. Cook, flipping occasionally for about 3-5 minutes or till golden brown from each side. 5. Transfer the fritters onto paper towel lined plate.

815. Chicken Popcorn

Yield: 2 servings Preparation Time: quarter-hour Cooking Time: 25 minutes

Ingredients:

½ pound chicken thigh, cut into bite-sized pieces • 7-ounce coconut milk • 1-2 teaspoons ground turmeric • Salt and freshly ground black pepper, to taste • 2 tablespoons coconut flour • 3 tablespoons desiccated coconut • 1 tablespoon coconut oil, melted

Directions:

1. In a large bowl, mix together chicken, coconut milk, turmeric, salt and black pepper. 2. Cover and refrigerate to marinate for overnight. 3. Preheat the oven to 390 degrees F. 4. In a shallow dish, mix together coconut flour and desiccated coconut. 5. Coat the chicken pieces in coconut mixture evenly. 6. Arrange chicken piece right into a baking sheet. 7. Drizzle with oil evenly. 8. Bake for around 20-25 minutes.

816. Quinoa & Veggie Croquettes

Yield: 12-15 servings Preparation Time: 15 minutes Cooking Time: 9 minutes

Ingredients:

1 tbsp essential olive oil • ½ cup frozen peas, thawed • 2 minced garlic cloves • 1 cup cooked quinoa • 2 large boiled potatoes, peeled and mashed • ¼ cup fresh cilantro leaves, chopped • 2 teaspoons ground cumin • 1 teaspoon garam masala • ¼ teaspoon ground turmeric • Salt and freshly ground black pepper, to taste • Olive oil, for frying

Directions:

1. In a frying pan, heat oil on medium heat. 2. Add peas and garlic and sauté for about 1 minute. 3. Transfer the pea mixture into a large bowl. 4. Add remaining ingredients and mix till well combined. 5. Make equal sized oblong shaped patties from your mixture. 6. In a large skillet, heat oil on medium-high heat. 7. Add croquettes and fry for about 4 minutes per side.

817. Lamb Burgers

Yield: 6 servings Preparation Time: 15 minutes Cooking Time: 8 minutes

Ingredients:

1½ pound ground lamb • 3 scallions, chopped • 1 tablespoon fresh ginger, grated finely • Salt and freshly ground black pepper, to taste

Directions:

1. Preheat the grill to medium heat. Grease the grill gate. 2. In a bowl, add all ingredients and mix till well combined. 3. Make equal sized small patties from your mixture. 4. Grill the patties for about 4 minutes from either side.

818. Quinoa & Beans Burgers

Yield: 12 servings Preparation Time: quarter-hour Cooking Time: 55 minutes

Ingredients:

½ cup dry quinoa • 1½ cups water • 1 cup cooked corn kernels • 1 (15-ounce) can black beans, rinsed and drained • 1 small boiled potato, peeled • 1 small onion, chopped • ½ teaspoon fresh ginger, grated finely • 1 teaspoon garlic, minced • ½ cup fresh cilantro, chopped • 1 teaspoon flax meal • 1 teaspoon ground cumin • 1 teaspoon paprika • 1 teaspoon chili flakes • ½ teaspoon ground turmeric • Salt and freshly ground black pepper, to taste

Directions:

1. In a pan, add water and quinoa on high heat and provide to a boil. 2. Reduce heat to medium and simmer for around 15-twenty or so minutes. 3. Drain excess water. 4. Preheat the oven to 375 degrees F. Line a sizable baking sheet with parchment paper. 5. In a sizable bowl, add quinoa and remaining ingredients. 6. With a fork, mix till well combined. 7. Make equal sized patties from mixture. 8. Arrange the patties onto prepared baking sheet in the single layer. 9. Bake for around 20-25 minutes. 10. Carefully, alter the side and cook for about 8-10 minutes.

819. Coconut & Banana Cookies

Yield: 7 servings Preparation Time: 15 minutes Cooking Time: 25 minutes

Ingredients:

2 cups unswee10ed coconut, shredded • 3 medium bananas, peeled • ½ teaspoon ground cinnamon • ½ teaspoon ground turmeric • Pinch of salt and freshly ground black pepper

Directions: 1. Preheat the oven to 350 degrees F. Line a cookie sheet having a lightly greased parchment paper. 2. In a mixer, add all ingredients and pulse till a dough like mixture forms. 3. Make small balls through the mixture and set onto prepared cookie sheet in a single layer. 4. With your fingers, gently press along the balls in order to create the cookies. 5. Bake for about 15-20 min or till golden brown.

820. Almond Scones

Yield: 6 servings Preparation Time: 10 minutes Cooking Time: twenty minutes

Ingredients:

1 cup almonds • 1 1/3 cups almond flour • ¼ cup arrowroot flour • 1 tablespoon coconut flour • 1 teaspoon ground turmeric • Salt and freshly ground black pepper, to taste • 1 egg • ¼ cup essential olive oil • 3 tablespoons raw honey • 1 teaspoon vanilla flavoring

Directions:

1. In a mixer, add almonds and pulse till chopped roughly 2. Transfer the chopped almonds in a big bowl. 3. Add flours and spices and mix well. 4. In another bowl, add remaining ingredients and beat till well combined. 5. Add flour mixture into egg mixture and mix till well combined. 6. Arrange a plastic wrap over cutting board. 7. Place the dough over cutting board. 8. With both your hands, pat into about 1-inch thick circle. 9. Carefully, cut the circle in 6 wedges. 10. Arrange the scones onto a cookie sheet in a single layer. 11. Bake for approximately 15-twenty minutes.

DESSERT

821. Raw Lime, Avocado & Coconut Pie

Yield: 8 servings Preparation Time: 20 minutes

Ingredients:

For Crust: • ¾ cup unswee10ed coconut flakes • 1 cup dates, pitted and chopped roughly • For Filing: • ¾ cup young coconut meat • 1½ avocados, peeled, pitted and chopped • 2 tablespoons fresh lime juice • ¼ cup raw agave nectar

Directions:

1. Lightly, grease an 8-inch pie pan. 2. In a sizable food processor, add all crust ingredients and pulse till smooth. 3. Transfer the crust mixture into prepared pan, pressing gently downwards. 4. With a paper towel, wipe out your blender completely. 5. In the same processor, add all filling ingredients and pulse till smooth. 6. Place filling mixture over crust evenly. 7. Freeze not less than 120 minutes or till set completely.

822. Pudding Muffins

Yield: 5 servings Preparation Time: fifteen minutes Cooking Time: 26 minutes

Ingredients:

For Muffins: • 12 dates, pitted and chopped • 10 tablespoons water • 2½-3 tablespoons coconut flour • ½ teaspoon baking powder • 2 organic eggs • 1½ bananas, peeled and sliced • 1 teaspoon organic honey • 1 tablespoon organic vanilla flavoring • For Topping: • 5-6, pitted and chopped • 3 tablespoons almond milk • Fresh juice of ½ orange • 1 teaspoon organic honey • 1 teaspoon organic vanilla flavoring • For Garnishing: • Fresh raspberries, as required

Directions:

1. Preheat the oven to 365 degrees F. Grease 5 cups of an large muffin tin. 2. For muffins in a very small pan, mix together dates and water on low heat. 3. Cook for approximately 3-4 minutes or till the dates break down and be thick. 4. Remove from heat and having a fork, mash the dates completely. 5. In a bowl, add remaining ingredients and beat till well combined. 6. Add mashed dates and stir to combine. 7. Transfer the mix in prepared muffin cups evenly. 8. Bake for about 20-22 minutes. 9. Meanwhile in a pan, add all topping ingredients on low heat. 10. Cook for about 3-4 minutes or till the dates break up and turn into thick. 11. Remove from heat and having a fork, mash the dates completely. Keep aside. 12. Remove muffins from oven and keep aside to cool for approximately 5 minutes. 13. Carefully, take away the muffins from cups. Top with date mixture evenly. 14. Garnish with raspberries and serve

823. Pineapple Sticks

Yield: 8 servings Preparation Time: 10 minutes

Ingredients:

¼ cup fresh orange juice • ¾ cup coconut, shredded and toasted • 8 (3x1-inch) fresh pineapple pieces

Directions:

Line a baking sheet with wax paper. 2. In a shallow dish, place pineapple juice. 3. In another shallow dish, squeeze pineapple. 4. Insert 1 wooden skewer in each pineapple piece through the narrow end. 5. Dip each pineapple piece in juice and then coat with coconut evenly. 6. Arrange the pineapple sticks onto prepared baking sheet inside a single layer. 7. Cover and freeze for around 1-2 hours.

824. Grilled Peaches

Yield: 6 servings Preparation Time: quarter-hour Cooking Time: 10 min

Ingredients:

3 medium peaches, halved and pitted • ½ cup coconut cream • 1 teaspoon vanilla flavoring • ¼ cup walnuts, chopped • Ground cinnamon, as required

Directions:

1. Preheat the grill to medium-low heat. Grease the grill grate. 2. Arrange the peach slices onto grill, cut-side down. 3. Grill for approximately 3-5 minutes per side or till desired doneness. 4. Meanwhile inside a bowl, add coconut cream and vanilla extract and beat till smooth. 5. Spoon the whipped cream over each peach half. 6. Top with walnuts and sprinkle with cinnamon and serve.

825. Stuffed Apples

Yield: 4 servings Preparation Time: fifteen minutes Cooking Time: 35 minutes

Ingredients:

4 large apples, peeled and cored • 2 teaspoons fresh lemon juice • 1 cup fresh blueberries • ½ cup fresh apple juice • ½ teaspoon ground cinnamon • ¼ cup almond meal • ¼ cup coconut flakes

Directions:

1. Preheat the oven to 375 degrees F. 2. Coat the apples with lemon juice evenly. 3. Arrange the apples inside a baking dish. 4. Stuff each apple with blueberries. 5. Scatter the rest of the blueberries around the apples. 6. Drizzle with apple juice. 7. Sprinkle each apple with cinnamon evenly. 8. Top with almond meal and coconut flakes evenly. 9. Bake approximately 30-35 minutes.

826. Citrus Strawberry Granita

Yield: 4 servings Preparation Time: quarter-hour Cooking Time: 5 minutes

Ingredients:

12-ounce fresh strawberries. hulled • 1 grapefruit, peeled, seeded and sectioned • 2 oranges, peeled, seeded and sectioned • ¼ of a lemon • ¼ cup raw honey

Directions:

1. In a juicer add strawberries, grapefruit, oranges and lemon and process based on manufacturer's directions. 2. In a pan, add 1½ cups from the fruit juice and honey on medium heat. 3. Cook, stirring approximately 5 minutes. 4. Remove from heat and stir within the remaining juice. 5. Keep aside to cool for approximately a half-hour. 6. Transfer the juice mixture into an 8x8-inch glass baking dish. 7. Freeze for approximately 4 hours, scraping after every 30 minutes.

827. Chocolaty Cherry Ice-Cream

Yield: 2 servings Preparation Time: 10 min

Ingredients:

1 cup raw cashews • 1 cup frozen cherries • ¼ cup coconut, shredded • 1 tablespoon raw honey • ¼ cup chocolate bars, chopped

Directions:

In a higher speed blender, add cashews and pulse till a flour like texture forms. 2. Add remaining ingredients except chocolate and pulse till smooth. 3. Add chocolate and pulse till just combined. 4. Transfer the ice-cream into airtight container and freeze for about 1-120 minutes or till set.

828. Chocolate Sorbet

Yield: 4-6 servings Preparation Time: fifteen minutes Cooking Time: 3-4 minutes

Ingredients:

1/3 cup chocolate bars, chopped • ½ cup unswee10ed cocoa powder • ½ cup coconut sugar • Pinch of salt • 2¼ cups water • 1 tablespoon plus 1 teaspoon extra-virgin olive oil

Directions:

1. Freeze ice-cream maker tub for around a day before making sorbet. 2. In a pan, add all ingredients except oil on medium heat. 3. Bring with a boil, beating continuously. 4. Reduce heat to low and simmer for approximately thirty seconds. 5. Remove from heat and transfer in a heat-proof bowl. 6. Refrigerate for about 2-8 hours. 7. Now, transfer into an ice-cream maker and process according to manufacturer's directions. 8. While motor is running, add 1 tablespoon of oil. 9. Return the ice-cream into airtight container and freeze for around couple of hours. 10. Serve using the drizzling of remaining oil.

829. Zesty Mousse

Yield: 4 servings Preparation Time: fifteen minutes

Ingredients:

2 cups bananas, peeled and chopped • 2 ripe avocados, peeled, pitted and chopped • 1 teaspoon fresh lime zest, grated finely • 1 teaspoon fresh lemon zest, grated finely • ½ cup fresh lime juice • ½ cup fresh lemon juice • 1/3 cup raw honey

Directions:

1. In a blender, add all ingredients and pulse till smooth. 2. Transfer the mousse in 4 serving glasses. 3. Refrigerate to relax approximately 3 hours.

830. Chocolaty Avocado Mousse

Yield: 4-6 servings Preparation Time: 10 minutes

Ingredients:

2 ripe avocados, peeled, pitted and chopped • ½ cup coconut milk • ½ cup cacao powder • 1 teaspoon ground cinnamon • ¼ teaspoon ground anchochile • 1/3 cup raw honey • 2 teaspoons vanilla extract

Directions:

1. In a blender, add all ingredients and pulse till smooth. 2. Transfer the mousse in serving glasses. 3. Refrigerate to relax completely.

831. Carrot Chia Pudding

Yield: 1 serving Preparation Time: 15 minutes Cooking Time: 7 minutes

Ingredients:

¾ cup carrot, peeled and chopped roughly • 2-3 tablespoons walnuts, chopped • ½ teaspoon ground cinnamon • ¼ teaspoon ground ginger • Pinch of ground nutmeg • Pinch of ground cloves • 1-2 tablespoons raw honey • 1 cup unswee10ed almond milk • ½ cup water • ½ teaspoon vanilla flavoring • 2 tablespoons chia seeds

Directions:

In a mixer, add carrot and walnuts and pulse till chopped finely. 2. Transfer the carrot mixture in the nonstick pan on medium heat. 3. Add spices and honey and cook, stirring occasionally for about 5-7 minutes. 4. Stir in almond milk, water and vanilla extract. 5. Transfer a combination into a serving bowl. 6. Add chia seeds and stir to blend well. 7. Cover and refrigerate for overnight.

832. Pumpkin Custard

Yield: 6 servings Preparation Time: 15 minutes Cooking Time: 1 hour

Ingredients:

1 cup canned pumpkin • 1 teaspoon ground cinnamon • ¼ teaspoon ground ginger • 2 pinches of nutmeg, grated freshly • Pinch of salt • 2 organic eggs • 1 cup coconut milk • 8-10 drops liquid stevia • 1 teaspoon vanilla Flavoring

Directions:

1. Preheat the oven to 350 degrees F. 2. In a big bowl, mix together pumpkin and spices. 3. In another bowl, add the eggs and beat well. 4. Add remaining ingredients and beat till well combined. 5. Add egg mixture into pumpkin mixture and mix till well combined. 6. Transfer a combination into 6 ramekins. 7. Arrange the ramekins in the baking dish, 8. Add enough water inside the baking dish about 2-inch high across the ramekins. 9. Bake for around 1 hour or till a toothpick inserted within the center comes out clean.

833. Spiced Egg Custard

Yield: 8 servings Preparation Time: fifteen minutes Cooking Time: 40 minutes

Ingredients:

5 organic eggs • Salt, to taste • ½ cup honey • 20-ounce coconut milk • ¼ teaspoon ground ginger • ¼ teaspoon ground cinnamon • ¼ teaspoon ground nutmeg • ¼ teaspoon ground cardamom • 1/8 teaspoon ground clove • 1/8 teaspoon ground allspice

Directions:

1. Preheat the oven to 325 degrees F. Grease 8 small ramekins. 2. In a bowl, add eggs and salt and beat well. 3. Arrange a sieve on the medium bowl. 4. Pour the eggs on the sieve to operate them through it by moving the sieve in a very circle. 5. Add the honey in eggs and stir to combine. 6. Add coconut milk and spices and beat till well combined. 7. Transfer a combination into prepared ramekins. 8. Arrange the ramekins in a big baking dish. 9. Add domestic hot water inside baking dish about 2-inch high across the ramekins. 10. Bake for about 30-40 minutes or till a toothpick inserted in the center happens clean.

834. Pumpkin Soufflé

Yield: 4 servings Preparation Time: quarter-hour Cooking Time: 35 minutes

Ingredients:

1 tablespoon coconut flour • ¼ tsp baking soda • 1 teaspoon pumpkin pie spice • 1 teaspoon ground cinnamon • Pinch of salt • 4 eggs • 1 cup canned pumpkin • 1/3 cup raw hone • ¼ cup coconut oil, melted • 2 tablespoons almond butter • ½ teaspoon vanilla flavor

Directions:

Preheat the oven to 350 degrees F. Arrange the rack inside the center from the oven. 2. In a bowl, sift together flour, baking soda, pumpkin pie spice, cinnamon and salt. 3. In another large bowl, add remaining ingredients and beat till well combined. 4. Add flour mixture into pumpkin mixture and mix till well combined. 5. Transfer the amalgamation into 4 ramekins evenly. 6. Bake for approximately 25-35 minutes or till the soufflé puffs up.

835. Cranberry & Apple Crisp

Yield: 4-6 servings Preparation Time: 20 min Cooking Time: 45 minutes

Ingredients:

For Filling: • 2 tablespoons coconut oil • 2 tablespoons raw honey • 2 teaspoons ground cinnamon • ½ teaspoon ground nutmeg • ¼ teaspoon ground ginger • ¼ teaspoon ground cloves • 1½ pound apples, peeled, cored and chopped • ½ cup fresh cranberries For Topping: • 1 cup coconut, shredded • ½ cup coconut palm sugar • ¼ cup coconut oil, sof10ed • 3 tablespoons tapioca starch • 2 tablespoons coconut flour • ½ teaspoon ground cinnamon • ¼ teaspoon ground nutmeg • Pinch of salt

Directions:

1. Preheat the oven to 350 degrees F. 2. For filling inside a pan, mix together coconut oil, honey and spices on low heat. 3. Cook for around 1-2 minutes. 4. Remove from heat and transfer the mixture into a bowl. 5. Add apples and cranberries and toss to coat well. 6. Transfer a combination into a 8x8-inch pie dish. 7. For topping in a very bowl, add all ingredients and mix till a crumbly mixture forms. 8. Place the topping over filling evenly. 9. Bake approximately 35-45 minutes or top becomes golden brown.

836. Pumpkin Pie

Yield: 6-8 servings Preparation Time: fifteen minutes Cooking Time: 1 hour 5 minutes

Ingredients:

For Crust: • 2½ cups walnuts • 1 tsp baking soda • Salt, to taste • 2 tablespoons coconut oil, melted For Filling: • 1 (15-ounce) pumpkin pie spice • 1 tablespoon arrowroot powder • ½ teaspoon ground nutmeg • ½ teaspoon ground cinnamon • ¼ teaspoon ground ginger • ¼ teaspoon ground cardamom • ¼ teaspoon ground cloves • Pinch of salt • 1 cup coconut milk • 3 eggs, bea10 • 3 tablespoons raw honey

Directions:

1. Preheat the oven to 350 degrees F. 2. For crust inside a blender, add walnuts, baking soda and salt and pulse till grounded finely. 3. Add coconut oil and pulse till well combined. 4. Place the crust mixture in a 9-inch pie dish. 5. With the back of spatula, smooth the outer lining of crust. 6. Arrange the pie dish in the baking sheet. 7. Bake for about quarter-hour. 8. Meanwhile for filling inside a bowl, add all ingredients and mix till well combined. 9. Remove the crust from your oven. 10. Place the mixture into crust. (Try to not overfill the crust) 11. Bake for approximately 50 minutes.

837. Cherry & Coconut Macaroons

Yield: 24 servings Preparation Time: 15 minutes Cooking Time: 25 minutes

Ingredients:

For Macaroons: • 1 cup dried cherries, soaked in water for thirty minutes • 1/3 cup raw honey • 1 tablespoon coconut oil, sof10ed • 1 teaspoon vanilla flavoring • 2 cups unswee10ed coconut, shredded • Salt, to taste For Chocolate Coating: • 3 tablespoons cacao powder • ½ tablespoon raw honey • ½ tablespoon coconut oil, melted

Directions:

Preheat the oven to 300 degrees F. Line a baking sheet with parchment paper. 2. Drain the cherries, reserving ¼ cup from the liquid. 3. In a blender, add cherries, reserved water, honey, coconut oil and vanilla flavor and beat till a paste forms. 4. Transfer the cherry paste into a large bowl. 5. Add coconut and salt and mix well. 6. With 1 tablespoon result in the balls from mixture. 7. Arrange the balls onto prepared baking sheet in a very single layer. 8. Bake for approximately 25 minutes. 9. Remove from oven whilst aside to cool down the for approximately half an hour. 10. Meanwhile for coating in the bowl, add all ingredients and beat till well combined. 11. Drizzle the coating over macaroons and serve.

838. Zucchini Brownies

Yield: 20-22 servings Preparation Time: 15 minutes Cooking Time: 45 minutes

Ingredients:

1½ cups zucchini, shredded • 1 cup chocolate bars chips • 1 organic egg • 1 cup almond butter • 1/3 cup raw honey • 1 teaspoon vanilla extract • 1 tsp baking soda • 1 teaspoon ground cinnamon • ½ teaspoon ground nutmeg

Directions:

1. Preheat the oven to 350 degrees F. Grease a 9x9-inch baking dish. 2. In a big bowl, add all ingredients and mix till well combined. 3. Transfer a combination into prepared baking dish evenly. 4. With the back of spatula, smooth the most notable surface. 5. Bake for approximately 35-45 minutes or till a toothpick inserted within the center comes out clean. 6. Remove from oven and keep aside to chill completely. 7. After cooling, cut into desired size squares and serve.

839. Mini Upside-Down Cherry Cakes

Yield: 6 servings Preparation Time: quarter-hour Cooking Time: 20 min

Ingredients:

¾ cup fresh cherries, pitted and chopped • ¼ teaspoon vanilla bean powder, divided • 1/3 cup raw honey, divided • 1¼ cups almond flour • ¼ tsp baking soda • Salt, to taste • ¼ cup coconut oil, melted • 2 organic eggs • 2 teaspoons almond extract

Directions:

1. Preheat the oven to 350 degrees F. Grease 6 cups of an muffin tray. 2. In a bowl, mix together cherries, 1/8 teaspoon of vanilla bean powder and two tablespoons of honey. 3. In an extra bowl, mix together flour, baking soda and salt. 4. In a third bowl, add oil, eggs, almond extract and remaining honey and vanilla bean powder and beat till well combined. 5. Add flour mixture into egg mixture and mix till well combined. 6. Place the cheery mixture into prepared muffin cups evenly. 7. Top with flour mixture evenly. 8. Bake for around twenty or so minutes. 9. Carefully invert the cakes onto serving plates.

840. Chocolaty Pumpkin Cake

Yield: 8 servings Preparation Time: fifteen minutes Cooking Time: 40 minutes

Ingredients:

For Cake: • 1 cup chocolates chips • 1/3 cup coconut oil, sof10ed • 1/3 cup coconut flour • 2 tablespoons coconut milk • ¼ cup raw honey • ¾ cup pumpkin puree • 3 organic eggs • ½ teaspoon ground nutmeg • ½ teaspoon ground cinnamon • ¼ teaspoon ground ginger For Frosting: • ½ (14-ounce) can coconut milk • 2 tablespoon pumpkin puree • 1 teaspoon raw honey • Pinch of ground cinnamon

Directions:

Preheat the oven to 350 degrees F. Grease an 8x8-inch glass baking dish. 2. In a microwave safe bowl, add chocolate chips and microwave on low for about 1 ½-2 minutes, stirring after every thirty minutes or till melted completely. 3. Remove the bowl from microwave. 4. Add coconut oil, flour and coconut milk and mix till a smooth mixture forms. 5. Keep aside to cool completely. 6. In another bowl, add honey, pumpkin puree, eggs and spices and beat till well combined. 7. Add chocolate mixture in egg mixture and mix till well combined. 8. Transfer the amalgamation into prepared cake pan evenly. 9. Bake for about 40 minutes. 10. Remove from oven and keep aside to chill completely. 11. For frosting in a very bowl, add all ingredients and mix till well combined. 12. Spread frosting over cake evenly and serve.

841. Chocolate Mug Cake

Yield: 1 serving Preparation Time: 10 min Cooking Time: 2 minutes

Ingredients:

1 tbsp olive oil • 3 tablespoons chocolates chips • 2 tablespoons coconut flour • 1/8 tsp baking soda • 2 tablespoons water • 1 organic egg

Directions:

1. In a microwave safe mug, add oil and chocolate chips and microwave on high for approximately 20-30 seconds. 2. Add the flour, baking soda and water and mix well. 3. Add egg and beat till well combined. 4. Microwave on high approximately 1½ minutes

842. Cherry Crisp

Yield: 8 serving Preparation Time: quarter-hour Cooking Time: 20 minutes

Ingredients:

3 cups fresh cherries, pitted and sliced • Coconut palm sugar, to taste • 1/3 cup unswee10ed almond milk • 2 teaspoons almond extract • ¼ cup almond flour • ¼ cup coconut flour • ¼ cup hemp seeds • 1 teaspoon ground cinnamon • Pinch of salt • 1 tablespoon water

Directions:

1. Preheat the oven to 375 degrees F. Grease a baking dish. 2. In a bowl, mix together cherries, coconut sugar, almond milk and almond extract. 3. In another bowl, add remaining ingredients and mix till a crumbly mixture forms. 4. Place the cherry mixture inside bottom of the prepared baking dish evenly. 5. Spread the crumb mixture over cherry mixture evenly. 6. Bake for around 20 min.

843. Almond Butter Balls Vegan

Time To Prepare: 10 Minutes Time to Cook: 0 0 Minute Yield: Servings 4

Ingredients:

12 dates, pitted and diced 2 and a ½ tablespoon of almond butter 1/3 cup of unsweetened shredded coconut

Directions:

Take a container and put in dates, almond butter, and coconut. Mix thoroughly Use the mixture to make small balls Store them in the refrigerator and chill them Enjoy!

844. Apricot Squares

Time To Prepare: twenty minutes Time to Cook: 0 minute Yield: Servings 8

Ingredients:

1 cup apricot, chopped 1 cup apricot, dried 1 cup macadamia nuts, chopped 1 cup shredded coconut, dried 1 teaspoon vanilla extract 1/3 cup turmeric powder

Directions:

Put all ingredients in a food processor Pulse until the desired smoothness is achieved Put the mixture into a square pan and press uniformly Best enjoyed chilled.

845. Avocado Brownies

Time To Prepare: 10 Minutes Time to Cook: 25 Minutes Yield: Servings 16

Ingredients:

¼ tsp. Sea Salt ½ cup Applesauce, unsweetened ½ cup Cocoa Powder, Dutch-processed & unsweetened ½ cup Coconut Flour ½ cup Maple Syrup 1 Avocado, big 1 tap. Vanilla Extract 1 tsp. Baking Soda 3 Eggs, large

Directions:

First, preheat your oven to 350 ° F. Next, place avocado, vanilla, applesauce, and maple syrup in a high-speed blender and blend for a couple of minutes or until the desired smoothness is achieved. After this, move the smooth mixture to a big mixing container. To this, mix in the eggs and mix until whisked well. Next, spoon in the coconut flour, sea salt, and cocoa powder to the mixture. Give a good stir until everything comes together. Now, pour the mixture to a greased baking dish and bake for 23 to twenty-five minutes or until cooked. Finally, take off from the oven and let it cool for fifteen to twenty minutes before you serve.

846. Avocado Choco Cake

Time To Prepare: ten minutes Time to Cook: twenty-five minutes Yield: Servings 8

Ingredients:

¼-tsp sea salt ½-cup applesauce, unsweetened ½-cup cocoa powder, unsweetened and Dutch-processed ½-cup coconut flour ½-cup maple syrup 1-pc big avocado 1-tsp baking soda 1-tsp vanilla extract 3-pcs big eggs

Directions:

Preheat the oven to 350°F. Grease a baking pan with coconut oil. Mix the avocado, vanilla, syrup, and applesauce in a food processor. Blend until meticulously blended. Move the mixture to a big mixing container. Whisk in the eggs. Put in the baking soda, cocoa powder, coconut flour, and sea salt. Mix thoroughly until meticulously blended. Put in the batter in the baking pan. Place the pan in your oven. Bake for about twenty-five minutes. Allow cooling for about twenty minutes before cutting the cake into 16 squares.

847. Banana & Avocado Mousse

Time To Prepare: ten minutes Time to Cook: 0 minutes Yield: Servings 4

Ingredients:

½ cup of fresh lemon juice ½ cup of fresh lime juice 1 teaspoon of fresh lemon zest, grated finely 1 teaspoon of fresh lime zest, grated finely 1/3 cup of raw honey 2 cups of bananas (peeled and chopped) 2 ripe avocados (peeled, pitted, and chopped)

Directions:

Combine all ingredients in a blender and pulse to puree. Move the mousse to four serving glasses. Place in your fridge for around three hours before eating.

848. Banana Cinnamon

Time To Prepare: two minutes Time to Cook: 8 minutes Yield: Servings 2-4

Ingredients:

1 big banana, chopped into ½ inch 1 tsp. cinnamon 2 tsp. honey

Directions:

In a small container, put the honey and cinnamon and mix well. Heat the olive oil in a pan. Cook banana slices for a couple of minutes or until browned all over. Pour honey and cinnamon mixture over the bananas and serve.

849. Beet Pancakes

Time To Prepare: ten minutes Time to Cook: twelve minutes Yield: Servings 3

Ingredients:

½ Cup Heavy Milk ½ Cup Melted Butter 1 Cup Flour 1 Large Egg 1 Tbsp. Baking Powder 1 Tsp. Vanilla Extract 1/3 Cup Plain Greek Yoghurt 1/4 Tsp Baking Soda 3 Cup Whole Wheat Flour 4 Cups Roasted Beet, Puree 6 Tsp. Brown Sugar Salt

Directions:

Combine the dry ingredients in a container. In another container, combine the wet ingredients. Mix both mixtures until the desired smoothness is achieved. Fry the batter on a pan to make pancakes. Serve with whip cream.

850. Grams Berry Parfait

Time To Prepare: 10 min Time to Cook: 10 min Yield: Servings 5

Ingredients:

14oz / 400g mixed berries 2 tsp honey 3.5oz / 100g Greek yogurt 7oz / 200g almond butter 7oz / 200g mixed nuts

Directions:

Combine the Greek yogurt, butter, and honey until its smooth. Put in a layer of berries and a layer of the mixture in a glass until it's full. Serve instantly with sprinkled nuts.

851. Tea Cake

Time To Prepare: ten minutes Time to Cook: thirty-five minutes Yield: Servings 10

Ingredients:

½ cup coconut butter ½ cup coconut oil 1 teaspoon baking soda 2 cups coconut milk 2 teaspoons vanilla extract 3 ½ cups almond flour 3 teaspoons baking powder 4 eggs 6 tablespoons black tea powder Chicory root powder to the taste

Directions:

Place the coconut milk in a pot and warm it up on moderate heat. Put in tea, stir thoroughly, take off the heat and cool down, In a container, mix the coconut butter with the chicory powder, eggs, vanilla, coconut oil, almond flour, baking soda, baking powder, and tea mix. Stir thoroughly, pour into a lined cake pan, and bake in your oven at 350 degrees F for half an hour Slice, split between plates, before you serve. Enjoy!

852. Blueberry Energy Bites

Time To Prepare: ten minutes Time to Cook: 0 minutes Yield: Servings 6

Ingredients:

¼ teaspoon of cinnamon ½ cup of gluten-free oat flour ½ cup of unsweetened almond milk ½ teaspoon of sea salt 2 tablespoons of dried blueberries 2 tablespoons of organic peanut butter 2 tablespoons of pure maple syrup

Directions:

Put the dry ingredients into a mixing container, including the peanut butter, and stir until blended. Put in the almond milk and maple syrup, and stir. Form into an inch balls, and place in your fridge to firm up before you serve.

853. Blueberry Tarts

Time To Prepare: 10 Minutes Time to Cook: 30 Minutes Yield: Servings 5

Ingredients:

To make the crust: ½ cup Raisins ½ tsp. Himalayan Salt 1 cup Cashews 1 cup Dates 1 cup Walnuts To make the filling: 1 tbsp. Maple syrup 1/8 tsp. Cinnamon 4 cups Blueberries

Directions:

To make this yummy dessert fare, keep all the nuts in a food processor and process the nuts until it becomes coarse flour. After this, spoon in the dates, salt, and raisin to the nuts mixture and process them once more. Next, spread this mixture onto a greased parchment paper-lined baking sheet and place it in your fridge until set. To make the filling, mix all the ingredients needed in a moderate-sized container and mix them well. To finish, spoon in the filling on to the crust and spread across uniformly on all sides. Top with blueberries if you wish

854. Fiber Caramelized Pears

Time To Prepare:twenty minutesTime to Cook: five minutes Yield:Servings 5

Ingredients:

¼ Cup Toasted Pecans, Chopped 1 Tablespoon Coconut Oil 1 Teaspoon Cinnamon 1/8 Teaspoon Sea Salt 2 Cups Yogurt, Plain 2 Tablespoon Honey, Raw 4 Pears, Peeled, Cored & Quartered

Directions:

Get out a big frying pan, and then heat the oil on moderate to high heat. Put in in your honey, cinnamon, pears, and salt. Cover, and let it cook for four to five minutes. Stir once in a while, and your fruit must be soft. Uncover it, and let the sauce simmer until it becomes thick. This will take a few minutes. Soon your yogurt into four dessert bowls. Top with pears and pecans before you serve

855. Chocolate Bananas

Time To Prepare: 5 Minutes Time to Cook: fifteen Minutes Yield: Servings 4

Ingredients:

1 tbsp. Coconut Oil 12 oz. Dark Chocolate 3 Bananas, big & cut into thirds

Directions:

Melt the chocolate and coconut oil in a twofold boiler for three to four minutes, till you get a smooth and shiny mixture. After this, keep the popsicles into the end of each of the banana by inserting it. Next, immerse the chocolate into the warm chocolate mixture. Shake off the surplus chocolate and put them on parchment paper. Drizzle with the topping of your choice. To finish, place them in the freezer for a few hours or until set.

856. Chocolate Chip Cookies

Time To Prepare: 10 Minutes Time to Cook: 20 Minutes Yield: Servings 16

Ingredients:

½ cup Almond Butter ½ cup Dark Chocolate Chips, sugar-free ½ cup Maple Syrup 2 cups Almond Flour, finely sifted

Directions:

Preheat your oven to 350 ° F. After this, mix the almond flour, almond butter, and maple syrup in a moderate-sized mixing container until combined well. To this, mix in the chocolate chips and mix once more. With the help of an ice cream scooper, scoop out the mixture to a greased baking sheet. Flatten the top slightly with your hand. To finish, bake them for ten to twelve minutes or until they are going to get browned.

857. Chocolate Covered Strawberries

Time To Prepare: fifteen Minutes Time to Cook: 0 Minute Yield: Servings 24

Ingredients:

16 ounces milk chocolate chips 1-pound fresh strawberries with leaves 2 tablespoons shortening

Directions:

In a bain-marie, melt chocolate and shorter, once in a while stirring until the desired smoothness is achieved. Hold them by the toothpicks and immerse the strawberries in the chocolate mixture. Put toothpicks in the top of the strawberries. Turn the strawberries and put the toothpick in the Styrofoam so that the chocolate cools.

858. Chocolate Mousse

Time To Prepare: 10 Minutes Time to Cook: 0 Minute Yield: Servings 4

Ingredients:

1 teaspoon of vanilla extract 3 tablespoons of Agave Nectar 4 tablespoons of cocoa Coconut cream scraped from the upper side of 2 pieces of 13.5-ounce chilled cans of full-fat coconut milk

Directions:

Take a big container and scoop out the thick coconut cream from the can to the container Put in nectar, vanilla extract and cocoa to the container Beat it well using an electric mixer, beginning from low and going to moderate until a foamy texture appears Split the mix uniformly amongst ramekins and chill to your desired level of cold Enjoy!

859. Citrus Cauliflower Cake

Time To Prepare: 5 hours and thirty minutes Time to Cook: 0 minutes Yield: Servings 10

Ingredients:

For the Crust: 1-cup dates, pitted 2½-cups pecan nuts 2-Tbsps maple syrup or agave For the Filling: ½-tsp lemon extract ½-tsp pure vanilla extract ¾-cup maple syrup or agave 1½-cups pineapple, crushed 1½-cups plain coconut yogurt 1-pc lemon, zest, and juice 1-tsp pure vanilla extract 3-cups cauliflower, riced 3-pcs avocados, halved and pitted 3-Tbsps maple syrup or agave A pinch of cinnamon For the Topping:

Directions:

For the Crust: Coat a baking tray using parchment paper. Set the outer ring of a 9-inch springform pan onto the baking tray. Pulse the pecans in a food processor to a thoroughly ground texture. Put in the remaining crust ingredients, and pulse further until the mixture holds together. Move and press the mixture to a uniform layer in the baking tray. For the Filling: Wipe the container of your food processor, and put in the avocado, cauliflower, pineapple, syrup, and lemon zest and juice. Process the mixture to a smooth consistency. Put in the cinnamon and the lemon and vanilla extracts. Pulse until meticulously blended. Pour the mixture over the crust. Put the tray in your freezer overnight, or for around five hours. Take the cake out from your freezer, and allow it to sit at room temperature for about twenty minutes. Take away the outer ring. For the Topping: Mix in all the topping ingredients in a mixing container. Pour the mixture over the cake and spread uniformly.

860. Coconut and Chocolate Cream

Time To Prepare: 2 hours Time to Cook: 0 minutes Yield: Servings 4

Ingredients:

½ teaspoon cinnamon powder 1 cup dark chocolate, chopped and melted 1 teaspoon vanilla extract 2 cups coconut milk 2 tablespoons ginger, grated 2 tablespoons honey

Directions:

Throw all the ingredients into a blender and blend. Split into bowls and store in the refrigerator for about two hours before you serve

861. Coconut Muffins

Time To Prepare: 5 Minutes Time to Cook: 25 Minutes Yield: Servings 8

Ingredients:

¼ cup of cocoa powder ¼ teaspoon vanilla extract ½ cup ghee, melted 1 cup coconut, unsweetened and shredded 1 teaspoon baking powder 3 tablespoons swerve eggs, whisked

Directions:

In a container, mix the ghee with the swerve, coconut, and the other ingredients, stir thoroughly and split it into a lined muffin pan. Bake at 370 degrees F for about twenty-five minutes, cool down before you serve.

862. Comforting Baked Rice Pudding

TimeTo Prepare: ten minutes Time to Cook: twenty minutes Yield:Servings 8

Ingredients:

¼ cup of almond flakes ¼ cup of raw honey ½ tsp. of ground cardamom ½ tsp. of ground ginger 1 peeled and cut banana 1 tsp. fresh lemon zest, finely grated 1 tsp. of ground cinnamon 2 big organic eggs 2 cups of cooked brown rice 2 cups of unsweetened almond milk

Directions:

Set the oven to 390 F, then grease a baking dish. Spread cooked rice at the bottom of the readied baking dish uniformly. In a big container, put together the coconut milk, eggs, honey, lemon zest, spices, and beat until well blended. Put the egg mixture over the rice uniformly. Position banana slices over egg mixture uniformly and drizzle with almonds. Bake for approximately twenty minutes. Serve warm.

863. Creamy & Chilly Blueberry Bites

Time To Prepare: 2 hours and five minutes Time to Cook: 0 minutes Yield: Servings 2

Ingredients:

1-pint blueberries 2-tsp lemon juice 8-oz. vanilla yogurt

Directions:

Coat the blueberries with the lemon juice and yogurt in a mixing container. Toss cautiously without squishing the berries. Scoop out each of the coated berries and arrange them on a baking sheet coated with parchment paper. Place the sheet in your freezer for a couple of hours before you serve.

864. Dark Chocolate Granola Bars

Time To Prepare: ten minutes Time to Cook: twenty-five minutes Yield: Servings 12

Ingredients:

¼ cup dark cocoa powder ¼ cup of flaxseed ½ cup dark chocolate chips 1 cup of walnuts 1 cup tart cherries, dried 1 teaspoon of salt 1 teaspoon of vanilla 2 cups buckwheat 2 eggs 2/3 cup honey

Directions:

Preheat the oven to 350 degrees F. Line with cooking spray your baking pan. Pulse together the walnuts, wheat, tart cherries, salt, and flaxseed in a food processor. Everything must be chopped fine. Mix together the honey, eggs, vanilla, and cocoa powder in a container. Put in the wheat mix to your container. Stir to blend well. Include the chocolate chips. Stir once more. Now pour this mixture into a baking dish. Drizzle some chocolate chips and tart cherries. Bake for about twenty-five minutes. Allow to cool before you serve.

865. Easy Peach Cobbler

Time To Prepare: five minutes Time to Cook: twenty minutes Yield: Servings 6

Ingredients:

¼ brown rice flour ¼ cup coconut palm sugar, divided ¼ cup extra virgin olive oil ¼ cup ground flaxseeds ½ cup gluten-free oats ½ teaspoon cinnamon ¾ cup chopped pecans 5 organic peaches, pitted and chopped

Directions:

Preheat your oven to 350°F. Grease the bottom of 6 ramekins. In a container, combine the peaches, ½ of the coconut sugar, cinnamon, and pecans. Distribute the peach mixture into the ramekins. In the same container, combine the oats, flaxseed, rice flour, and oil. Put in in the rest of the coconut sugar. Mix until a crumbly texture is formed. Top the mixture over the peaches. Put for about twenty minutes.

866. Fennel and Almond Bites

Time To Prepare: ten minutes + three hours freezing time Time to Cook: twenty-five minutes Yield: Servings 10

Ingredients:

¼ cup almond milk ¼ cup of cocoa powder ½ cup almond oil 1 teaspoon fennel seeds 1 teaspoon vanilla extract A pinch of sunflower seeds

Directions:

Take a container and mix the almond oil and almond milk Beat until the desired smoothness is achieved and shiny by using an electric beater Stir in the remaining ingredients Take a piping bag and pour into a parchment paper-lined baking sheet Freeze for around three hours and stored in your refrigerator

867. Fried Pineapple Slice

Time To Prepare: ten minutes Time to Cook: 8 minutes Yield: Servings 8

Ingredients:

¼ cup of coconut oil ¼ cup of coconut palm sugar ¼ teaspoon of ground cinnamon 1 fresh pineapple (peeled and slice into big slices)

Directions:

Warm a huge cast-iron frying pan on moderate heat. Put in oil and sugar and cook until the coconut oil has melted while stirring constantly. Put in the pineapple slices into two batches and cook for roughly 1-2 minutes. Flip the medial side and cook for approximately one minute. Carry on cooking for one more minute. Repeat the steps with the rest of the slices. Drizzle with cinnamon before you serve.

868. Grams Fruit Salad

Time To Prepare: 10 Minutes Time to Cook: 20 Minutes Yield: Servings 2-3

Ingredients:

½ of 1 Watermelon, chopped into little pieces 1 Pineapple, cut into little pieces 1 Pomegranate, small 1 Red Papaya, cut into little pieces 1 tsp. Ginger, freshly grated 4 Strawberries, chopped Dash of Turmeric

Directions:

To start with, place all the fruits in a large-sized container. Next, spoon in the turmeric and ginger over the fruits. Toss thoroughly before you serve.

869. Glorious Blueberry Crumble

Time To Prepare: ten minutes Time to Cook: thirty minutes Yield: Servings 6

Ingredients:

½ cup of softened coconut oil ½ tsp. of ground cinnamon 1 cup of almond meal 1 cup of toasted and finely crushed almonds 2 tbsp. of coconut sugar 4 cups of fresh blueberries

Directions:

Set the oven to 350F then lightly, grease a pie dish. In a huge container, combine all ingredients apart from blueberries. Split half of the almond mixture at the bottom of the prepared pie dish. Put blueberries over almond mixture uniformly. Top with the rest of the almond mixture uniformly. Bake for minimum 30 minutes or till the top becomes golden brown. Serve warm.

870. Grilled Peaches

Time To Prepare: ten minutes Time to Cook: ten minutes Yield: Servings 6

Ingredients:

¼ cup of walnuts, chopped ½ cup of coconut cream 1 teaspoon of organic vanilla extract 3 medium peaches (halved and pitted) Ground cinnamon

Directions:

Preheat the grill on moderate to low heat. Grease the grill grate. Position the peach slices on the grill with the cut-side down. Grill each side for three to five minutes or until the desired doneness is attained. .In the meantime, mix coconut cream with vanilla extract in a container. Beat until the desired smoothness is achieved. Ladle the whipped cream over each peach half. Top with walnuts and drizzle with cinnamon. Serve instantly.

871. Lemon Sorbet

Time To Prepare: ten minutes Time to Cook: 0 minutes Yield: Servings 2

Ingredients:

½ cup of raw honey ½ cups of fresh lemon juice 2 cups of filtered water 2 tablespoons of fresh lemon zest, grated

Directions:

Put into your freezer the ice-cream maker tub for a day before making the sorbet. Combine all ingredients in a pan, excluding the freshly squeezed lemon juice and cook on moderate heat. Simmer for minimum 1 minute, up to the sugar dissolves while stirring constantly. Take away the mixture from the heat and put in lemon juice. Move the combination to an airtight container and place in your fridge for around 2hours. Put it into an ice-cream maker and process according to the manufacturer's instructions. Put in one tablespoon of oil when the motor is running. Return the ice-cream into the airtight container and freeze for roughly 2 hours.

872. Lemonade Ice Pops

Time To Prepare: 4 hours and ten minutes Time to Cook: 0 minutes Yield: Servings 4

Ingredients:

1 cup hot water 2 cups cold water 2 iced tea and lemonade tea bags

Directions:

Put hot water in a container, put in tea bags, cover, and set aside for about ten minutes to steep. Squeeze the tea bags to take off all the water and then discard them. Put in cold water, split into your ice pop maker, freeze for around six hours, before you serve. Enjoy!

873. Mediterranean Rolled Baklava With Walnuts

Time To Prepare: twenty minutes Time to Cook: forty minutes Yield: Servings 12

Ingredients:

1 cup Cream of wheat or plain breadcrumbs 1 Lemon zest 1 medium Lemon 1/3 cup Milk 2 cups Walnuts 3 cups Granulated sugar 3 cups Water 3 sticks Melted Unsalted butter 3 tbsp. Sugar 8 sheets Thawed phyllo dough Syrup:

Directions:

Mix 3 cups of sugar, 3 cups of water and lemon slices in a pan and leave to boil Reduce the heat, then allow it to simmer until the sugar completely dissolves. It should take fifteen minutes. You should have a nice smooth syrup now. Now allow to cool for a bit. Cut the walnuts in a blender into bits using short pulses. Pour the walnuts in a container together with the cream of wheat, lemon zest and 4 tablespoons of sugar. Mix in milk and save for later. Now, preheat the oven to 375°F. Spread out the phyllo dough and fit it into a baking pan. Trim off the edges that do not fit with scissors. Cover the rest of the phyllo sheets while you work so they do not dry out. Put a sheet on a clean flat surface and glaze with melted butter. Do this for all the sheets until it's finished. Position the walnut mixture on one side of the sheets and roll them up like you're trying to make a sausage. Do this for all the sheets and walnuts. Position the walnut rolls on an ungreased baking pan and glaze with the leftover butter. Bake for approximately 45 minutes. It's ready when it looks golden. Turn off the oven then pull out the baking pan. Sprinkle syrup over the baklava, ensuring the syrup gets everywhere. Bring back the baking pan into the oven then let sit for five minutes. Remove from the oven and allow to cool for a few hours. Cut the rolls into small amounts before you serve.

874. No-Bake Carrot Cake Bites

Time To Prepare: fifteen minutes Time to Cook: 0 minutes Yield: Servings 6

Ingredients:

½ teaspoon of ground ginger ¾ cup of shredded coconut 1 and a ½ cups of carrots 1 cup of pitted Medjool dates 1 cup of walnuts 1 tablespoon of pure maple syrup 1 teaspoon of cinnamon

Directions: Put all together the ingredients into a high-speed blender or food processor, and blend until the mixture comes together, putting in a teaspoon of water at a time if required. Take the carrot mixture and press down into a cupcake tin, and place in your fridge until firm. Pop the carrot cakes out of the muffin tin, and enjoy!

875. Paleo Raspberry Cream Pie

Time To Prepare: twenty minutes Time to Cook: 0 minutes Yield: Servings 12

Ingredients:

For the crust: ½ cup Unsweetened shredded coconut 1 ½ tbsp. Maple syrup 1 cup Roasted or salted cashews 1 tsp. Vanilla extract Pinch Salt Raspberry filling: ¼ cup & 2 tsp. Fresh lemon juice ¼ cup Coconut cream from the top solid part of a can of coconut milk that has been placed in the fridge overnight ½ cup & 1 tbsp. Maple syrup ¾ cup Unrefined coconut oil 1 ½ cup Roasted or salted cashews 2 tsp. Vanilla extract 3 cups Fresh raspberries Pinch Salt

Directions: Prepare 12 muffin pans, line them with muffin liners, and set them aside. Make the crust. Set a pan on moderate heat and the coconut and stir until it's completely toasted. Stay by the pan because coconuts tend to burn very easily. Move the toasted coconuts to a container and leave to cool for five minutes or so. Honestly, this toasting step isn't particularly necessary, but I feel it adds amazing flavor to the crust. To make the crust, put all the ingredients in a blender and pulse at the lowest speed until the mix gets all clumpy. Also, do not pulse for too long, or you might end up with a paste. To know if it's ready, put a small amount of the mixture on your fingers and pinch. If it gets clumpy, you're on track, if not, put in a little water and pulse at the lowest speed for further minutes. Scoop the mix into the lined tins using your fingers to pack the mix firmly inside the pan. Place the pans to place in your fridge while you get to make the filling. In a tiny pot set using low heat, mix in all the ingredients until the oil and coconut cream melts completely. Clean the blender using a paper towel and pour in the filling. Pulse at high-speed for like 60 seconds or until it's super smooth. The only clumps we can forgive are the raspberry seeds. Sprinkle a quarter of the filling over the top of each crust. There must be extra filling; you can store and use that in a different dish. Put the coated muffins in your refrigerator to cool. This will take a few hours, like 6 hours, so if you do not have time for that, put it in the freezer. To serve, allow them to defrost for 80 minutes or until obviously creamy.

876. Peanut Butter Cookies

Time To Prepare: fifteen Minutes Time to Cook: 0 Minute Yield: Servings 9

Ingredients:

½ a cup of peanut butter (creamy and unsalted) 1 and a ¼ teaspoon of vanilla extract 1 cup of pitted Medjool dates 1 cup of raw almonds Sea salt as required

Directions:

Take a food processor and put in almonds, peanut butter, vanilla, dates and blend the whole mixture until a dough-like texture comes (should take a few minutes) If you desire, put in some more peanut butter to make the dough sticker. Form balls using the dough and press down using a fork to create a criss-cross pattern Drizzle salt liberally Serve instantly.

877. Pineapple Pie

Time To Prepare: fifteen minutes Time to Cook: 50 minutes Yield: Servings 8

Ingredients:

½-tsp baking powder 1-cup almond flour 1-tsp pure vanilla extract 2-pcs eggs 2-pcs fresh pineapple, peeled, cored, and cut into rings 3-Tbsps liquid coconut oil 5-Tbsps raw honey (divided) fifteen-pcs sweet cherries, fresh or frozen

Directions:

Preheat the oven to 350 °F. Pour 1½-tablespoon of the honey in a round baking tin. Position the cherries and pineapple rings on the bed of honey in a decorative pattern. Put the pan in your oven, then bake for minimum fifteen minutes. Meanwhile, mix in all the rest of the ingredients in a mixing container. Mix thoroughly until forming the mixture into dough. Set aside. Take the pan out from the oven. Push down the batter over the pineapple rings, smoothing it at the top. Return the pan in your oven, and bake further for a little more than half an hour

878. Pumpkin Ice Cream

Time To Prepare: fifteen minutes Time to Cook: 0 minutes Yield: Servings 6

Ingredients:

½ cup of dates (pitted and chopped) ½ teaspoon of ground cinnamon ½ teaspoon of vanilla flavor 1 (fifteen-ounce) can of sugar-free pumpkin puree 1 ½ teaspoon of pumpkin pie spice 2 (14-ounce) cans of unsweetened coconut milk Pinch of salt

Directions:

Combine all ingredients in a high-speed blender and pulse. Move the puree to an airtight container and freeze for roughly 1-2 hours. Move the frozen puree to an ice-cream maker and process following the manufacturers. Return the ice-cream to the airtight container and freeze for approximately 1-2 hours before you serve

879. Raspberry Diluted Frozen Sorbet

Time To Prepare: 10 min Time to Cook: 20 min Yield: Servings 4

Ingredients:

1 tsp honey 14oz / 400g frozen raspberry fl oz / 50g almond milk Mint

Directions:

Place the almond milk and raspberry in a mixer till it's smooth and leave the consistency in the freezer for about twenty minutes. When serving, place them in ice cream bowls and serve with mint on top.

880. Raspberry Gummies

Time To Prepare: five minutes Time to Cook: fifteen minutes Yield: Servings 6

Ingredients:

¼ cup of grass-fed gelatin ¾ cup of cold water 1 cup of frozen raspberries 3 tablespoons of raw honey

Directions:

Pour water into a blender followed by frozen raspberries. Puree and move them to a deep cooking pan on moderate heat. Put in honey and gelatin. Whisk. Reduce the heat, then whisk constantly for five minutes. Place the mixture on a baking dish or molds and place in your fridge for 60 minutes or until it firms. If you used a baking dish, chop the gelatin into squares. Pop the gelatin out with the molds.

881. Refreshing Raspberry Jelly

Time To Prepare: ten minutes+ 1 hour freezing Time to Cook: thirty minutes Yield: Servings 4

Ingredients:

¼ cup of water 1 tbsp. of fresh lemon juice 2 pound of fresh raspberries

Directions:

In a moderate-sized pan, put in raspberries and water on low heat and cook for approximately 8-ten minutes until done completely. Put in lemon juice and cook for approximately 30 minutes, stirring once in a while. Turn off the heat and put the mixture into a sieve. Position a strainer over a container. Through strainer, strain the mixture by pushing using the backside of a spoon. Place the mixture into a blender then pulse till a jelly-like texture is formed. Move into serving glass bowls and place in your fridge for minimum for approximately 1 hour.

882. Rum Butter Cookies

Time To Prepare: ten minutes + chilling time Time to Cook: five minutes Yield: Servings 12

Ingredients:

½ cup coconut butter ½ cup confectioners' Swerve 1 stick butter 1 teaspoon rum extract 4 cups almond meal

Directions:

Melt the coconut butter and butter. Mix in the Swerve and rum extract. Afterward, put in in the almond meal and mix to blend. Roll the balls and put them on a parchment-lined cookie sheet. Keep in your fridge until ready to serve.

883. Spiced Tea Pudding

Time To Prepare: ten minutes Time to Cook: ten minutes Yield: Servings 3

Ingredients:

½ cup coconut flakes ½ teaspoon cloves 1 ½ cups berries 1 can coconut milk 1 cup almond milk 1 tablespoon chia seeds 1 tablespoon ground cinnamon 1 tablespoon raw honey 1 teaspoon allspice 1 teaspoon cardamom 1 teaspoon green tea powder 1 teaspoon nutmeg 2 tablespoons pumpkin seeds 2 teaspoons ground ginger

Directions:

In your blender, puree tea powder with coconut milk, almond milk, cinnamon, coconut flakes, nutmeg, allspice, cloves, honey, cardamom, and ginger split into bowls. Heat a pan on moderate heat, put in berries until bubbling, then move to your blender and pulse well. Split the berries into the bowls with the coconut milk mix, top with chia seeds and pumpkin seeds before you serve. Enjoy!

884. Strawberry Granita

Time To Prepare: ten minutes Time to Cook: ten minutes Yield: Servings 8

Ingredients:

¼ teaspoon balsamic vinegar ½ teaspoon lemon juice 1 cup of water 2 lb. strawberries, halved & hulled Agave to taste Just a small pinch of salt

Directions:

Wash the strawberries in water. Keep in a blender. Put in water, agave, balsamic vinegar, salt, and lemon juice. Pulse multiple times so that the mixture moves. Blend until smooth. Pour into a baking dish. The puree must be 3/8 inch deep only. Place in your fridge the dish uncovered till the edges start to freeze. The center must be slushy. Stir crystals from the edges lightly into the center. Stir thoroughly to mix. Chill till the granite is nearly fully frozen. Scrape loose the crystals like before and mix. Place in your fridge once more. Using a fork, stir 3-4 times till the granite has become light.

885. Strawberry Orange Sorbet

Time To Prepare: five minutes Time to Cook: 0 minutes Yield: Servings 3

Ingredients:

1 cup Orange juice or coconut water 1 pound Frozen strawberries

Direction:

Pour strawberries in a blender and pulse until all you have left are flakes. two minutes tops. Now put in the coconut water or orange juice and pulse until you get a nice and smooth puree. Have a spatula handy because you might need to scrape some of the puree off the walls of the blender sometimes. Serve the moment you're done or put in the freezer for about forty-five minutes for a sorbet feel. Also, you can pour the smoothie into popsicle molds and freeze for hours or even overnight. Enjoy!

886. Strawberry Soufflé

Time To Prepare: fifteen minutes Time to Cook: twelve minutes Yield: Servings 6

Ingredients:

18 ounces of fresh strawberries, hulled 5 organic egg whites, divided 4 teaspoons of fresh lemon juice 1/3 cup of raw honey, divided

Directions:

Preheat your oven to 350F. Place the strawberries in a blender then pulse until a puree form. Strain the strawberry puree using a strainer while discarding the seeds. Mix the strawberry puree to three tablespoons of honey, two egg whites, and fresh lemon juice. Pulse until a frothy and light-weight develops. Beat the eggs in a separate container up to it becomes frothy. Put in the remaining honey and beat until a stiff peak forms. Gently- fold the egg whites into the strawberry mixture. Move the mixture toto six big ramekins and place them on a baking sheet. Bake for around 10-twelve minutes. Take out of the oven and serve instantly.

887. The Most Elegant Parsley Soufflé Ever

Time To Prepare: five minutes Time to Cook: six minutes Yield: Servings 5

Ingredients:

1 fresh red chili pepper, chopped 1 tablespoon fresh parsley, chopped 2 tablespoons coconut cream 2 whole eggs Sunflower seeds to taste

Directions:

Preheat the oven to 390 degrees F Almond butter 2 soufflé dishes Place the ingredients to a blender and mix thoroughly Split batter into soufflé dishes and bake for about six minutes Serve and enjoy!

888. Tropical Popsicles

Time To Prepare: 10 Minutes Time to Cook: 10 Minutes Yield: Servings 6

Ingredients:

½ tsp. Black Pepper 2 Kiwi, cut 2 tbsp. Coconut Oil 2 tsp. Turmeric 3 cups Pineapple, chopped

Directions:

First, place all the ingredients needed to make the popsicles excluding the kiwi in a high-speed blender for a couple of minutes or until you get a smooth mixture. After this, pour the smoothie into the popsicle molds. Next, insert the kiwi slices into the molds and then put the frames in the freezer until set. Tip: If you desire texture, you can blend it less

889. Vanilla Cakes

TimeTo Prepare: ten minutes Time to Cook: fifteen minutes Yield:Servings 8

Ingredients: .

5 tsp. Baking soda .5 tsp. Salt 1 cup Agave sweetener 1 cup Almond milk 1 tbsp. Apple cider vinegar 2 cup Whole wheat flour 2 tsp. Baking powder C.5 cup warmed coconut oil tsp. Vanilla extract

Directions: Ensure the oven is set to 350F. Prepare two muffin pans (12 c) for use by greasing them. Put in the apple cider vinegar into a measuring c that is big enough to hold minimum 2 c. Put in in the almond milk for a total of 1.5 c. Allow the results to curdle roughly five minutes or until done. Put together the salt, baking soda, baking powder, sugar, and flour together in a big container and whisk well. Separately, mix the vanilla, coconut oil, and curdled almond in its container before combining the two bowls and blending well. Put in the results to the muffin pans, dividing uniformly. Put the muffin pans in your oven and allow them to cook for approximately fifteen minutes. You will know if it's all already cook when you can press down on the tops and spring back when pressed lightly. Allow the cake pans to cool on a wire rack before removing the cakes for the best results.

890. Watermelon Sorbet

Time To Prepare: 5 Minutes Time to Cook: fifteen Minutes Yield: Servings 4

Ingredients:

1 Seedless Watermelon, cubed

Directions: To start with, put the watermelon cubes in a baking sheet in a uniform layer. Next, keep the sheet in the freezer for about two hours or until the watermelon is solid. After this, move the frozen watermelon cubes in the high-speed blender and puree them until you get a smooth puree. Next, pour the puree among the two loaf pans.

891. No-Bake Strawberry Cheesecake

Yield: 8 servings Preparation Time: twenty minutes Cooking Time: 5 minutes

Ingredients:

For Crust: • 1 cup almonds • 1 cup pecans • 2 tablespoons unswee10ed coconut flakes • 6 Medjool dates, pitted, soaked for 10 min and drained • Pinch of salt • For Filling: • 3 cups cashews, soaked and drained • ¼ cup organic honey • ¼ cup fresh lemon juice • 1/3 cup coconut oil, melted • 1 teaspoon organic vanilla flavor • ¼ teaspoon salt • 1 cup fresh strawberries, hulled and sliced • For Topping: • 1/3 cup maple syrup • 1/3 cup water • Drop of vanilla flavor • 5 cups fresh strawberries, hulled, sliced and divided

Directions: 1. Grease a 9-inch spring foam pan. 2. For crust in the small mixer, add almonds and pecans and pulse till finely grounded. 3. Add remaining all ingredients and pulse till smooth. 4. Transfer the crust mixture into prepared pan, pressing gently downwards. Freeze to create completely. 5. In a large blender, add all filling ingredients and pulse till creamy and smooth. 6. Place filling mixture over crust evenly. 7. Freeze for at least couple of hours or till set completely. 8. In a pan, add maple syrup, water, vanilla and 1 cup of strawberries on medium-low heat. 9. Bring to a gentle simmer. Simmer for around 4-5 minutes or till thickens. 10. Strain the sauce and allow it to go cool completely. 11. Top the chilled cheesecake with strawberry slices. Drizzle with sauce and serve.

892. Blackberry & Apple Skillet Cake

Yield: 4 servings Preparation Time: 20 minutes Cooking Time: 25 minutes

Ingredients:

For Filling: • 2 tablespoons coconut oil • 1 tablespoon coconut sugar • 3 sweet apples, cored and cut into bite sized pieces • ½ teaspoon ground cinnamon • ¼ teaspoon ground cardamom • 1/8 teaspoon ground cloves • 1/8 teaspoon ground ginger • 1 cup frozen blackberries • For Cake Mixture: • ¾ cup ground almonds • ½ teaspoon baking powder • 2 tablespoons coconut sugar • Pinch of salt • ¼ cup full- Fat coconut milk • 1 tablespoon coconut oil, melted • 1 organic egg, bea10 • ½ teaspoon organic vanilla extract

Directions:

1. Preheat the oven to 40 degrees F. 2. In an ovenproof skillet, add butter and coconut sugar on high heat. 3. Cook, stirring for approximately 2-3 minutes. 4. Stir in apples and spices and cook, stirring approximately 5 minutes. 5. Remove from heat and stir in blackberries. 6. Meanwhile in a bowl, mix together ground almonds, baking powder, coconut sugar and salt. 7. In another bowl, add remaining ingredients and beat till well combined. 8. Add egg mixture into ground almond mixture and mix till well combined. 9. Place a combination over fruit mixture evenly. 10. Transfer the skillet into oven. 11. Bake approximately 15-20 min. Serve warm.

893. Black Forest Pudding

Yield: 2 servings Preparation Time: 15 minutes Cooking Time: 2 minutes

Ingredients:

1 teaspoon coconut cream • 1 teaspoon coconut oil • 3-4 squares 70% chocolate bars, chopped • 1 cup coconut cream, whipped till thick and divided • 2 cups fresh cherries, pitted and quartered • 70% chocolate bars shaving, for garnishing • Shredded coconut, for garnishing

Directions:

1. In a smaller pan, add 1 teaspoon coconut cream, coconut oil and chopped chocolate on low heat. 2. Cook, stirring continuously for about 2 minutes or till thick and glossy. Immediately, remove from heat. 3. In 2 serving glasses, divide chocolate sauce evenly. 4. Now, place ½ cup of cream over chocolate sauce in the glasses. 5. Divide cherries in glasses evenly. 6. Top with remaining coconut cream. 7. Garnish with chocolate shaving and shredded coconut.

894. Fried Pineapple Slices

Yield: 6-8 servings Preparation Time: quarter-hour Cooking Time: 6 minutes

Ingredients

1 fresh pineapple, peeled and cut into large slices • ¼ cup coconut oil • ¼ cup coconut palm sugar • ¼ teaspoon ground cinnamon

Directions:

Heat a large surefire skillet on medium heat. 2. Stir in oil and sugar till coconut oil is very melted. 3. Add pineapple slices in batches and cook for approximately 1-2 minutes. 4. Carefully flip the side and cook for around 1 minute. 5. Cook for approximately 1 minute more. 6. Repeat with remaining slices. 7. Sprinkle with cinnamon and serve.

895. Baked Apples

Yield: 4 servings Preparation Time: quarter-hour Cooking Time: 18 minutes

Ingredients:

4 tart apples, cored • ¼ cup coconut oil, sof1oed • 4 teaspoons ground cinnamon • 1/8 teaspoon ground ginger • 1/8 teaspoon ground nutmeg

Directions:

1. Preheat the oven to 350 degrees F. 2. Fill each apple with 1 tablespoon of coconut oil. 3. Sprinkle with spices evenly. 4. Arrange the apples onto a baking sheet. 5. Bake for around 12-18 minutes.

896. Rhubarb & Blueberry Granita

Yield: 8 servings Preparation Time: 15 minutes Cooking Time: 10 min

Ingredients:

1 cup fresh blueberries • 3cups rhubarb, sliced • ½ cup raw honey • 2½ cups water • Fresh mint leaves, for garnishing

Directions:

1. In a pan, add all ingredients on medium heat. 2. Cook, stirring occasionally for around 10 minutes. 3. Strain the mix through a strainer by pressing a combination. 4. Discard the pulp of fruit. 5. Transfer the strained mixture right into a 13x9-inch glass baking dish. 6. Freeze for around 20-a half-hour. 7. Remove from freezer and with a fork scrap the mix. 8. Cover and freeze for approximately 60 minutes, scraping after every half an hour.

897. Pumpkin Ice-Cream

Yield: 6-8 servings Preparation Time: quarter-hour Ingredients: • 1 (15-ounce) can pumpkin puree • ½ cup dates, pitted and chopped • 2 (14-ounce) cans coconut milk • ½ teaspoon vanilla extract • 1½ teaspoons pumpkin pie spice • ½ teaspoon ground cinnamon • Pinch of salt

Directions:

1. In an increased speed blender, add all ingredients and pulse till smooth. 2. Transfer into an airtight container and freeze for approximately 1-couple of hours. 3. Now, transfer into an ice-cream maker and process based on manufacturer's directions. 4. Return the ice-cream into airtight container and freeze for approximately 1-couple of hours.

898. Pineapple & Banana Ice-Cream

Yield: 6 servings Preparation Time: 15 minutes Cooking Time: 20 min

Ingredients:

1(14-ounce) can coconut milk • 1 cup frozen pineapple chunks, thawed • 4 cups frozen banana slices, thawed • 2 tablespoons fresh lime juice • Pinch of salt

Directions:

Line a glass baking dish with plastic wrap. 2. In a higher speed blender, add all ingredients and pulse till smooth. 3. Transfer the amalgamation into prepared baking dish evenly. 4. Freeze approximately 35-40 minutes.

899. Lemon Sorbet

Yield: 2 servings Preparation Time: 10 minutes

Ingredients:

2 tablespoons fresh lemon zest, grated • ½ cup raw honey • 2 cups water • 1½ cups freshly squeezed lemon juice

Directions:

1. Freeze ice-cream maker tub for about one day prior to sorbet. 2. In a pan, add all ingredients except fresh lemon juice on medium heat. 3. Simmer, stirring for approximately 1 minute or till sugar dissolves. 4. Remove from heat and stir in fresh lemon juice. 5. Transfer into an airtight container. 6. Refrigerate approximately 2 hours. 7. Now, transfer into an ice-cream maker and process according to manufacturer's directions. 8. While motor is running, add 1 tablespoon of oil. 9. Return the ice-cream into airtight container and freeze approximately 120 minutes.

900. Chocolate & Coffee Mousse

Yield: 4 servings Preparation Time: quarter-hour Cooking Time: twenty minutes

Ingredients:

¼ cup chocolate brown chips • ½ cup coconut milk • ¼ cup boiling water • 1 tablespoon ground coffees • Raw honey, to taste • ¼ teaspoon almond extract • 1 tablespoon vanilla flavor

Directions:

1. In a nonstick pan, add chocolate chips on medium-low heat. 2. Cook, stirring continuously for around 2-3 minutes or till chocolate chips are melted. 3. Add coconut milk and beat till well combined. 4. Cook, stirring continuously for around 1-2 minutes. 5. Meanwhile in a small bowl, mix together hot water and coffee beans. 6. In a sizable bowl, add chocolate mixture, coffee mixture, honey and both extracts and mix till well combined. 7. Transfer the mousse in 4 serving glasses. 8. Refrigerate to relax for approximately 2-3 hours.

901. Chocolaty Chia Pudding

Yield: 4 servings Preparation Time: 10 min

Ingredients:

6-9 dates, pitted and chopped • 1½ cups unswee10ed almond milk • 1/3 cup chia seeds • ¼ cup unswee10ed cocoa powder • ½ teaspoon ground cinnamon • Salt, to taste • ½ teaspoon vanilla flavor

Directions:

1. In a mixer, add all ingredients and pulse till smooth. 2. Transfer the mixture into serving bowls. 3. Refrigerate to chill completely before serving.

902. Apple Chia Pudding

Yield: 1 serving Preparation Time: fifteen minutes Cooking Time: 20 minutes

Ingredients:

½ cup unswee10ed almond milk • 2 tablespoons chia seeds • ½ teaspoon ground cinnamon, divided • 1/8 teaspoon vanilla extract • 1 apple, cored and chopped finely • ½ teaspoon raw honey • 1½ teaspoons water • 2 tablespoons golden raisins

Directions:

1. In a bowl, mix together almond milk, chia seeds, ¼ teaspoon of cinnamon and vanilla flavoring. 2. Refrigerate for around 1-120 minutes. 3. In a microwave safe bowl, mix together apple, honey, water and remaining cinnamon and microwave on high for around 1-2 minutes, stirring once. 4. Remove from microwave and stir in raisins. 5. Add 50 % of apple mixture in chia seeds mixture and stir to blend. 6. Refrigerate before serving. 7. Top with remaining apple mixture and serve.

903. Chocolate Custard

Yield: 4-8 servings Preparation Time: 15 minutes Cooking Time: 35 minutes

Ingredients:

1½ (14-ounce) cans coconut milk • 5 large organic eggs • ½ cup raw honey • 1 tablespoon vanilla flavor • 3 tablespoons powered cocoa • 2 tablespoons trouble • Pinch of ground cinnamon • Pinch of ground nutmeg

Directions:

1. Preheat the oven to 325 degrees F. Grease a casserole dish. 2. In a bowl, add coconut milk, eggs and honey and beat till well combined. 3. In a tiny bowl, add cocoa powder and warm water and mix till a paste forms. 4. Add chocolate paste in eggs mixture and stir to blend. 5. Transfer the mixture into prepared casserole dish evenly. 6. Sprinkle with cinnamon and nutmeg. 7. Arrange the casserole dish in a large baking dish. 8. Pour the boiling water in baking dish about midway of the casserole dish. 9. Bake for about 35 minutes or till a toothpick inserted inside the center comes out clean.

904. Strawberry Soufflé

Yield: 6 servings Preparation Time: quarter-hour Cooking Time: 12 minutes

Ingredients:

18-ounce fresh strawberries, hulled • 1/3 cup raw honey, divided • 5 organic egg whites, divided • 4 teaspoons fresh lemon juice

Directions:

1. Preheat the oven to 350 degrees F. 2. In a blender, ad strawberries and pulse till a puree forms. 3. Through a strainer, strain the seeds. 4. In a bowl, add strawberry puree, 3 tablespoons of honey, 2 egg whites and lemon juice and pulse till frothy and light-weight. 5. In another bowl, add remaining egg whites and beat till frothy. 6. While beating gradually, add remaining honey and beat till stiff peaks form. 7. Gently, fold the egg whites into strawberry mixture. 8. Transfer the amalgamation into 6 large ramekins evenly. 9. Arrange the ramekins in a baking sheet. 10. Bake approximately 10-12 minutes.

905. Mango & Pineapple Crisp

Yield: 6 servings Preparation Time: quarter-hour Cooking Time: fifteen minutes

Ingredients:

For Filling: • 2 tablespoons coconut oil • 2 tablespoons coconut sugar • 1 large mango, peeled, pitted and cut into chunks • 1 large pineapple, peeled and cut into chunks • 1/8 teaspoon ground cinnamon • 1/8 teaspoon ground ginger For Topping: • ¾ cup almonds • 1/3 cup coconut, shredded • ½ teaspoon ground allspice • ½ teaspoon ground cinnamon • ½ teaspoon ground ginger

Directions:

Preheat the oven to 375 degrees F. 2. For filling in the pan, melt coconut oil on medium-low heat. 3. Add coconut sugar and cook, stirring approximately 1-2 minutes. 4. Stir in remaining ingredients and cook approximately 5 minutes. 5. Remove from heat and transfer the mixture in a baking dish. 6. Meanwhile for topping in a blender, add all ingredients and pulse till a coarse meal forms. 7. Place the topping over filling evenly. 8. Bake for approximately fifteen minutes or top becomes golden brown.

906. Cherry Cobbler

Yield: 4 servings Preparation Time: fifteen minutes Cooking Time: 25 minutes

Ingredients:

2 cups fresh cherries, pitted • ¼ cup plus 1 tablespoon coconut palm sugar, divided • ¼ cup pecans, chopped • ¼ cup unswee10ed coconut, shredded • ¼ cup coconut flour • 1 tablespoon arrowroot flour • ½ teaspoon ground cinnamon • Pinch of salt

Directions:

1. Preheat the oven to 375 degrees F. 2. In a 7x5-inch baking dish, position the cherries. 3. Place ¼ cup of coconut sugar over cherries evenly. 4. Inna bowl, add 1 tablespoon of coconut sugar and remaining ingredients. 5. Spread pecan mixture over cherries evenly. 6. Bake for around 20-25 minutes.

907. No-Bake Lemony Cheesecake

Yield: 12 servings Preparation Time: twenty minutes

Ingredients:

For Crust: • 1 cup dates, pitted and chopped • 1 cup raw almonds • 2-3 tablespoons unswee10ed coconut, shredded For Filling: • 3½ cups cashews, soaked for overnight • ½ cup coconut oil, melted • 2 tablespoons fresh lemon rind, grated finely • ¾ cup fresh lemon juice • ¾ cup raw honey • 10 drops liquid stevia • 1 teaspoon vanilla flavoring • Salt, to taste • 1 lemon, sliced thinly

Directions:

1. In a blender, add dates, almonds and coconut and pulse till mixture just starts to blend. 2. Transfer the amalgamation in a greased spring foam pan. 3. With the back of spatula, smooth the top of crust. 4. In a food processor, add cashews and oil and pulse till well combined. 5. Add remaining ingredients except lemon slices and pulse till creamy and smooth. 6. Place the mixture over crust evenly. 7. With the back of spatula, smooth the surface of filling. 8. Refrigerate for about 60 minutes.

908. Banana Mug Cake

Yield: 1 serving Preparation Time: 10 minutes Cooking Time: 2 minutes

Ingredients:

1 banana, peeled a mashed • 3 tablespoons almond meal • ½ teaspoon baking powder • 1 tablespoon coconut sugar • ½ teaspoon ground cinnamon • Pinch of ground ginger • Pinch of salt • 1 tablespoon coconut oil, sof10ed • ½ teaspoon vanilla extract

Directions: 1. In a bowl, add all ingredients and mix till well combined. 2. Transfer the amalgamation right into a microwave safe mug. 3. Microwave on high for about 2 minutes.

909. Brown Rice Pudding

Yield: 6-8 servings Preparation Time: quarter-hour Cooking Time: twenty minutes

Ingredients:

2 cups cooked brown rice • 2 cups coconut milk • 2 large organic eggs • ¼ cup raw honey • 1 teaspoon fresh lemon zest, grated finely • 1 teaspoon ground cinnamon • ½ teaspoon ground ginger • ½ teaspoon ground cardamom • ¼ teaspoon fresh ginger, grated finely • 1 banana, peeled and sliced • ¼ cup almond flakes

Directions:

1. Preheat the oven to 390 degrees F. Grease a baking dish. 2. Place cooked rice inside bottom of prepared baking dish evenly. 3. In a big bowl, add coconut milk, eggs, honey, lemon zest and spices and beat till well combined. 4. Place the egg mixture over rice evenly and top with banana slices and almonds. 5. Bake for around 20 minutes.

910. Pineapple Upside-Down Cake

Yield: 6 servings Preparation Time: 15 minutes Cooking Time: 50 minutes

Ingredients:

5 tablespoons raw honey, divided • 2 (½-inch thick) fresh pineapple slices • 15 fresh sweet cherries • 1 cup almond flour • 12 teaspoon baking powder • 2 organic eggs • 3 tablespoons coconut oil, melted • 1 teaspoon vanilla extract • Fresh cherries, for garnishing

Directions:

1. Preheat the oven to 350 degrees F. 2. In an 8-inch round cake pan, place about 1½ tablespoons of honey evenly. 3. Arrange the pineapple slices and 15 cherries over honey within your desired pattern. 4. Bake for approximately 15 minutes. 5. In a bowl, mix together almond flour and baking powder. 6. In another bowl, add eggs and remaining honey and beat till creamy. 7. Add coconut oil and vanilla extract and beat till well combined. 8. Add flour mixture into egg mixture and mix till well combined. 9. Remove the wedding cake pan from oven. 10. Place the flour mixture over pineapple and cherries evenly. 11. Bake approximately 35 minutes. 12. Remove from oven and make aside to chill for approximately 10 min. 13. Carefully invert the dessert onto serving plate. 14. Garnish with cherries and serve.

911. Fudge Brownies

Yield: 9 servings Preparation Time: 15 minutes Cooking Time: 26 minutes

Ingredients:

2-ounce unsweet10ed dark chocolate, chopped roughly • ½ cup cocoa powder • ½ cup coconut oil, melted • ¾ cup raw honey • 2 organic eggs • 1 teaspoon vanilla extract • ¼ cup coconut flour • Salt, to taste

Directions:

1. Preheat the oven to 350 degrees F. Line a 9x9-inch baking dish using a greased parchment paper. 2. In a medium nonstick pan, mix together the chocolate, powered cocoa and coconut oil on medium heat. 3. Cook, beating continuously approximately 2-3 minutes or till the amalgamation becomes smooth. 4. Remove from heat and immediately, stir in honey. 5. Add the eggs and vanilla flavoring and beat till well combined. 6. Transfer the amalgamation into prepared baking dish evenly. 7. With the back of spatula, smooth the very best surface. 8. Bake for around 20-23 minutes or till a toothpick inserted inside the center happens clean. 9. Remove from oven and make aside to cool completely. 10. After cooling, cut into desired size squares and serve.

912. Lemony Tarts

Yield: 4 servings Preparation Time: 15 minutes Cooking Time: quarter-hour

Ingredients:

For Crust: • 1 cup almond meal • 4 teaspoon dates, pitted • 3 tablespoons fresh lemon juice For Filling: • 2 teaspoons fresh lemon zest, grated finely • 1/3 cup fresh lemon juice • 1 tablespoon raw honey • 2 organic eggs, bea10

Directions:

Preheat the oven to 350 degrees F. Line 4 muffin cups with paper liners. 2. For crust inside a food processor, add all ingredients and pulse till well combined. 3. Place the amalgamation into prepared muffin cups and press firmly inside the bottom or more sides. 4. Bake approximately 10-12 minutes. 5. Meanwhile in a pan, mix together the all filling ingredients except egg on low heat. 6. Simmer for about 2 minutes. 7. Slowly, add the eggs, beating continuously till well combined. 8. Remove from heat and make aside to cool for around 5 minutes. 9. Place the filling inside the shells and refrigerate to cool.

913. Chocolaty Cherry Truffles

Yield: 10-11 serving Preparation Time: twenty minutes

Ingredients:

2½ cups canned cherries in natural juice, drained • 2 cups almond meal • 1½ tablespoons coconut oil, sof10ed • 2 tablespoons raw honey • 3 cups unswee10ed coconut (desiccated) • 1 teaspoon flaxseed oil • 2/3 bar of dark chocolate bar, grated finely

Directions:

1. In a food processor, add cherries, almond meal, coconut oil and honey and pulse till a thick mixture forms. 2. Transfer a combination in to a bowl. 3. Add coconut and flaxseed oil and mix till well combined. 4. With your hands, make small equal sized balls through the mixture. 5. In a shallow dish, place the grated chocolate. 6. Roll the balls in chocolate evenly. 7. Arrange the balls onto a parchment paper lined baking sheet. 8. With a plastic wrap, cover the baking sheet and refrigerate for about 2-3 hours.

914. Almond Cookies

Time To Prepare: fifteen min Time to Cook: fifteen min Yield: Servings 12

Ingredients:

½ tsp honey ½ tsp vanilla 1.7oz / 50g coconut butter 14oz / 400g non-wheat flour 1tsp baking powder 1tsp baking soda 3.5oz / 100g tahini Salt

Directions:

Combine the flour, soda, salt, baking powder together. Mix tahini and coconut butter together and put in 2 tbsp. water in the same container. Put in honey, vanilla to the tahini mixture and blend it well with a mixer. Preheat the oven (180C/356F) and place a baking sheet on it. Put in 24 tablespoons of the mixture onto the baking sheet and allow it to bake in your oven for 11-fifteen minutes. Allow it to get cold a little bit before you serve.

915. Apple Fritters

Time To Prepare:fifteen minutes Time to Cook: ten minutes Yield:Servings 4

Ingredients:

½ cup cashew milk 1 apple, cored, peeled, and chopped 1 cup all-purpose flour 1 egg 1½ teaspoons of baking powder 2 tablespoons of stevia sugar

Directions: Preheat the air fryer to 175 degrees C or 350 degrees F. Place parchment paper at the bottom of your fryer. Line with cooking spray. Mix together ¼ cup sugar, flour, baking powder, egg, milk, and salt in a container. Mix well by stirring. Drizzle 2 tablespoons of sugar on the apples. Coat well. Mix the apples into your flour mixture. Use a cookie scoop and drop the fritters with it to the air fryer basket's bottom. Now air fry for five minutes. Flip the fritters once and fry for another three minutes. They must be golden.

916. Avocado Chia Parfait

Time ToPrepare:five minutes Time to Cook: twenty minutes Yield:Servings 2

Ingredients:

⅛ teaspoon nutmeg powder ½ teaspoon cinnamon powder ¾ teaspoon cinnamon powder 1 banana, mashed 1 tablespoon cashew nuts, chopped 1¼ cups almond milk 2 avocados, diced 2 tablespoons chia seeds 2 tablespoons pumpkin seeds For the Avocado Jam For the Parfait Base Pinch of sea salt

Directions: In a container, mix almond milk, banana, nutmeg powder, cinnamon powder, and pumpkin seeds. Mix until well blended. Chill in your refrigerator. In the meantime, put the deep cooking pan on moderate heat. Mix avocados, nutmeg powder, cinnamon powder, and salt. Bring to its boiling point. Allow simmering for about twenty minutes. Remove the heat. Mash half of the jam using a wooden spoon. Allow to cool. Set aside. Ladle 2 tablespoons of parfait base and apple jam into parfait glasses. Decorate using cashew nuts and serve

917. Avocado Chocolate Mousse

Time To Prepare: ten minutes Time to Cook: 0 minute Yield: Servings 9

Ingredients:

¼ cup espresso beans, ground ¼ cup of cocoa powder ½ teaspoon salt 1 bar dark chocolate 1 teaspoon vanilla extract 1/8 cup almond milk, unsweetened 2 tablespoons raw honey 3 ripe avocado, pitted and flesh scooped out 6 ounces plain Greek yogurt

Directions:

Put all ingredients in a food processor Pulse until the desired smoothness is achieved Best enjoyed chilled.

918. Banana Bars

Time To Prepare: ten minutes Time to Cook: 60 minutes Yield: Servings 4

Ingredients:

½ Cup Coconut Milk ½ Cup Melted Butter 1 Cup Chocolate Chips 1 Tsp. Baking Soda 1 Tsp. Pure Vanilla Extract 1/4 Tbsp. Cinnamon 2 Cup Brown Sugar 2 Cup Whole Wheat Flour 2 Eggs 5 Cup Ripe Mashed Banana Salt

Direction:

Preheat your oven to 170C. Mix all together the ingredients to make the batter. Put the batter in a wide tray and bake for about twenty minutes at 170C. Serve with liquid chocolate or fruits

919. Banana Cinnamon Cookies

Time To Prepare: five minutes Time to Cook: ten minutes Yield: Servings 2

Ingredients:

2 ripe bananas, peeled ¼ cup almond milk, unsweetened 4 pitted dates 1 tablespoon cinnamon 1 teaspoon vanilla 1 ½ teaspoon lemon juice 3 tablespoons dried and chopped cranberries 1 teaspoon baking powder 2 tablespoons dried and chopped raisins 2/3 cup applesauce, unsweetened 2/3 cup coconut flour

Directions:

Preheat your oven to 350 degrees F. Use a food processor to mix almond milk, applesauce, dates, and bananas. Blend until you achieve a smooth consistency. Put in in coconut flour, baking powder, cinnamon, vanilla, and lemon juice. Blend for a minute. Fold in cranberries and raisins. Pour a baking sheet with the cookie dough. Put inside the oven for about twenty minutes. Let sit for five minutes and allow it to harden and serve.

920. Berry Ice Pops

Time To Prepare:3 Hours 5 Minutes Time to Cook: 0 minutes Yield:Servings4

Ingredients:

¼ Cup Water 1 Cup Blueberries, Fresh or Frozen 1 Cup Strawberries, Fresh or Frozen 1 Teaspoon Lemon Juice, Fresh 2 Cups Whole Milk Yogurt, Plain 2 Tablespoons Honey, Raw

Directions:

Put all together the ingredients in a blender, and blend until the desired smoothness is achieved. Pour into your molds, and freeze for minimum three hours before you serve

921. Berry-Banana Yogurt

Time To Prepare: ten minutes Time to Cook: 0 minute Yield: Servings 1

Ingredients:

¼ cup collard greens, chopped ¼ cup quick-cooking oats ½ banana, frozen fresh ½ cup blueberries, fresh and frozen 1 container 5.3ounes Greek yogurt, non-fat 1 cup almond milk 5-6 ice cubes

Directions:

Take microwave-safe cup and put in 1 cup almond milk and ¼ cup oats Put the cups into your microwave on high for 2.5 minutes When oats are cooked and 2 ice cubes to cool Combine them well Put in all ingredients in your blender Blend until smooth and creamy Best enjoyed chilled.

922. Blueberry Crisp

Time To Prepare: five minutes Time to Cook: thirty minutes Yield: Servings 4

Ingredients:

¼ cups pecans, chopped ¼ teaspoon nutmeg ½ teaspoon ginger 1 cup buckwheat 1 lb. blueberries 1 teaspoon of cinnamon 1 teaspoon of honey 2 tablespoons olive oil

Directions:

Preheat the oven to 350 degrees F. Grease a baking dish. Mix together the pecans, wheat, oil, spices, and honey in a container. Put in the berries to your pan. Layer the topping on your berries. Bake for thirty minutes at 350 F.

923. Blueberry Sour Cream Cake

Time To Prepare: twenty minutes Time to Cook: 70 minutes Yield:Servings 4

Ingredients:

1 Cup Blueberry 1 Cup Of Melted Butter 1 Cup Sour Cream 1 Tsp Vanilla Extract 1 Tsp. Baking Powder 1 Tsp. Cinnamon Powder 2 Cups Of Brown Sugar 2 Large Eggs 2 Tbsp. All-Purpose Flour Salt

Direction:

Preheat oven on 175C. Mix together the butter and sugar till light and fluffy. Put sour cream, vanilla extract, and eggs into the mixture. In another container, put all together the dry ingredients then mix. Place the dry mixture into the butter mixture, putting in blueberries, then mix well. Put the batter into a greased pan then bake for about fifty minutes at 170C. Serve with sour cream and blueberries.

924. Café-Style Fudge

Time To Prepare: ten minutes + chilling time Time to Cook: 0 minutes Yield: Servings 6

Ingredients:

½ teaspoon vanilla extract 1 stick butter 1 tablespoon instant coffee granules 4 tablespoons cocoa powder 4 tablespoons confectioners' Swerve

Directions:

Beat the butter and Swerve at low speed. Put in in the cocoa powder, instant coffee granules, and vanilla and continue to stir until well blended. Ladle the batter into a foil-lined baking sheet. Place in your fridge for two to three hours. Enjoy!

925. Grams Choco Chia Cherry Cream

Time To Prepare: 4 hours and five minutes Time to Cook: 0 minutes Yield: Servings 4

Ingredients:

¼-cup chia seeds, powdered ½-cup cherries, pitted and cut + extra for plating 1½-cups almond milk 2-Tbsps pure maple syrup or honey 3-Tbsps raw cacao, powdered Additional toppings: extra raw cacao nibs, cherries, and 70% or higher dark chocolate shavings

Directions:

Mix in all the ingredients, excluding the cherries in a mason jar. Mix thoroughly until meticulously blended. Place in your fridge overnight or for 4 hours. Before you serve, split the pudding equally among four serving plates. Top each plate with the cherries. Decorate using the additional toppings.

926. Chocolate Cherry Chia Pudding

Time To Prepare: 4 hours and five minutes Time to Cook: 0 minutes Yield: Servings 4

Ingredients:

¼ cup Chia seeds You can also use chia seed powder. ½ cup Sliced pitted cherries 1 ½ cup Any non-dairy milk like coconut or almond milk 3 tbsp. Maple syrup or honey 3 tbsp. Raw cacao powder Additional toppings: Dark chocolate shavings (Preferably 70% dark chocolate or more) Extra cherries Raw cacao nibs

Directions:

Use a mason jar or a container. If you're using a container, just pour in the milk, maple syrup, chia seeds or powder, and raw cacao. Stir meticulously and place in your fridge for 4 hours or more. If you decide to use a mason jar, just pour in the same ingredients, screw the lid on and shake vigorously! Serve in separate dishes and top with any or all of the toppings I listed above. Enjoy!

927. Chocolate Chip Quinoa Granola Bars

Time To Prepare: five minutes Time to Cook: ten minutes Yield: Servings 16

Ingredients:

¼ teaspoon salt ½ cup flax seed ½ cup of chia seeds ½ cup of chocolate chips ½ cup of honey ½ cup walnuts, chopped 1 cup buckwheat 1 cup uncooked quinoa 1 teaspoon of cinnamon 1 teaspoon of vanilla 2/3 cup dairy-free margarine

Directions:

Preheat the oven to 350 degrees F. Spread the walnuts, quinoa, wheat, flax, and chia on your baking sheet. Bake for about ten minutes. Coat a baking dish using plastic wrap. Line with cooking spray. Keep aside. Melt the margarine and honey in a saucepot. Mix together the vanilla, salt, and cinnamon into the margarine mix. Keep the wheat mix and quinoa in a container. Pour the margarine sauce into it. Mix the mixture. Coat well. Let it cool. Mix in the chocolate chips. Spread your mixture into the baking dish. Push tightly into the pan. Plastic wrap. Place in your fridge overnight. Cut into bars and serve.

928. Chocolate Fudge Bites

TimeTo Prepare:ten minutes Time to Cook: three minutes Yield: Servings 10

Ingredients:

½ cup of coconut milk powder ½ cup of cold water ½ cup of raw cocoa powder 1 and a ¼ cup of boiling water 1 cup of coconut oil 1/3 cup of pure maple syrup 3 tablespoons of grass-fed gelatin

Directions:

Mix one and a quarter cup of boiling water with the gelatin, and boil for about three minutes. Next, put the gelatin mixture into a blender with the cold water and rest of the ingredients. Blend for about 2 minutes to help the gelatin solidify. Put the mixture into the bottom of a greased baking dish, then place in your fridge until firm. Cut into little serving squares.

929. Cinnamon Apple Chips

Time To Prepare: 10 Minutes Time to Cook: 2 Hours Yield: Servings 3

Ingredients:

¾ tsp. Cinnamon, grounded 3 Honey crisp Apple, big & sweet

Directions:

For making this dessert fare, preheat your oven to 200 °F. Next, keep a parchment paper-lined baking sheet in the center and lower rack. With the help of an apple corer, core the apples and then slice the apples into 1/8-inch-thick rounds. Next, position the apples in the preheated baking sheet in a single layer. After this, drizzle the cinnamon over the apples. Once sprinkled, bake them for an hour. Take away the baking sheet and then switch their position. Bake them for another one to 1 ½ hour or until the chips are crunchy. To finish, once they are crisp in accordance with your liking, remove the apple chips from the oven. Let the chips cool for one hour before you serve.

930. Citrus Strawberry Granita

Time To Prepare: fifteen minutes Time to Cook: 0 minutes Yield: Servings 4

Ingredients:

¼ cup of raw honey ¼ lemon 1 grapefruit (peeled, seeded, and sectioned) 12 ounces of fresh strawberries, hulled 2 oranges (peeled, seeded and sectioned)

Directions:

Put strawberries, grapefruit, oranges, and lemon in a juicer and extract juice according to the manufacturer's instructions. Put 1½ cups of the veggie juice and honey to a pan and cook on moderate heat for five minutes while stirring constantly. Remove it from heat and put in it to the rest of the juice. Set aside for roughly thirty minutes. Move the juice mixture into an 8x8-inch glass baking dish. Freeze for 4 hours while scraping after every thirty minutes

931. Coconut Butter Fudge

Time To Prepare: ten minutes Time to Cook: 0 minutes Yield: Servings 6

Ingredients:

¼ teaspoon of salt 1 cup of coconut butter 1 teaspoon of pure vanilla extract 2 tablespoons of raw honey

Directions:

Start by lining an 8 x 8 inch baking dish using parchment paper. Melt the coconut butter, honey, and vanilla using low heat. Place the mixture into the baking pan, and place in your fridge for about two hours before you serve.

932. Coffee Cream

TimeTo Prepare: ten minutes Time to Cook: fifteen minutes Yield:Servings 4

Ingredients:

¼ cup brewed coffee 1 teaspoon vanilla extract 2 cups heavy cream 2 eggs 2 tablespoons ghee, melted 2 tablespoons swerve

Directions:

In a container, mix the coffee with the cream and the other ingredients, whisk well and split it into 4 ramekins and whisk well. Introduce the ramekins in your oven at 350 degrees F and bake for fifteen minutes. Serve warm

933. Cookie Dough Bites

Time To Prepare: 10 Minutes Time to Cook: 5 Minutes Yield: Servings 2

Ingredients:

¼ cup Almond Flour ¼ cup Chocolate Chips, dairy-free & sugar-free ½ cup Almond Butter or any nut butter ½ tsp. Salt 1 ½ cups Chickpeas, cooked 1 tsp. Vanilla Extract 2 tbsp. Maple Syrup

Directions:

First, place all the ingredients excluding the chocolate chips in a high-speed blender for about three minutes or until you get a thick, smooth mixture. After this, move the mixture to a moderate-sized container. Next, fold in the chocolate chips into the batter. Check for sweetness and put in more maple syrup if required. Serve and enjoy.

934. Creamy Frozen Yogurt

Time To Prepare: ten minutes + 2-three hours freezing Time to Cook: Yield: Servings 3

Ingredients:

½ cup of coconut yogurt ½ cup of unsweetened almond milk 1 tbsp. of raw honey 1 tsp. of fresh mint leaves 1 tsp. of organic vanilla extract 2 peeled, pitted and chopped medium avocados 2 tbsp. of fresh lemon juice

Directions:

Throw all the ingredients into a blender apart from mint leaves and pulse till creamy and smooth. Put into an airtight container then freeze for minimum 2-three hours. Take off from the freezer and keep aside for about fifteen minutes. With a spoon stir thoroughly. Top with fresh mint leaves before you serve.

935. Date Dough & Walnut Wafer

Time To Prepare: fifteen minutes Time to Cook: eighteen minutes Yield: Servings 8

Ingredients:

¼-cup coconut oil ¼-tsp sea salt ½-cup coconut, unsweetened ½-cup walnuts ½-tsp baking soda ½-tsp sea salt 1½-cup oats (divided) 18-pcs Medjool dates, pitted 1-pc egg 1-tsp lemon juice 2-Tbsps ground flaxseed 6-pcs Medjool dates, pitted and cut into four equivalent portions For the Date Layer:

Directions: Preheat the oven to 325°F. Coat a baking pan using parchment paper. Pulse a cup of oats in a food processor until making a flour consistency. Put in in the dates, coconut, baking soda, and sea salt. Pulse again until the dates completely break up. Put in the remaining oats and walnuts, and pulse until the nuts break, but still a bit lumpy. Put in the flaxseed, egg, and oil. Pulse the mixture further until meticulously blended. Set aside ½-cup of the date mixture to use as a topping later. Push down the rest of the mix to a uniform layer in the pan. Wash your food processor, and put in all the date layer ingredients. Pulse the mixture until the dates completely break up and take on a light caramel color. With wet hands, press the mixture down, smoothing it on the date mixture. Crumble and drizzle the reserved date mixture over the top. Place the pan in your oven. Bake for eighteen minutes. Allow the wafer to cool to room temperature before cutting into 16 pieces.

936. Fall-Time Custard

Time To Prepare: fifteen minutes Time to Cook: 60 minutes Yield: Servings 6

Ingredients:

¼ tsp. of ground ginger 1 cup of canned pumpkin 1 cup of coconut milk 1 tsp. of ground cinnamon 1 tsp. of organic vanilla extract 2 organic eggs 2 pinches of freshly grated nutmeg 8-10 drops of liquid stevia Pinch of salt

Directions: Preheat your oven to 350 degrees F. In a big container, put together pumpkin and spices then mix. In another container, put in the eggs and beat thoroughly. Put in the rest of the ingredients then whisk till well blended. Put in egg mixture into pumpkin mixture and mix till well blended. Move the mixture toto 6 ramekins. Position the ramekins in a baking dish, Put in sufficient water in the baking dish about two-inch high around the ramekins. Bake for approximately 1 hour or till a toothpick inserted in the middle comes out clean

937. Flourless Sweet Potato Brownies

Time To Prepare: ten minutes Time to Cook: thirty minutes Yield: Servings 9

Ingredients:

¼ cup Unsweetened Cocoa powder ½ cup Almond butter ½ cup Cooked sweet potato ½ tsp. Baking soda 1 big Whole egg 2 tsp. Vanilla extract 3 tbsp. Dairy-free chocolate chips, optional. 6 tbsp. Honey

Directions:

Prep the oven by preheating to 350°F. Coat a baking pan using parchment paper leaving a few extra inches on the sides to make it easier to discard or remove Blend all the ingredients, excluding the chocolate chips until you get a super smooth and tender batter. Move the creamy batter to your readied baking pan and use a spatula to spread it around, so it looks almost even. Slide it in your oven, then bake for thirty minutes or until a knife inserted into the pan comes out clean. Remove from the oven and leave to cool in the pan for fifteen minutes before putting it up on a wire rack. If you decide to use the chocolate chip topping, put the chips in a microwave-safe dish and heat until it completely melts. Remove from the microwave and sprinkle over the brownies. Serve or store!

938. Fruit Cobbler

Time To Prepare: ten minutesTime to Cook: twenty minutes Yield:Servings 8

Ingredients:

¼ Cup Coconut Oil, Melted ¼ Cup Coconut Sugar ½ Teaspoon Vanilla Extract, Pure ¾ Cup Almond Flour ¾ Cup Rolled Oats 1 Teaspoon Coconut Oil 1 Teaspoon Ground Cinnamon 2 Cups Nectarines, Fresh & Sliced 2 Cups Peaches, Fresh & Sliced 2 Tablespoons Lemon Juice, Fresh Dash Salt Filter Water for Mixing

Directions:

Begin by heating the oven to 425. Get out a cast-iron frying pan, coating it with a teaspoon of coconut oil. Mix your lemon juice, peaches, and nectarines together in the frying pan. Prepare your food processor, mixing your almond flour, oats, coconut sugar, and remaining coconut oil. Put in in your cinnamon, vanilla, and salt, pulsing until the oat mixture looks like a dry dough. If you need more moisture, put in filtered water a tablespoon at a time, and then break the dough into chunks, spreading it across the fruit. Bake for 20 minutes before you serve warm.

939. Glazed Banana

Time To Prepare: ten minutes Time to Cook: five minutes Yield: Servings 2

Ingredients:

1 peeled and cut under-ripened banana 1 tbsp. of filtered water 1 tbsp. of olive oil 1 tbsp. of raw honey 1/8 tsp. of ground cinnamon

Directions: In a nonstick frying pan, warm oil on moderate heat. Put in banana slices and cook for approximately 1-2 minutes per side. In the meantime, in a small container, put in water and honey and beat thoroughly. Move the banana slices on a serving plate. Instantly, pour honey mixture over banana slices. Keep aside to cool to room temperature. Serve with the drizzling of cinnamon

940. Green Tea Pudding

Time To Prepare: twenty minutesTime to Cook: ten minutes Yield:Servings 3

Ingredients:

1 Tsp. Matcha Green Tea Powder 1/4 Cup Brown Sugar 1/4 Cup Corn Starch 1/8-Tbsp. Cinnamon Powder 100g Butter 2 Cup Heavy Milk 3 Eggs Salt

Directions: In a big pot, mix brown sugar, milk, cornstarch, and matcha powder. In moderate heat, keep whisking until combined. Combine the hot batter with whisked eggs slowly. Cook for three to five minutes. Strain the mixture and put in butter. Place the mixture in a container, place in your fridge for a few hours before you serve.

941. Hot Chocolate

Time To Prepare: 5 Minutes Time to Cook: 5 Minutes Yield: Servings 2

Ingredients:

¼ tsp. Turmeric ½ tsp. Cinnamon 1 tbsp. Coconut Oil 1 tbsp. Honey, raw 2 cups Almond Milk 2 tbsp. Cocoa Powder, unsweetened

Directions:

To start with, bring the almond milk to its boiling point in a deep deep cooking pan on moderate heat. Now, bring this mixture to a simmer and then mix in the cocoa powder to it. Next, spoon in the turmeric powder and cinnamon to it. Mix thoroughly/ Next, put in honey to it and once blended well, put in the coconut oil Give the drink a good stir until everything comes together. Serve instantly.

942. Lemon Vegan Cake

Time To Prepare: ten minutes Time to Cook: ten minutes Yield: Servings 3

Ingredients:

½ lemon extract 1 cup of pitted dates 1 lemon juice and zest 1½ cup agave 1½ cups of dairy-free yogurt 1½ cups pineapple, crushed 1½ teaspoon vanilla extract 2½ cups pecans ½ 3 avocados, halved & pitted 3 cups of cauliflower rice, prepared Pinch of cinnamon

Directions:

Coat your baking sheet using parchment paper. Pulse the pecans in a food processor. Put in the agave and dates. Pulse for one minute. Move this mix to the baking sheet. Wipe the container of your processor. Combine the pineapple, agave, avocados, cauliflower, lemon juice, and zest in a food processor. Pulse till smooth Now put in the lemon extract, cinnamon, and vanilla extract. Pulse. Pour this mix into your pan, on the crust. Place in your fridge for around five hours at least. Take out the cake and keep it at room temperature for about twenty minutes. Take out the cake's outer ring. Mix together the vanilla extract, agave, and yogurt in a container. Pour on your cake

943. Matcha and Blueberries Pudding

Time To Prepare: three hours Time to Cook: 0 minutes Yield: Servings 2

Ingredients:

1 banana, cut 1 cup blueberries 1 cup matcha green tea powder 2 cups almond milk 4 tablespoons chia seeds

Directions:

Put chia seeds, milk and matcha powder in a container. Stir, cover, then place in your fridge for around three hours. Split into bowls, top with banana slices and blueberries before you serve. Enjoy!

944. Mint Chocolate Chip Ice-cream

Time To Prepare: five minutes Time to Cook: 0 minutes Yield: Servings 2

Ingredients:

½ cup Raw cashews or coconut cream, optional. 1/8 tsp. Pure peppermint extract 2 Frozen overripe bananas 3 tbsp. Chocolate chips or sugar-free chocolate chips Pinch Salt Pinch Spirulina or any natural food coloring, optional.

Directions:

Mint or imitation peppermint won't be a substitute for this. Use pure peppermint extract and pour in slowly. Peel and chop the bananas first. Put the slices in a Ziplock bag then freeze. For the ice cream, put all the ingredients in a blender and pulse. You can skip the chocolate chips and just put in them after blending. Serve the moment it's ready or freeze until it's firm enough, then serve

945. No-Bake Cheesecake

Time To Prepare: twenty minutes Time to Cook: 0 minutes Yield: Servings 12

Ingredients:

For Crust: 1 cup of dates (pitted and chopped) 1 cup of raw almonds two to three tablespoons of unsweetened coconut, shredded For Filling: ½ cup of coconut oil, melted ¾ cup of fresh lemon juice ¾ cup of raw honey 1 teaspoon of organic vanilla extract 10 drops of liquid stevia 2 tablespoons of fresh lemon rind, grated finely 3½ cups of cashews, soaked overnight A thinly cut lemon Salt

Directions: Put together the dates, almonds, and coconut in a blender and pulse. Move the puree a greased springform pan. Smooth the outer lining of the crust using a spatula. Put cashews and oil in a food processor and pulse. Put in the rest of the ingredients except for lemon slices and pulse until it turns creamy and smooth. Put the combination over the crust uniformly. Smooth the counter of filling using the corner of a spatula. Place in your fridge for one hour. Take it off from the fridge and decorate with lemon slices. Chop it into desired sized slices before you serve

946. Peanut Butter Balls

Time To Prepare: twenty minutes Time to Cook: thirty minutes Yield: Servings 5

Ingredients:

1 Tsp. Vanilla Extract 2 Tbsp. Peanut Oil. 200g Powdered Sugar 250g Chocolate 250g Creamy Peanut Butter 90g Melted Butter

Direction: Mix everything apart from the oil and chocolates to make a batter Place in your fridge the batter for about forty-five minutes. Make small balls with the batter using and put them on a parchment paper. Place in your fridge for one more hour. Melt some dark chocolate. Place the peanut balls into the chocolate and place in your fridge for about twenty minutes. Serve with strawberry

947. Pineapple Cake

Time To Prepare: fifteen minutes Time to Cook: 50 minutes Yield: Servings 8

Ingredients:

½ tsp. Baking powder 1 tbsp. Almond flour 1 tsp. Vanilla extract 2 slices Fresh pineapples 2 Whole medium eggs 3 tbsp. Melted coconut oil 5 tbsp. Raw honey fifteen pcs. Frozen sweet cherries

Directions: Preheat your oven to 350°F. Take away the skin and core of the pineapples. Set aside. Sprinkle 1½ tablespoons of raw honey in a round cake tin. Layer the pineapple rings and sweet cherries on the honey in a decorative fashion. Bring the cake tin in your oven then bake for fifteen minutes. While all that is going on, mix in the almond and baking powder. In a different container, mix the eggs and leftover honey. Sprinkle in coconut oil and stir. Now put in the almond mix to the egg mix and stir meticulously. Take out the cake tin and sprinkle batter over the top of the partly baked pineapple rings and use a spatula to spread it uniformly. Place the cake tin back in your oven and bake for an additional thirty-five minutes. When it's all set, take it out of the oven and leave it to sit for about ten minutes before place it to a plate. Serve with extra cherries if you prefer.

948. Pistachioed Panna-Cotta Cocoa

Time To Prepare: eighteen minutes Time to Cook: two minutes Yield: Servings 6

Ingredients:

12-oz. dark chocolate 1-Tbsp coconut oil 3-pcs big bananas, cut into thirds Cocoa nibs, chopped Salted pistachios, chopped Spiced or smoked almonds, chopped

Directions: Coat a baking pan using parchment paper. Melt the dark chocolate with oil in your microwave. Set aside. Pierce a Popsicle stick midway into one end of each banana. Immerse each banana into the melted chocolate. Put dipped bananas into the baking sheet. Drizzle liberally with the cocoa nibs, almonds, and pistachios. Put the sheet in your freezer to harden and set.

949. Pure Avocado Pudding

Time To Prepare: three hours Time to Cook: 0 minutes Yield: Servings 4

Ingredients:

¼ teaspoon cinnamon ¾ cup cocoa powder 1 cup almond milk 1 teaspoon vanilla extract 2 avocados, peeled and pitted 2 tablespoons stevia Walnuts, chopped for serving

Directions:

Put in avocados to a blender and pulse well Put in cocoa powder, almond milk, stevia, vanilla bean extract and pulse the mixture well Put into serving bowls then top with walnuts Chill for two to three hours and serve!

950. Raspberry Gummies

TimeTo Prepare:five minutes Time to Cook: fifteen minutes Yield: Servings 6

Ingredients:

¼ cup of grass-fed gelatin ¾ cup of cold water 1 cup of frozen raspberries 3 tablespoons of raw honey

Directions:

Put the water and frozen raspberries into a blender, and blend until the desired smoothness is achieved. Put into a big deep cooking pan on moderate heat. Put in the honey and gelatin and whisk together. Reduce the heat, then whisk for another five minutes. Pour into molds or a baking dish, and place in your fridge for minimum 1 hour until firm. If you use a baking dish, chop the gelatin into squares; if not, just pop the gelatin out of the molds.

951. Raw Black Forest Brownies

Time To Prepare: 2 hours and ten minutes Time to Cook: 0 minute Yield: Servings 6

Ingredients:

¼ teaspoon salt ½ cup almonds, chopped ½ cup dates pitted 1 and ½ cups cherries, pitted, dried and chopped 1 cup raw cacao powder 2 cups walnuts, chopped

Directions:

Put all ingredients in a food processor Pulse until small crumbs are formed Push the brownie batter in a pan Freeze for a couple of hours Slice before you serve and enjoy

952. Roasted Bananas

Time To Prepare: two minutes Time to Cook: seven minutes Yield:Servings 1

Ingredients:

1 banana, cut into diagonal pieces Avocado oil cooking spray

Directions:

Take parchment paper and line the air fryer basket with it. Preheat the air fryer to 190 degrees C or 375 degrees F. Keep your slices of banana in the basket. Make sure they do not touch Apply avocado oil to mist the slices of banana. Cook for five minutes. Take out the basket. Flip the slices cautiously. Cook for two more minutes. The slices of banana must be caramelized and brown. Remove them from the basket.

953. Pineapple

Time To Prepare: 20 Minutes Time to Cook: 0 Minute Yield: Servings 4

Ingredients:

1 can of 8-ounce pineapple chunks ¼ teaspoon of ground ginger ¼ teaspoon of vanilla extract 1 can of 11-ounce orange sections 2 cups of pineapple, lemon or lime sherbet 1/3 cup of orange marmalade

Directions:

Drain the pineapple, ensure you reserve the juice. Take a moderate-sized container and put in pineapple juice, ginger, vanilla and marmalade to the container Put in pineapple chunks, drained mandarin oranges as well Toss thoroughly and coat everything Free them for fifteen minutes and let them chill Ladle the sherbet into 4 chilled stemmed sherbet dishes Top each of them with fruit mixture Enjoy!

954. Spicy Popper Mug Cake

Time To Prepare: five minutes Time to Cook: five minutes Yield: Servings 2

Ingredients:

¼ teaspoon sunflower seeds ½ a jalapeno pepper ½ teaspoon baking powder 1 bacon, cooked and cut 1 big egg 1 tablespoon almond butter 1 tablespoon cashew cheese 1 tablespoon flaxseed meal 2 tablespoons almond flour

Directions:

Take a frying pan then place it on moderate heat Put cut bacon and cook until they have a crunchy texture Take a microwave proof container and mix all of the listed ingredients(including cooked bacon), clean the sides Microwave for 75 seconds making to put your microwave to high power Take out the cup and slam it against a surface to take the cake out Decorate using a bit of jalapeno and serve!

955. Strawberry Ice Cream

Time To Prepare: 5 Minutes Time to Cook: 5 Minutes Yield: Servings 2-3

Ingredients:

1 Banana, frozen & cut 1 cup Strawberries, frozen 1 tsp. Vanilla extract 2 tbsp. Coconut Milk

Directions:

Begin by placing strawberries and banana in a high-speed blender and blend it for two to three minutes. While you blend, spoon in the coconut milk, and the vanilla extract. Carry on blending until the mixture is thick and smooth. Serve the ice-cream instantly since it does not keep well in the freezer

956. Strawberry Shortcake

Time To Prepare: fifteen minutes Time to Cook: 0 minutes Yield: Servings 4

Ingredients:

.25 cup Semi-sweet chocolate chips 1 tbsp. Low-calorie margarine 12 hulled Strawberries 2.3-inch Shortcake, quartered

Directions:

Using waxed paper, line a cookie sheet. Thread 2 shortcake pieces and 3 strawberries on 4 skewers. In a small deep cooking pan, mix together the margarine and chocolate chips before placing the deep cooking pan on the stove over a burner turned to low heat. Stir until the ingredients are well mixed. Sprinkle the chocolate onto the kabobs and then put them in your fridge for about four minutes to cool.

957. Sweet Almond And Coconut Fat Bombs

Time To Prepare: ten minutes + twenty minutes chill time Time to Cook: 0 minutes Yield: Servings 4

Ingredients:

¼ cup melted coconut oil 3 tablespoons cocoa 9 and ½ tablespoons almond butter 9 tablespoons melted almond butter, sunflower seeds 90 drops liquid stevia

Directions:

Take a container and put in all of the listed ingredients Combine them well Pour scant 2 tablespoons of the mixture into as many muffin molds as you prefer Chill for about twenty minutes and pop them out Serve and enjoy!

958. Tropical Fruit Crisp

Time To Prepare: ten minutesTime to Cook: fifteen minutes Yield:Servings 6

Ingredients:

For the Filling: 1 big mango (cut into chunks) 1 big pineapple (cut into chunks) 1/8 teaspoon of ground cinnamon 1/8 teaspoon of ground ginger 2 tablespoons of coconut oil 2 tablespoons of coconut sugar For the Topping: ¾ cup of almonds ½ teaspoon of ground allspice ½ teaspoon of ground cinnamon ½ teaspoon of ground ginger 1/3 cup of unsweetened coconut, shredded

Directions:

Preheat your oven to 375 degrees F. To make the filling: melt the coconut oil in a pan on medium-low heat and cook the coconut sugar for a couple of minutes while stirring. Put in the rest of the ingredients then cook for minimum five minutes. Stir. Take away the contents from heat and move it to a baking dish. For the topping: Combine all ingredients in a mixer and pulse until a coarse meal forms. Put the topping over the filling. Bake for minimum fifteen minutes or until the top becomes golden brown.

959. Turmeric Milkshake

Time To Prepare: five minutes Time to Cook: 0 minutes Yield: Servings 2

Ingredients:

1 tablespoon of ground flaxseeds 1 teaspoon of turmeric 2 cups of unsweetened almond milk 2 frozen bananas 2 tablespoons of raw cocoa powder 3 tablespoons of raw honey

Directions:

Combine all ingredients into a high-speed blender, and blend until the desired smoothness is achieved. Split between two serving glasses, and enjoy straight away.

960. Watermelon and Avocado Cream

Time To Prepare: 2 hours Time to Cook: 0 minutes Yield: Servings 4

Ingredients:

1 tablespoon honey 1 watermelon, peeled and chopped 2 avocados, peeled, pitted and chopped 2 cups coconut cream 2 teaspoons lemon juice

Directions:

Throw all the ingredients into a blender. Split it into bowls, and keep in your refrigerator for about two hours before you serve.

961. Yummy Fruity Ice-Cream

Time To Prepare: twenty minutes + 3-4 hours freezing Time to Cook: 0 minutes Yield: Servings 4

Ingredients:

½ cup of coconut cream   ½ peeled and cut small banana   1 cup fresh strawberries, hulled and cut   2 tbsp. of shredded coconut

Directions:

In a powerful blender, put all together the ingredients and pulse till smooth. Put it into an ice cream maker, then process in accordance with the manufacturer's directions. Now, move into an airtight container. Freeze to set for minimum 3-4 hours, stirring after every thirty minutes.

SAUCES, DRESSINGS & CONDIMENTS

962. Tomato Sauce (Ketchup)

Yield: 4-6 servings Preparation Time: 15 minutes Cooking Time: couple of hours 22 minutes

Ingredients:

1 tbsp organic olive oil • 1 yellow onion, chopped • 1 (1-inch) piece fresh ginger, minced • 4 garlic cloves, minced • 3 tablespoons tomato paste • 1 teaspoon ground mustard • ½ teaspoon red pepper cayenne • ½ teaspoon paprika • ¼ teaspoon ground coriander • 1/8 teaspoon ground cloves • 2 bay leaves • 1 (28-ounce) can diced tomatoes • ¼ cup coconut crystals • ½ cup coconut vinegar • Salt, to taste

Directions:

1. In a pan, heat oil on medium-high heat. 2. Add onion and sauté approximately 5 minutes. 3. Add ginger and garlic and sauté for around 1 minute. 4. Stir in tomato paste and spices and sauté for around 1 minute. 5. Stir in remaining ingredients minimizing the temperature to medium. 6. Simmer, stirring occasionally for about fifteen minutes. 7. Remove from heat and make aside to cool down the slightly. 8. In a blender, add tomato mixture and pulse till smooth. 9. Return the amalgamation into pan on low heat. 10. Simmer, stirring occasionally for around 120 minutes.

963. Beet Sauce

Yield: 6 servings Preparation Time: 15 minutes Cooking Time: one hour

Ingredients:

2 pound beets, peeled and cubed • 1 tablespoon coconut oil, melted • 2 garlic cloves, chopped • 2 tablespoons fresh lemon juice • 1 tablespoon using apple cider vinegar • ¼ cup water • Salt, to taste • 1/3 cup extra-virgin olive oil

Directions:

1. Preheat the oven to 400 degrees F. 2. Coat the beet cubes with coconut oil evenly. 3. Place the beet cubes in the baking dish. 4. Bake approximately 60 minutes, stirring after every twenty minutes. 5. Remove from oven and make aside to chill approximately 10 min. 6. In a food processor, add beets and remaining ingredients except extra virgin olive oil and pulse till well combined. 7. While motor is running slowly, add oil pulsing continuously till smooth.

964. Apple & Coconut Sauce

Yield: 8 servings Preparation Time: quarter-hour Cooking Time: 7 minutes

Ingredients:

For Sauce: • 1 Granny Smith apple, cored and chopped roughly • 2 tablespoons onion, chopped • 1/8 teaspoon fresh ginger, chopped • 1 green chile, chopped • ½ cup raw coconut, grated • 1 cup plain Greek yogurt • 1 teaspoon freshly squeezed lemon juice For Seasoning: • 1 tbsp essential olive oil • 1 teaspoon mustard seeds • 1 curry leaf • 1 teaspoon onion, sliced thinly • Salt, to taste

Directions:

For sauce in a blender, add all ingredients and pulse till smooth. 2. Transfer the sauce into a bowl. 3. In a frying pan, heat oil on medium-high heat. 4. Add mustard seeds and sauté for around 2 minutes. 5. Add curry leaf and onion and sauté for about 5 minutes. 6. Place the onion mixture over sauce with salt and stir to blend.

965. Nutty Basil Sauce (Pesto)

Yield: 4 servings Preparation Time: 10 minutes

Ingredients:

¾ cup fresh basil leaves • 1 garlic clove, chopped • 3 tablespoons pine nuts, toasted • ¾ teaspoon fresh lemon juice • Sat, to taste • 3 tablespoons extra-virgin essential olive oil

Directions:

1. In a blender, all ingredients except oil and pulse till well combined. 2. While motor is running slowly, add oil pulsing continuously till smooth.

966. Veggie Sauce

Yield: 8 servings Preparation Time: fifteen minutes

Ingredients:

1 cup zucchini, peeled and chopped • ¾ cup pumpkin puree • ¼ cup tahini • 2 tablespoons extra-virgin organic olive oil • 2 tablespoons fresh lemon juice • 1 teaspoon ground cumin • 1 teaspoon garlic powder • ½ teaspoon smoked paprika • Salt, to taste • Olive oil, for drizzling

Directions:

1. In a blender, all ingredients except extra virgin olive oil and pulse till smooth. 2. Serve with the drizzling of extra virgin olive oil.

967. Moroccan Spice Rub

Yield: 4 servings Preparation Time: 5 minutes

Ingredients:

1 teaspoon Hungarian sweet paprika • ½ teaspoon ground cinnamon • ½ teaspoon ground cumin • ¼ teaspoon ground red pepper • ¼ teaspoon ground ginger • Salt and freshly ground black pepper, to taste

Directions:

1. In a bowl, mix together all ingredients. 2. Store in an airtight jar.

968. Taco Seasoning

Yield: 10 servings Preparation Time: 5 minutes

Ingredients:

1 tablespoon red chili powder • 1½ teaspoons ground cumin • ½ teaspoon paprika • ¼ teaspoon dried oregano, crushed • ¼ teaspoon red pepper flakes, crushed • ¼ teaspoon garlic powder • ¼ teaspoon onion powder • Salt and freshly ground black pepper, to taste

Directions:

1. In a bowl, mix together all ingredients. 2. Store in the airtight jar.

969. Pumpkin Pie Spice

Yield: 3 servings Preparation Time: 5 minutes Ingredients: • 1 teaspoon ground cinnamon • ¼ teaspoon ground ginger • ¼ teaspoon ground nutmeg • 1/8 teaspoon ground cloves

Directions:

1. In a bowl, mix together all ingredients. 2. Store within an airtight jar.

970. Turmeric Paste

Yield: 16 servings Preparation Time: 5 minutes

Ingredients:

1 cup raw honey • 1 tablespoon coconut oil, sof10ed • 3 tablespoons ground turmeric • ¼ teaspoon freshly ground black pepper

Directions:

1. In a sealable jar, add all ingredients and which has a butter knife, mix well. 2. Refrigerate to store

971. Basic Mustard

Yield: 10-12 servings Preparation Time: 10 minutes

Ingredients:

¼ cup black mustard seeds • ¼ cup yellow mustard seeds • 1/3 cup freshly squeezed lemon juice • 1/3 cup water • 1½ teaspoons raw honey • ¼ teaspoon ground turmeric • Salt, to taste

Directions:

1. In a bowl, mix together mustard seeds, fresh lemon juice and water whilst aside covered for approximately 24-36 hours. 2. In an increased speed blender, add mustard seeds mixture and remaining ingredients and pulse till smooth. 3. Transfer the mustard in a airtight jar and store in refrigerator.

972. Cashew Cheese

Yield: 12-14 servings Preparation Time: 10 minutes

Ingredients:

1½ cups raw cashews, soaked in water for approximately 1-2 hours and drained • 1-2 garlic cloves, chopped • 2 tablespoons freshly squeezed lemon juice • ¼ cup water • ½ teaspoon salt

Directions:

1. In a blender, add all ingredients and pulse till smooth and creamy. 2. Transfer the cashew cheese in an airtight jar and store in refrigerator.

973. Worcestershire Sauce

Yield: 10 servings Preparation Time: 5 minutes Cooking Time: 4 minutes

Ingredients:

½ cup apple cider vinegar treatment • 2 tablespoons coconut aminos • 2 tablespoons water • ¼ teaspoon ground mustard • ¼ teaspoon ground ginger • ¼ teaspoon garlic powder • ¼ teaspoon onion powder • 1/8 teaspoon ground cinnamon • 1/8 teaspoon freshly ground black pepper

Directions:

In a tiny pan, mix together all ingredients on medium heat. 2. Bring with a boil. 3. Reduce the temperature to low and simmer approximately 1-2 minutes. 4. Remove from heat and keep aside to cool completely. 5. Transfer the sauce within an airtight glass jar and store in refrigerator for approximately 4-6 months.

974. Hot Sauce

Yield: 48 servings Preparation Time: fifteen minutes Cooking Time: quarter-hour

Ingredients:

1 tbsp organic olive oil • ½ cup onion, chopped • 1 cup carrot, peeled and chopped • 5 garlic cloves, minced • 6 habanero peppers, stemmed • 1 tomato, chopped • 1 tablespoon fresh lemon zest • ¼ cup fresh lemon juice • ¼ cup white vinegar • ¼ cup water • Salt and freshly ground black pepper, to taste

Directions:

1. In a pan, heat oil on medium heat. 2. Add onion, carrot and garlic and sauté for about 10 minutes. 3. Remove from heat and make aside to cool slightly. 4. In a mixer, add onion mixture and remaining ingredients and pulse till smooth. 5. Return the amalgamation to pan on medium-low heat. 6. Simmer, stirring occasionally approximately 3-5 minutes. 7. Remove from heat and keep aside to cool completely. 8. Transfer the sauce within an airtight glass jar and store in refrigerator for around 4-6 months.

975. Teriyaki Sauce

Yield: 16 servings Preparation Time: 5 minutes

Ingredients:

2 teaspoons fresh ginger, grated • 2 garlic cloves, chopped finely • ½ cup coconut aminos • ¼ cup raw honey • ¼ teaspoon red pepper flakes, crushed

Directions:

1. In a bowl, add all ingredients and mix till well combined. 2. Transfer the sauce in the airtight glass jar and store in refrigerator for about 4-6 months

976. Dressing Recipes Creamy Cashew

Yield: 4 servings Preparation Time: 10 minutes

Ingredients:

1 tablespoon white chia seeds • ¼ cup raw cashews • 2/3 cup unswee10ed cashew milk, divided • 1 tablespoon raw honey • 1 tablespoon apple cider vinegar treatment • 12 teaspoon fresh ginger, minced • ½-¾ teaspoon curry powder • ½ teaspoon ground turmeric • 1/8 teaspoon mustard powder • Salt and freshly ground black pepper, to taste

Directions:

1. In a spice grinder, add chia seeds and cashews and grind till a powdered finely. 2. In a blender, add cashew mixture and 50 % of cashew milk and pulse till smooth. 3. Add remaining milk and remaining ingredients and pulse till smooth. 4. Refrigerate to relax for around a half-hour before serving.

977. Lemony Egg Dressing

Yield: 3-4 servings Preparation Time: quarter-hour

Ingredients:

1 organic egg yolk • ¼ teaspoon Dijon mustard • Salt, to taste • 2 tablespoons essential olive oil • 1 tablespoon fresh lemon juice • 1 tablespoon coconut milk • 2 teaspoons using apple cider vinegar • ¼ teaspoon dried parsley, crushed • ¼ teaspoon ground turmeric • Freshly ground black pepper, to taste

Directions:

1. In a bowl, add egg yolk, Dijon mustard along with a pinch of salt and beat till mixture becomes a little thick. 2. Slowly, add oil, beating continuously till well combined. 3. Add remaining ingredients and mix till well combined.

978. Sunflower Seeds Dressing

Yield: 4 servings Preparation Time: 10 minutes

Ingredients:

½ cup sunflower seeds • 1/3 cup apple cider vinegar treatment • ½ cup water • 1 tablespoon Dijon mustard • 1 teaspoon ground turmeric • Salt and freshly ground black pepper, to taste • ¼ cup extra-virgin essential olive oil

Directions:

1. In a blender, all ingredients except oil and pulse till well combined. 2. While motor is running slowly, add oil pulsing continuously till smooth.

979. Tahini Dressing

Yield: 4-6 servings Preparation Time: 10 min

Ingredients:

½ cup tahini • 2/3-¾ cup water • 2 tablespoons coconut aminos • 2 tablespoons apple cider vinegar treatment • 1 teaspoon raw honey • 2 teaspoons ground turmeric

Directions:

1. In a blender, add all ingredients and pulse till smooth. 2. Refrigerate before serving.

980. Feta & Olives Dressing

Yield: 16 servings Preparation Time: 10 min

Ingredients:

3 tablespoons feta cheese, crumbled • 3 tablespoons kalamata olives, pitted and chopped • 2 tablespoons red onion, chopped • 1 garlic oil, chopped • 1 tablespoon raw honey • 1 tablespoon Dijon mustard • 3 tablespoons fresh lemon juice • 3 tablespoons extra-virgin essential olive oil • 1 teaspoon dried oregano, crushed • Salt and freshly ground black pepper, to taste

Directions:

1. In a blender, add all ingredients and pulse till smooth.

981. Sauces Sweet Potato Sauce

Yield: 24 servings Preparation Time: 15 minutes Cooking Time: 16 minutes

Ingredients:

2 tablespoons coconut oil • 1 onion, chopped • 2 minced garlic cloves • 1 (2-inch) piece fresh ginger, minced • 2 cups white sweet potato, peeled and cubed • 1 cup bone broth • 2 tablespoons ground turmeric • ½ tablespoon ground ginger • ¼ teaspoon ground cinnamon • Salt, to taste • 1 (13½-ounce) can coconut milk • 2 tablespoons fresh lemon juice

Directions:

In a pan, melt coconut oil on medium heat. 2. Add onion and sauté for approximately 5minutes. 3. Add garlic and ginger and sauté for around 1 minute. 4. Add sweet potato, broth and spices and bring to your boil. 5. Reduce heat to low and simmer, covered for around 10 minutes. 6. Remove from heat and aside to cool down the for approximately 5 minutes. 7. In a blender, add sweet potato mixture and remaining ingredients and pulse till smooth.

982. Scallion Sauce

Yield: 4-6 servings Preparation Time: fifteen minutes Cooking Time: 5 minutes

Ingredients:

2 cups scallions, chopped finely • 1/3 cup fresh ginger, minced • 1 teaspoon Aleppo pepper • Salt, to taste • ¼ cup coconut oil • 2 tablespoons extra-virgin olive oil

Directions:

1. In a sizable glass bowl, mix together all ingredients except both oils. 2. In a little pan, melt coconut oil approximately 3-5 minutes. 3. Place the Protein over scallion mixture evenly. 4. After 1-2 minutes, add organic olive oil and stir to combine well.

983. Eggplant Sauce

Yield: 8 servings Preparation Time: fifteen minutes Cooking Time: 35 minutes

Ingredients:

2 large eggplants • 2 garlic cloves, chopped • 2 tablespoons tahini • 2 tablespoons freshly squeezed lemon juice • 3 teaspoons extra-virgin extra virgin olive oil • 1 teaspoon ground cumin • Salt and freshly ground black pepper, to taste • Olive oil, for drizzling • Chopped fresh parsley leaves, for garnishing

Directions:

1. Preheat the oven to 400 degrees F. Grease a baking dish. 2. Place the eggplants in prepared baking dish. 3. Bake for around 35 minutes. 4. Remove from oven and immediately, devote bowl of cold water to cool down the slightly. 5. Peel off your skin of eggplants. 6. In a blender, add eggplants and remaining ingredients except extra virgin olive oil and parsley and pulse till smooth. 7. Refrigerate to relax before serving. 8. While serving, drizzle with olive oil and garnish with parsley.

984. Cherry & Cranberry Sauce

Yield: 6-8 servings Preparation Time: quarter-hour Cooking Time: 10 min

Ingredients:

6-ounce frozen cherries • 6-ounce frozen cranberries • ½ teaspoon fresh ginger, minced • ¾ cup fresh apple juice • Pinch of salt • ¼ teaspoon ground cinnamon • 1-2 tablespoons raw honey

Directions:

1. In a pan, mix together cherries, cranberries, ginger, apple juice and salt on high heat. 2. Bring to some boil and lower the warmth to medium. 3. Simmer, stirring occasionally for approximately 8-10 minutes. 4. Stir in cinnamon and honey and take off from heat.

985. Avocado Sauce

Yield: 6 servings Preparation Time: quarter-hour

Ingredients:

2 avocados, peeled, pitted and chopped • ½ cup onion, chopped • 1 cup fresh cilantro leaves • 2 garlic cloves, chopped • 1 jalapeño pepper, chopped • 1 cup vegetable broth • 2 tablespoons freshly squeezed lemon juice • 2 teaspoons balsamic vinegar • 1 teaspoon ground cumin • Pinch of red pepper cayenne • Salt, to taste

Directions:

In a blender, all ingredients and pulse till smooth.

986. Condiments Curry Paste

Yield: 6-8 servings Preparation Time: 5 minutes

Ingredients:

2 shallots, chopped roughly • 1 tablespoon fresh ginger, chopped roughly • 4 garlic cloves, chopped roughly • 1 fresh lemongrass stalk • 2 teaspoons fresh lime zest • 3-6 Serrano peppers, seeded and chopped • ¾ cup fresh cilantro, chopped roughly • ½ cup fresh basil leaves, chopped • 1 teaspoon ground coriander • 1 teaspoon ground cumin • 2 teaspoons paprika • 1 teaspoon salt • 1 tablespoon fresh lime juice • 1 tablespoon coconut aminos

Directions:

1. In a food processor, add all ingredients and pulse till an even paste forms. 2. Preserve within an airtight container. Curry Powder A nice composition of spice mix... This homemade curry powder will bring a delish aroma inside your dishes. Yield: 20 servings Preparation Time: 5 minutes Ingredients: • 2 tablespoons ground coriander • 2 tablespoons ground cumin • 2 teaspoons ground turmeric • ½ teaspoon ground turmeric • ½ teaspoon mustard seeds • ½ teaspoon red pepper flakes, crushed Directions: 1. In a spice grinder, add all ingredients and pulse till powdered finely. 2. Store in an airtight jar.

987. Garam Masala

Yield: 12 servings Preparation Time: 5 minutes

Ingredients:

1 tablespoon ground cumin • 1½ teaspoons ground cardamom • 1½ teaspoons ground coriander • 1 teaspoon ground cinnamon • ½ teaspoon ground nutmeg • ½ teaspoon ground cloves • 1½ teaspoons freshly ground black pepper

Directions:

1. In a bowl, mix together all ingredients. 2. Store in the airtight jar.

988. Adobo Seasoning

Yield: 40 servings Preparation Time: 10 minutes

Ingredients:

3 tablespoons garlic powder • 1 teaspoon dried oregano, crushed • ½ teaspoon ground cumin • 2½ teaspoons salt • 2 teaspoons freshly ground black pepper

Directions:

1. In a bowl, mix together all ingredients. 2. Store in the airtight jar.

989. Ginger-Garlic Paste

Yield: 24 servings Preparation Time: 10 minutes

Ingredients:

4-ounce fresh cinnamon, chopped • 4-ounce garlic, chopped • 1 tbsp organic olive oil

Directions:

In a mixer, add ginger and garlic and pulse till chopped finely. 2. While motor is running slowly, add oil and pulse till smooth. 3. Transfer the paste in a airtight jar and store in refrigerator.

990. Garlicky Harissa

Yield: 16 servings Preparation Time: quarter-hour Cooking Time: 4 minutes

Ingredients:

8 dried New Mexico chiles, stemmed and seeded • 8 dried guajillochiles, stemmed and seeded • Boiling water, as required • ½ teaspoon caraway seeds • ¼ teaspoon cumin seeds • ¼ teaspoon coriander seeds • 1 teaspoon dried mint leaves • 5 garlic cloves, chopped • 3 tablespoons extra-virgin organic olive oil and many more, as needed • 2 tablespoons fresh lemon juice • Salt, to taste

Directions:

1. In a bowl, add chiles and cover with boiling water. 2. Keep aside for around 20 minutes. 3. Meanwhile, heat a nonstick skillet on medium heat. 4. Add spice seeds and toast for about 4 minutes, swirling the skillet continuously. 5. In a grinder, add spice mixture and mint and pulse till powdered finely. 6. Drain the chiles completely. 7. In a food processor, add chiles, spice mixture and remaining ingredients and pulse till an even paste forms. 8. Transfer the Harissa in a1-pint glass jar. 9. Add enough oil which will submerge the Harissa completely.

991. Sweet Almond Butter

Yield: 6 servings Preparation Time: 15 minutes Cooking Time: 15 minutes

Ingredients:

2¼ cups raw almonds • 1 tablespoon coconut oil • ¾ teaspoon salt • 2 tablespoons raw honey • ½ teaspoon ground cinnamon

Directions: 1. Preheat the oven to 325 degrees F. 2. Arrange the almonds onto a rimmed baking sheet. 3. Bake approximately 12-quarter-hour. 4. Remove from oven and keep aside to chill completely. 5. In a food processor, fitted with metal blade, add almonds and pulse till a fine meal forms. 6. Add coconut oil and salt and pulse for approximately 6-9 minutes. 7. Add honey and cinnamon and pulse for approximately 1-2 minutes. 8. Transfer the almond butter in an airtight jar and store in refrigerator

992. Mayonnaise

Yield: 10 servings Preparation Time: 10 minutes

Ingredients:

2 organic egg yolks • 3 teaspoons freshly squeezed lemon juice, divided • 1 teaspoon mustard • ½ cup coconut oil, melted • ½ cup organic olive oil • Salt and freshly ground black pepper, to taste (optional)

Directions: 1. In a blender, add egg yolks, 1 tablespoon of lemon juice and mustard and pulse till combined. 2. While motor is running slowly, add both oils and pulse till a thick mixture forms. 3. Add freshly squeezed lemon juice, salt and black pepper and pulse till well combined.

993. Fish Sauce

Yield: 28 servings Preparation Time: quarter-hour

Ingredients:

1 teaspoon fresh lemon zest, grated finely • 6 garlic cloves, chopped finely • 3 tablespoons salt • 1½ pound small herring, cut into ½-inch pieces • 2-3 teaspoons black peppercorns • 6 bay leaves • 2 tablespoons sauerkraut brine • 1-2 cups non-chlorine water

Directions: 1. Place lemon peel, garlic and salt onto a cutting board. 2. Place a wide blade knife over lemon peel and garlic and press down hardly till a crushed finely. 3. In a bowl, add garlic mixture and fish and toss to coat well. 4. Transfer the fish mixture in a sizable mason jar. 5. Add peppercorn, bay leaves, sauerkraut brine and enough water that submerges the fish mixture completely. 6. Cover the jar tightly and aside in room temperature for about 2-3 days. 7. Now, refrigerate for around 4-6 weeks. 8. Through a fine sieve, strain the fish mixture twice and discard the solids. 9. Transfer the sauce within an airtight glass jar and store in refrigerator approximately 4-6 months.

994. Hoisin Sauce

Yield: 16 servings Preparation Time: quarter-hour Cooking Time: 20-a few seconds

Ingredients:

1 tablespoon fresh ginger, grated • 1 teaspoon garlic, chopped finely • 2 tablespoons almond butter • 1 teaspoon raw honey • 1 teaspoon tomato paste • ¼ cup fresh orange juice • 5 tablespoons coconut aminos • 1 teaspoon sesame oil • 1 teaspoon apple cider vinegar treatment • ½ teaspoon five spice powder • ½ teaspoon red pepper flakes, crushed

Directions:

1. In a pan, add all ingredients on medium heat and convey with a boil. 2. Reduce the heat to low and simmer approximately 5 minutes, stirring occasionally. 3. Remove from heat and aside to cool down the completely. 4. Transfer the sauce in the airtight glass jar and store in refrigerator for around 4-6 months.

995. BBQ Sauce

Yield: 16 servings Preparation Time: fifteen minutes Cooking Time: fifteen minutes

Ingredients:

½ of Habanero pepper • 1 cup mango, peeled, pitted and chopped • ½ tablespoon fresh ginger, chopped • 2 tablespoons garlic, chopped • ½ cup dates, pitted and chopped roughly • 1 cup tomato sauce • ¼ cup apple cider vinegar treatment • 2 teaspoons curry powder • Salt and freshly ground black pepper, to taste

Directions:

1. Reheat the broiler of oven to high. 2. Arrange the Habanero pepper half onto a baking sheet, cut side down. 3. Broil for around 5-10 minutes. 4. Remove the pepper rom broiler and chop it. 5. Inna pan, add pepper and remaining ingredients and stir to blend on medium-high heat. 6. Bring to your boil, stirring occasionally. 7. Reduce the warmth to medium, and simmer for around 10 minutes, stirring occasionally. 8. Remove from heat and make aside for cooling slightly. 9. In a food processor, add the mango mixture and pulse till smooth. 10. Transfer the sauce in a airtight glass jar and store in refrigerator.

996. Lemony Dressing

Yield: 6 servings Preparation Time: 10 minutes

Ingredients:

3 garlic cloves, minced • ½ cup extra-virgin olive oil • ½ cup fresh lemon juice • Salt and freshly ground black pepper, to taste

Directions:

1. In a bowl, add all ingredients and beat till well combined.

997. Lemony Avocado Dressing

Yield: 4 servings Preparation Time: quarter-hour

Ingredients:

¼ of avocado, peeled, pitted and chopped • 1 tablespoon fresh lemon zest, grated • 1 garlic herb, chopped • ¼ cup fresh lemon juice • ¼ cup extra-virgin essential olive oil • 1 tablespoon raw honey • 1 tablespoon ground turmeric • Pinch of salt

Directions:

In a blender, add all ingredients and pulse till smooth.

998. Sesame Dressing Such

Yield: 2 servings Preparation Time: 10 minutes

Ingredients:

½ tablespoon fresh ginger, minced • ½ tablespoon garlic, minced • 2 tablespoons sesame seeds • 2 tablespoons sesame oil, toasted • 2 tablespoons coconut aminos • ½ teaspoon red pepper flakes, crushed • Salt and freshly ground black pepper, to taste

Directions:

1. In a bowl, add all ingredients and beat till well combined

999. Lemony Tomato Dressing

Yield: 4 servings Preparation Time: 10 min

Ingredients:

1 large tomato, chopped roughly • 2 garlic cloves, chopped • ½ cup extra virgin olive oil • 2 tablespoons fresh lemon juice • 1 packet stevia • 1 tablespoon dried thyme, crushed • 1 tablespoon dried tarragon, crushed • ½ teaspoon paprika • Salt, to taste

Directions:

1. In a blender, add all ingredients and pulse till smooth

1000. Carrot Dressing

Yield: 6 servings Preparation Time: 15 minutes

Ingredients:

¼ cup onion, chopped • ¼ cu carrot, peeled and chopped • 1 tablespoon celery stalk, chopped • 1 garlic cloves, chopped • 1 tablespoon fresh ginger, chopped • 1 tablespoon tomato paste • 1½ teaspoons coconut sugar • 3 tablespoons balsamic vinegar • 3 tablespoons coconut aminos • 1 teaspoon fresh lemon juice • Salt and freshly ground black pepper, to taste

Directions:

1. In a blender, add all ingredients and pulse till smooth. 2. Refrigerate for just two-3 hours before serving.

Conclusion

A healthy diet always helps healing one's body to make it healthier plus much more energetic. In this regard, anti-inflammatory diet plays vital role in not simply keeping your system from chronic inflammation but in addition helps gaining good health. All you need to do is to persistly keep to the diet and try not falling off of the wagons. A whole lot of healthy anti-inflammatory recipes within this book will give you a good launch in this regime. Just discard off inflammatory foods from the pantry and fill it with only anti-inflammatory foods to get succeeded.

I am extremely glad and happy that you were able to go through the whole book. I sincerely hope that you enjoyed the contents of the book and found it useful.

I wish you luck in your future ventures and hope that you stay safe and healthy.

Made in the USA
Monee, IL
16 February 2021